D0874051

HYPNOSIS AND HYPNOTHERAPY WITH CHILDREN
Third Edition

HYPNOSIS AND HYPNOTHERAPY WITH CHILDREN

Third Edition

KAREN OLNESS, M.D.
DANIEL P. KOHEN, M.D.

THE GUILFORD PRESS
New York   London

©1996 The Guilford Press
A Division of Guilford Publications, Inc.
72 Spring Street, New York, NY 10012

Printed in the United States of America

This book is printed on acid-free paper.

Last digit is print number: 9   8   7

Library of Congress Cataloging-in-Publication Data

Olness, Karen.
    Hypnosis and hypnotherapy with children / Karen Olness, Daniel P.
Kohen. — 3rd ed.
      p.   cm.
    Includes bibliographical references and indexes.
    ISBN 1-57230-054-X
    1. Hypnotism — Therapeutic use.   2. Child psychotherapy.
I. Kohen, Daniel P. II. Title.
    [DNLM: 1. Hypnosis — in infancy & childhood. 2. Psychotherapy — in
infancy & childhood. WM 415 051hb 1996]
RJ505.H86046 1996
615.8′512′083 — dc20
DNLM/DLC
for Library of Congress   95-26800
                                              CIP

In the Children's Room, Public Library

The little Japanese boy comes in ahead
of his mother,
moves toward the playhouse,
throwing tiny fierce karate chops.

A golden-haired girl with blue-moon eyes
looks up, says in a lisping soft voice,
Um . . . do you have any books about
princesses?

And Fred comes in,
a tiny dark braid in back of his short hair.
His young sweaty body steams.
He's ridden here alone
on his bike, which
hopefully will still be down on the street
when he leaves.
He goes for the computer,
before placing at least 15 books in
his backpack.

Then slowly the children circle
the storyteller
who sits on the floor now,
ready to bring words to life.

And soon
in the back of the room
something stirs
on the shelves,
as spirits silently climb down from
the book stacks.

Curious George tumbles and leaps over
chairs and tables—
Merlin suddenly appears,
his robe of stars shining—
Mother Hubbard comes charging out,
her face red with work and worry.
Even the butterflies and bees, sheep
and unicorn
slip out of their hardcovers,
roam the room freely.

—KAREN KENYON

From *Christian Science Monitor* (April 15, 1994). With permission.

Note to the Third Edition

The burgeoning research in this area makes it mandatory to revise the second edition of *Hypnosis and Hypnotherapy with Children*. Over the past 25 years, I have observed the increased application of hypnosis and related clinical strategies in child health care delivery. One of the new leaders in this field and a friend and colleague for many years is Daniel Kohen, whom I have asked to coauthor this edition. I consider Dr. Kohen to be one of the most talented clinicians in the application of cyberphysiologic methods in the world. I am grateful that this book will be enriched by his rich clinical insights and clinical research experience in hypnotherapy with children.

Once again, I give thanks to those on whose shoulders we stand and whose clinical observations have now been validated in many research studies.

I also acknowledge the value to this field of the professional hypnosis societies—the American Society of Clinical Hypnosis and the Society for Clinical and Experimental Hypnosis (SCEH)—and also of the Society for Developmental and Behavioral Pediatrics. Marion Kenn was the administrator for the SCEH for 35 years until her death in 1994. She had hoped to retire and to write about hypnosis. In recognition of her dedication to the SCEH and her commitment to furthering education about hypnosis, I dedicate this third edition to Marion Kenn.

KAREN OLNESS, M.D.

In my 18th year of applying hypnotherapeutic strategies toward the improvement of children's health and well-being I feel privileged to coauthor this third edition of *Hypnosis and Hypnotherapy with Children*. A brief expression of my feelings about my dear friend and colleague Karen Olness is inadequate to convey the profound sense of gratitude and pride I have for our association. I continue to learn from the joy of watching, listening, and sharing perspectives with Dr. Olness as her vast, world-wide clinical experience, humility, creativity, and vision have made her the world's premier thinker and researcher in pediatric hypnosis and hypnotherapy and related cyberphysiologic techniques.

I echo Dr. Olness's thanks to our colleagues, to the Society for Developmental and Behavioral Pediatrics, and to the American Society of Clinical Hypnosis and the Society for Clinical and Experimental Hypnosis for their continued and valuable contributions; and, most importantly, to all of the children and their families who, through their learning of hypnosis, have taught me so much about what is really possible.

Finally, I would like to dedicate this third edition to my family: To the memory of my beloved father, Benjamin L. Kohen (*Z'L'*), who always supported me, and who allowed me to teach him self-hypnosis to ease his breathing; to my loving mother, Roselea Kohen, for her love and unwavering confidence in this second book; to my sons, Joshua and Aaron, for their creativity, love, confidence, and ongoing contributions to my knowledge and joy; and to my partner and wife of 25 years, Harriet, for her love, tolerance, enduring spirit, and continued belief in my energy and ability.

DANIEL P. KOHEN, M.D.

Introduction

More than 25 years ago G. Gail Gardner, a clinical child psychologist, and Karen Olness, a pediatrician, separately became interested in the possibilities of using therapeutic hypnosis with children. They were impressed with the lack of knowledge in the area of child hypnosis, not only among child health professionals but also among hypnotherapists, most of whom worked only with adults. Among child health professionals there were beliefs that children were not responsive to hypnotherapy and/or that this was not an appropriate treatment for them.

Drs. Gardner and Olness scoured the literature, found a few people who did use hypnotherapy successfully and appropriately with children, discarded all the wrong information given to them, and began to use hypnotherapy with child patients. Soon they met each other, and they began teaching together in the early 1970s. Interest and knowledge expanded, both in the United States and in other countries. Eventually they decided that the available information warranted a comprehensive text on the topic and published the first edition of *Hypnosis and Hypnotherapy with Children* in 1981. This was followed with a second edition published in 1988. Coauthor of this third edition is Daniel P. Kohen, M.D., a pediatrician who has applied hypnotherapy in pediatric practice since 1977, has participated in many controlled studies of hypnotherapy, and is well known as an author and lecturer about hypnosis.

We still hear that child hypnotherapy is a recent development. This is not true; it is only the breadth of interest that is recent. Hypnotherapy has been used with children for more than 200 years. In 1959, Dr. André Weitzenhoffer published *A Bibliography of Hypnotism in Pediatrics* containing 86 references — many in French and German — spanning the years 1886 to 1959. In 1980, Gardner published a bibliography of 114 references dating from 1955 to 1980, almost entirely limited to publications in American journals.

The growth of interest in child hypnotherapy is also reflected in expanded opportunities for training in this subspecialty. For example, in 1971, Dr. Gardner was invited to lecture for an hour on child hypnosis as part of an advanced-level workshop sponsored by the Society for Clinical and Experimental Hypnosis. In 1976, the same society initiated a full 3-day workshop on clinical hypnosis with children, which has been conducted annually since then. In 1988, the Society for Behavioral Pediatrics began offering a 3-day workshop on clinical hypnosis with children. Each year since then, the maximum attendance limit has been reached. Seminars on hypnosis, including child hypnosis, are now included in many medical school curricula and in graduate programs in clinical psychology, social work, and nursing. Teachers of child hypnotherapy are often asked to present hospital grand rounds on this subject. As a result, hypnotherapeutic methods with children are used in many hospitals, clinics, and in private practices.

A generic term for self-regulation, cyberphysiology, was coined by Earl Bakken (1988), founder of Medtronic, about a decade ago. *Cyber* derives from the Greek *kybernan,* meaning the helmsman or steersman. "To govern" evolved from this. Hence, cyberphysiology refers to self-regulation or self-governance of physiological processes. It is useful to think of hypnotherapy, relaxation-imagery training, or biofeedback as strategies facilitating cyberphysiologic controls.

In line with the heightened interest in child hypnotherapy, three broad topics are discussed in this book. First, the early history of therapeutic hypnosis with children is reviewed. This historical review emphasizes the 19th-century literature so as to collect in one place those intriguing reports that predated modern scientific method. Second, issues especially important in child hypnosis are discussed. The normative studies of the 1960s and 1970s are reviewed in detail. These uniformly conclude that, in general, children have a higher level of hypnotic responsiveness than adults. This section also includes developmental issues, and hypnotic induction techniques appropriate for children of different ages and abilities, including biofeedback as an important adjunct in child and adolescent hypnotherapy. The third broad topic is hypnotherapy with children and adolescents, including chapters devoted to the treatment of specific psychological, medical, and surgical problems. A critical review of the literature and samples of clinical experience are included.

It is important to distinguish between hypnosis and hypnotherapy, terms too often confused. *Hypnosis is an altered state of consciousness or awareness.* No scientiest claims fully to understand its parameters, but most people in the field agree that it is a state of consciousness different both from the normal waking state and from any of the stages of sleep. It resembles in some ways various kinds of meditative states, especially with respect to characteristics of narrowly focused attention, primary process thinking, and ego receptivity (Fromm, 1977, 1979). There are also characteristic alterations in cognition associated especially with deeper levels of hypnosis, and those forms of "trance logic" may be elicited by careful experimental methods (Orne, 1959). Hypnosis is sometimes indistinguishable from simple physical and mental relaxation, and both adults and children may enter an altered state of consciousness or awareness spontaneously, in the course of daily activities.

Hypnotherapy is a treatment modality in which the patient is in the altered state of hypnosis at least part of the time. The patient in hypnosis is then treated with any number of methods ranging from simple suggestion to psychoanalysis. Strictly speaking, no patient is treated by "hypnosis," that is, by the mere fact of having entered a certain altered state of consciousness, although this confusion of terms is very common in the literature. A patient who merely goes into hypnosis may experience reduced tension and even reduced tension-related pain, but there is no specific therapeutic intervention. Hypnotherapy, by definition, implies therapeutic intervention either by a therapist or by the patient. In the latter case, the term "self-hypnosis" is so widespread that we have chosen to retain it rather than coin a new term. We acknowledge the inconsistency.

Inasmuch as there is disagreement, confusion, and imperfect knowledge about hypnosis, these problems are greatly multiplied in the case of hypnotherapy. There are very few cases of "successful hypnotherapy" in which one can be absolutely certain that the results are due to hypnotherapy and not to something else. On the other hand, the usual clinical applications of medications do not take into account issues of placebo effect and/or suggestibility. With respect to hypnotherapy, some people are overly enthusiastic and make claims about hypnotherapy far in excess of the bounds of scientific responsibility. We take a middle position on this issue. We believe that when some patients are treated for some problems while in the state of hypnosis, changes occur that would not have occurred had the patients been in the usual state of awareness.

We do not claim to be writing the *dernier cri* on hypnosis and hypnotherapy with children. We fully expect that future research will prove some of the statements made in this book to be wrong. There may be a time when "hypnosis" will be subsumed under cyberphysiologic methods or strategies. We hope that this book might stimulate more clinical reports and sophisticated research that will allow us to make a greater contribution to the children with whom we work.

This book is not intended to be a "how-to-do-it" guide for persons with no previous training in hypnotherapy. One does not learn these skills from a textbook any more than one learns psychotherapy or pediatrics by reading a book. We hope our readers will avail themselves of opportunities for training in hypnotherapy and child hypnotherapy. We recommend workshops and courses sponsored by the Society for Clinical and Experimental Hypnosis, the American Society of Clinical Hypnosis, and the Society for Developmental and Behavioral Pediatrics, as well as courses offered by approved medical and graduate schools.* We intend this book to complement these courses.

The recommended workshops are limited to persons already trained in the health professions. We cannot overemphasize the point that a hypnotherapist first must be a competent therapist, and a person doing research in hypnosis must first have a solid background in research techniques. This book is directed to child health professionals who assume primary responsibility for child patients and to researchers in related areas. We hope that it will provide our colleagues with new ideas and will stimulate creative approaches to understanding children and adolescents and helping them develop their potential to the fullest extent.

---

*Detailed information about training opportunities in child hypnosis and hypnotherapy may be obtained from the following organizations: *American Society of Clinical Hypnosis* (2200 East Devon Avenue, Suite 291, Des Plaines, IL 60018-4534; phone 708-297-3317; fax 708-297-7309); *Society for Clinical and Experimental Hypnosis* (3905 Vincennes Road, Suite 304, Indianapolis, IN 46268; phone 800-214-1738; fax 317-872-7133); *Society for Developmental and Behavioral Pediatrics* (19 Station Lane, Philadelphia, PA 19118; phone 215-248-9168; fax 215-248-1981).

Contents

PART ONE

HYPNOSIS WITH CHILDREN

CHAPTER ONE

Scenes of Childhood

To help the reader more fully understand our approach to hypnotherapy, we present some themes of child development that form the rationale for our methods with children.

THE URGE FOR EXPERIENCE

Beginning at birth, babies seek stimulation. In the first days of life, they prefer to focus their gaze on something and prefer a more complex visual stimulus (e.g., a striped pattern) to a simple one (e.g., a solid red square). Most of all, they enjoy gazing at a human face. Very soon, children define all objects as things-to-find-out-about, and they make maximal use of sensory and motor development to experience themselves and their world. They do this first with mouths and eyes, then with hands, and finally with their whole bodies. If the results of such experiences are generally pleasurable, they continue to explore in more complex ways, using to their own advantage such developing ego functions as motility and coordination, language, perceptual skills, memory, ability to distinguish between reality and fantasy, and social skills. Temperamental and environmental factors combine to shape and often to put limits on the child's urge for experience, but only rarely can these cancel the urge altogether. For example, in the case of the frightened child who retreats to a corner on the first day of school, a patient teacher usually finds that the child prefers to stand facing the room rather than facing the wall. For such children, visual exploration often leads to good school adjustment as efficiently as motor exploration for other children. As Fromm (1972) pointed out, it is very important not to confuse behavioral passivity with ego passivity. On the other hand, Kagan's work (Kagan, 1994) has documented that there is substantial capacity for change in temperament and behavior between 2 and 7 years. Evidence of an inhibited personality in infancy does not necessarily predict the adolescent or adult personality.

3

THE URGE FOR MASTERY

Right on the heels of the urge for experience comes the urge for mastery, both of the self and of the environment. Objects and people become things-to-do-something-with. Ego activity and behavioral activity join forces, sometimes to the dismay of parents who find the contents of the dresser drawers on the floor. It is sheer pleasure to share with young children in the mastery process. As children grow older, they continue to experience the same drive for mastery, unless this aspect of ego functioning is seriously derailed by environmental or physical or mental handicaps.

THE URGE FOR SOCIAL INTERACTION

Children are social creatures. Even at birth, their favorite visual stimulus is a human face. Children develop language not only for its own reward of mastery but because it vastly increases possibilities for social interaction. The endless "why" questions of the toddler are often less a request for information than for social play, just as endless requests for peek-a-boo or chase-around-the-tree serve to exercise social as much as sensory and motor needs. Social interaction is more than social control, more than merely a way to have needs satisfied; for the child, it is a pleasure in itself. Children progress from interaction with parents to interaction with peers, and in this way they develop social skills that may provide pleasure for the rest of their lives. Again, socialization skills can be derailed by physical or mental handicaps or by abusive adults, but most children manage to remember that at least some relationships are safe and may be a means to pleasure. Although some children may be slow to warm up in new relationships, very few choose to remain totally isolated.

THE URGE FOR THE INNER WORLD OF IMAGINATION

Just as children enjoy increasing the range of their experiences in and with their everyday external world, so they also delight in the realms of their inner experience, that is, what they call pretending, daydreaming, or imagination, and what we call fantasy. These internal activities serve useful functions. Children may explore unconsciously several possible actions in their fantasies before selecting the apparent best behavioral choice, thus saving time and energy. They spontaneously may use such fantasy to modify unpleasant situations, to gratify unmet needs, or to prepare for creative activities and new achievements (J. R. Hilgard, 1970; Olness, 1985b). Imaginative involvement, of course, may be pleasurable in its own right. For example, a group of 15 4-year-olds were asked to report dreams. After the first child described what was probably a nocturnal "monster" dream, the rest excitedly jumped in with variations. It was obvious that, for the most part, these other reports were not dreams, but instead were entries into a quite conscious competition to see who could create the wildest monster story; all had happy, masterful endings, again following the lead of the first child who managed to throw her dream monster out the window. Such fantasies are typical of countless stories and fairy tales that have existed for many centuries throughout different cultures. The development of imagery in the thinking processes of children is an important part of child development, related to play patterns and creativity as well as, ultimately, to adult activity. Image-generated effects on physiology, nutrition, behavior, performance, and disease, formerly not understood to be subject to voluntary modulation, are under investigation by many researchers today (Felt et al., 1994; Hall, Minnes, Tosi, & Olness, 1992; Olness, 1985b; Wang & Morgan, 1992). For example, in our laboratory, we (Lee & Olness, 1995) have documented changes in cardiac rate dependent on shifts in the imagining of children.

Inasmuch as we recognize a basic need for nocturnal dreams, we could postulate a similar need and value for waking fantasy and imaging. There is valid current concern that the images provided by television have negative effects on childhood development and that violent images may impact negatively on a young child's value system. Part of the damage of television may be that it steals from spontaneous, creative imagining time for children and adolescents. In fact, we wonder whether Western culture's devaluation of fantasy during adolescence may not contribute to some of the conflict and strife typical of that developmental period.

THE URGE FOR WELLNESS

Under most circumstances, children choose to be healthy rather than sick, comfortable rather than distressed. Children like to be well. When physically stressed, the body automatically adapts in an effort to restore integration. Thus, platelets and white cells rush to the site of a wound to stop bleeding and prevent infection. Likewise, when psychologically distressed, the individual uses various defense mechanisms and coping devices to handle the situation as adaptively as possible. Maladaptive behavior serves a purpose, conscious or unconscious or both. But almost always there is some part of the person that would gladly trade maladaptive behavior for behavior that serves the same purpose in a more constructive and truly self-satisfying way. In the case of maladaptive behavior in children, there is the added advantage of a higher degree of ego resiliency and flexibility than is often seen with adults. Children have still another advantage in their search for wellness, namely their generally greater comfort in seeking help, learning new skills, and in allowing a certain degree of adaptive regression that is inherent in a successful helping relationship.

IMPLICATIONS FOR HYPNOTHERAPY

In our therapeutic work, we recognize that we are not treating problems; we are treating and helping children who happen to have problems. No matter how severe the problems of our child patients, we address ourselves to their striving for experience, for mastery, for social interaction, for the inner world of imagination, and for wellness. Thus, we gain an ally in that part of the child that wants to experience life to the fullest, and this alliance forms the foundation of treatment.

When we select hypnotherapy as the treatment of choice for a particular child's problem, we emphasize specific therapeutic techniques that enhance and strengthen healthy strivings. Induction techniques are selected partly on the basis of experiential satisfaction as well as the developmental stage and learning style of each child. Treatment is conducted in the context of a safe, comfortable relationship in which the child is invited to capitalize on imagery skills to enhance and promote feelings of control and mastery and, in so doing, to recover a state of wellness to the greatest extent possible. Treatment should not require passive submission but, rather, active and joyful participation. In the final analysis, we see ourselves as guides, coaches, and teachers. It is the children who bring healing to themselves.

CHAPTER TWO

Early Uses of Hypnosis with Children

The use of hypnotic-like techniques with children goes back to ancient times. Both the Old and New Testaments contain accounts of ill children responding to healing methods based on suggestion and faith (I Kings XVII:17–24; Mark IX:17–27). Children in primitive cultures have employed trance phenomena in initiation rites and other ceremonies (Mead, 1949).

FRANZ ANTON MESMER (1734–1815)

The modern history of hypnosis begins with Mesmer, an Austrian physician whose interest in the healing power of magnetic influence was a logical extension of attention to magnetic forces among astronomers and physicists of that time. In 1766, Mesmer wrote a dissertation entitled *The Influences of the Planets on the Human Body* (cited in Tinterow, 1970).

During the next decade, Mesmer developed his theory of animal magnetism. Briefly, the theory held that all objects in the universe are connected by and filled with a physical fluid having magnetic properties. When the fluid is out of balance in the human body, disease occurs. Certain techniques can be employed to restore the fluid to proper equilibrium and thus heal the patient. Mesmer's techniques included staring into his patients' eyes and making various "hand movements" over their bodies, using his own "magnetic influence" to promote a cure. While living in Vienna, Mesmer (Tinterow, 1970) reported his use of animal magnetism to cure several patients, including children and adolescents. Though details of his methods with specific patients are sketchy, verbal instructions and suggestions seem to have been minimized in favor of the "hand movements" that supposedly restored the patient's own magnetic fluid to proper balance.

One of Mesmer's patients was Miss Ossine, an 18-year-old girl whose problems included tuberculosis, melancholia, fits, rage, vomiting, spitting up blood, and fainting. She recovered after treatment with animal magnetism. Another patient, also 18 years old at the time of treatment, was Miss Paradis, who had been blind since age 4 and who suffered melancholia "accompanied by stoppages in the spleen and liver" that often brought on fits of delirium and rage. Most significant is Mesmer's awareness of the extent to which parental interference can sabotage treatment. Following restoration of the girl's sight by animal magnetism, a public dispute developed over whether she could really see or was just faking. Moreover, the father became fearful that his daughter's disability pension might be stopped. He terminated her treatment, whereupon she soon relapsed into frequent seizures and later into blindness. The father then changed his mind and asked that Mesmer resume treatment. Intensive treatment for 15 days again controlled the seizures and restored the girl's vision, after which she returned home. Subsequently, the family claimed that she had again relapsed. Mesmer thought the girl was being forced to imitate her maladies, but he could not obtain further follow-up.

At the same time, Mesmer described his treatment of Miss Wipior, age 9, who had a tumor on one cornea, rendering her blind in that eye. He stated that animal magnetism resulted in partial removal of the tumor so that the child could read sideways. He anticipated a full cure, but circumstances interrupted the treatment.

Following his work with these and other patients, Mesmer became discouraged by his colleagues' repeated charges that animal magnetism was no more than quackery. In 1778, Mesmer moved to Paris where he initially enjoyed good favor and, in 1779, published his famous *Dissertations on the Discovery of Animal Magnetism*. His fame spread rapidly, and he began treating patients in large groups, using more and more dramatic methods. His colleagues again charged quackery, and local scientific societies refused to acknowledge his discoveries. Once more discouraged, Mesmer left Paris, but "mesmerism" continued to flourish in the hands of his disciples, especially Charles d'Eslon.

THE FRANKLIN COMMISSION

In 1784, King Louis XVI appointed a commission to investigate mesmerism and, particularly, the claims of the disciple d'Eslon (Tinterow, 1970). The president of the commission was Benjamin Franklin, then the American Ambassador to France. Other distinguished members included the chemist Lavoisier and the physician Guillotin. The commissioners agreed that some patients were cured by mesmerism, but they questioned the underlying theory of the existence of magnetic fluid.

In experiments designed to test the theory, the commissioners took pains to include several children, particularly from the lower classes, so as to minimize the effects of prior knowledge and expectation. One of these was Claude Renand, a 6-year-old boy with tuberculosis. Unlike other patients, who had usually experienced pain, perspiration, and convulsions during mesmeric treatment, little Claude reported no sensation at all. Another child subject was Geneviève Leroux, age 9, suffering convulsions and chorea; she, too, felt no sensation. Procedures used with these and other subjects included passes made with iron rods and hand or finger pressure on various body parts, sometimes for several hours. An assistant played rapid piano music for the purpose of enhancing the likelihood of a "convulsive crisis."

Since Mesmer had claimed that he could transfer magnetic influence to inanimate objects and that patients could then be healed merely by touching these objects, the commission tested this aspect of the theory, again with a naive child as subject. On the extensive grounds of Franklin's estate outside Paris, d'Eslon magnetized a certain apricot tree. A 12-year-old boy, known to be susceptible to the more common methods of animal magnetism, remained indoors, unaware of which tree was magnetized. The commissioners reported their observations in detail.

> The boy was then brought into the orchard, his eyes covered with a bandage, and successively taken to trees upon which the procedure had not been performed, and he embraced them for the space of two minutes, the method of communication which had been prescribed by M. d'Eslon.
>
> At the first tree, the boy, being questioned at the end of a minute, declared that he had perspired in large drops, he coughed, spit, and complained of a slight pain in his head; the distance of the tree which had been magnetized was about twenty-seven feet.
>
> At the second tree he felt the sensations of stupefaction and pain in his head; the distance was thirty-six feet.
>
> At the third tree, the stupefaction and headache increased considerably, and he said that he believed he was approaching the tree which had been magnetized. The distance was then about thirty-eight feet.
>
> In line with the fourth tree, one which had not been rendered the object of the procedure, and at a distance of about twenty-four feet from the tree which had, the boy fell into a crisis, he fainted, his limbs stiffened, and he was carried on to a plot of grass, where M. d'Eslon hurried to his side and revived him.
>
> The result of this experiment is entirely contrary to the theory of animal magnetism. M. d'Eslon accounted for it by observing that all the trees, by their very nature, participated in the magnetism, and that their magnetism was reinforced by his presence. But in that case, a person, sensitive to the power of magnetism, could not hazard a walk in the garden without the risk of convulsions, an assertion which is contradicted by the experience of every day. The presence of M. d'Eslon had no greater influence here than

in the coach, in which the boy came along with him. He was placed opposite the coach and he felt nothing. If he had experienced no sensation even under the tree which was magnetized, it might have been said that at least on that day he had not been sufficiently susceptible. However, the boy fell into a crisis under a tree which was not magnetized. The crisis was therefore the effect of no physical or exterior cause, but is to be attributed solely to the influence of imagination. The experiment is therefore entirely conclusive. The boy knew that he was about to be led to a tree upon which the magnetical operation had been performed, his imagination was struck, it was increased by the successive steps of the experiment, and at the fourth tree it was raised to the height necessary to produce the crisis. (quoted in Tinterow, 1970, pp. 108–109)

The commissioners thus rejected the theory of animal magnetism and concluded that the results of these and other experiments "are uniform in their nature, and contribute alike to the same decision. They authorize us to conclude that the imagination is the true cause of the effects attributed to the magnetism" (p. 114).

JOHN ELLIOTSON (1791–1868)

Charges and countercharges raged between Mesmer's disciples and others who agreed with the Franklin Commission report. The controversy between proponents of animal magnetism and those of imagination spread to England where the defense of animal magnetism was led by John Elliotson, a distinguished physician whose achievements included introducing the stethoscope to his country. Hoping to convince his colleagues, Elliotson decided in 1842 to edit a journal, *The Zoist,* concerned with information about cerebral physiology and mesmerism. The 13 volumes of this journal, published from 1842 to 1856, contain several references to the use of mesmerism in the management of childhood problems. Apparently Elliotson lacked the scientific sophistication of the 1784 Commission, for much of his argument in support of the theory rested on evidence that patients could be cured after mesmerism, a point never contested by the Commission. Like Mesmer and d'Eslon, Elliotson was denounced by the medical profession, and the practice of mesmerism was prohibited in many English hospitals. The doctor and his pupils, unwilling to submit papers to traditional medical journals where they would not have been accepted, reported many successful cases in *The Zoist.* Failures were not reported.

Elliotson (1843a) reported an 18-year-old boy with rheumatism and delirium with convulsions, probably associated with fever. The boy made little progress during the first month of medical treatment, which included bleeding, opium, purgatives, head shaving and application of lotions to the scalp, quinine, musk, creosote, iron, prussic acid, and arsenic. His behavior was so violent that he was tied with ropes across his bed and further restrained by three strong men. At this point, Elliotson visited the patient. In the first session, 45 minutes of mesmeric passes had no effect. Elliotson turned the case over to one of his former pupils. The following evening's session lasted over 2 hours; the doctor noted that the convulsive attack, which usually occurred in the evening, ended a bit sooner than usual. Medication was continued in reduced doses. Mesmeric treatment continued each evening, with gradual improvement noted. After 1 week, the doctor reported that the boy was becoming attached to him. To our knowledge, this is the earliest reference to the transference aspects of the hypnotherapeutic relationship. The transference was reported almost in passing, and its role in the curative process was not fully recognized. Eleven days after mesmeric treatment began, the patient's violent attacks ceased, and treatment stopped. The patient continued to sleep poorly for several weeks, a problem which Elliotson attributed to premature termination of treatment.

In the same paper, Elliotson reported successful mesmeric treatment in eight cases of chorea, of which six were children ranging in age from 9 to 17 years. Duration of treatment ranged from 1 day to 2 months. With the exception of iron, other medications were discontinued, most of them doing more harm than good.

In 1843, Elliotson published a book entitled *Numerous Cases of Surgical Operations Without Pain in the Mesmeric State* (1843b), describing both his own work and that of his colleagues. Here he mentioned several cases of painless dental extractions in children. He reported that after 5 minutes of mesmeric passes a colleague had opened a large abscess behind the ear of a 12-year-old boy. The patient was comfortable throughout the procedure. He also reported a colleague's operation on a 17-year-old girl to release knee contractures while she was in a mesmeric trance. She experienced no pain and was unaware that the procedures had been accomplished until she saw spots of blood on the sheets of her hospital bed.

Elliotson concluded from his clinical experience that his favorable results were attributable to mesmeric passes, and he continued to deny most vehemently that imagination played any role in the cures. He apparently never understood that his methods could not provide any evidence in favor of one theory or the other.

JAMES BRAID (1795–1860)

Braid was an English surgeon, a contemporary of Elliotson, who began investigating mesmerism as a complete skeptic. Unlike Elliotson, when he saw that such phenomena as induced catalepsy and analgesia were real, he elected

to avoid diatribes and to be open-minded with regard to the underlying theoretical explanation, although he leaned toward imagination as a good possibility.

In 1843, Braid wrote of his techniques:

> I feel we have acquired in this process a valuable addition to our cura-
> tive means; but I repudiate the idea of holding it up as a universal remedy;
> nor do I even pretend to understand, as yet, the whole range of diseases
> in which it may be useful. . . . Whether the extraordinary physical effects
> are produced through the imagination chiefly, or by other means, it ap-
> pears to me quite certain, that the imagination has never been so much un-
> der our control, or capable of being made to act in the same beneficial and
> uniform manner, by any other mode of management hitherto known.
> (1843/1960)

However, Braid rejected the idea that imagination alone could produce trance.

Both for theoretical and for practical reasons, Braid discarded the whole
idea of animal magnetism, and he avoided the world mesmerism. Thinking
of trance phenomena as some sort of nervous sleep, he coined the term "hypnosis" from the Greek word hypnos, meaning sleep. He abandoned use of
passes and, instead, required his subjects to fix their gaze on an object and
concentrate attention on a single idea (monoideism). Braid's elucidation of
the psychological aspects of hypnosis was a major contribution, and his theories were subsequently adopted by Broca, Charcot, Liébault, and Bernheim.

Braid was impressed by the ease and rapidity with which trance could
be induced, and he took careful notice of instances in which some individuals went into a trance state without any formal induction. In an 1855 work,
he reported an anecdote in which an elderly man discovered a boy who had
climbed up into one of his apple trees and was in the midst of stealing an
apple.

> At this moment the gentleman addressed the boy in a *stern* manner,
> declaring that he would *fix* him there in the position he was then in. Hav-
> ing said so, the gentleman left the orchard and went off to church, not doubt-
> ing that the boy would soon come down and effect his escape when he knew
> the master of the orchard was gone. However, it turned out otherwise; for,
> on going into the orchard on his return from church, he was not a little
> surprised to find that the boy had been spell-bound by his declaration to
> that effect—for there he still remained, *in the exact attitude in which he
> left him, with his arm outstretched, and his hand ready to lay hold of the
> apple.* By some farther remarks from this gentleman the spell was broken,
> and the boy allowed to escape without further punishment. (Braid, 1855)

In this and other anecdotes, Braid recognized the power mind has over
body, and he pointed out that children were frequently "sensitive" in this

regard. He failed to recognize these instances as spontaneous hypnosis, describing them instead as waking phenomena. Holding to the idea that hypnotic phenomena were produced by formal visual and mental fixation, he said, "In cases of children, and those (adults) of weak intellect, or of restless and excitable minds whom I could not manage so as to make them comply with these simple rules, I have always been foiled, although most anxious to succeed" (Braid, 1843/1960). He made this comment in spite of the fact that, in the same paper, he reported inducing light hypnosis with arm catalepsy in 32 children at once by making them stand and sit over a period of 10 to 12 minutes. It seems that, like Mesmer and Elliotson before him, Braid made the mistake of defining hypnotic phenomena by the techniques he used to produce them.

Braid seemed tantalizingly close to the step of recognizing the independence of trance phenomena from particular induction methods. He fully recognized that the operator involved in trance production did not communicate any magnetic, electrical, or other force from his own body but, rather, acted as an engineer, using various modes to direct vital forces within the patient's body. He recognized the importance of the patient's faith and confidence in the process. He even recognized the possibility of self-hypnosis, using it to manage his own pains. But it would be several more years before his speculations about the role of imagination in hypnosis would be deliberately applied to child patients.

JEAN-MARTIN CHARCOT (1835–1893)

Charcot, a distinguished French neurologist, began his investigation of hypnosis at the School of the Salpêtrière in 1878. His descriptions of hypnosis in neurological terms gave it a new measure of scientific respectability. By 1882, the subject appeared regularly in the best medical journals as well as in the lay press. Scientific journals devoted entirely to hypnosis sprang up in both France and Germany (Tinterow, 1970).

In spite of—or perhaps because of—Charcot's having his own clinic with ample numbers of assistants to work with patients, he really did little to advance understanding of hypnosis, especially in the case of children. He conceived of hypnosis as a pathological state, a form of hysterical neurosis, able to be produced more easily in women than in men. He considered all children insusceptible. According to a biography by Guillain (cited in Tinterow, 1970), Charcot failed to check the work of his assistants and never personally hypnotized a single patient. Having developed a theory, he unwittingly restricted his experimental work in such a way that the data could only support his ideas. Late in his life, in the face of increasing criticism, he saw the need to revise his theory, but by this time he was quite ill, and he died without beginning the actual work of revision.

AUGUSTE AMBROSE LIÉBAULT (1823–1904) AND HIPPOLYTE BERNHEIM (1840–1919)

At about the same time that Charcot founded the School of the Salpêtrière, Liébault founded another French school devoted to the investigation of hypnosis, the School of Nancy. He was soon joined by Bernheim, and together they developed the theories and gathered data that opposed those of Charcot and have since proved to be more accurate. Specifically, they conceived of hypnosis as an entirely normal phenomenon based chiefly on suggestion and imagination, thus clarifying and extending the earlier speculation of Braid. In 1888, Bernheim wrote, "I define hypnotism as the induction of a peculiar physical condition which increases the susceptibility to suggestion. Often, it is true, the sleep that may be induced facilitates suggestion, but it is not the necessary preliminary. It is suggestion that rules hypnotism" (in Tinterow, 1970, p. 454). He concluded that hypnosis occurs as a result of various induction methods "acting upon imagination."

As might be expected on the basis of their theories, Liébault and Bernheim found that most children were quickly and easily hypnotized, so long as they were able to pay attention and understand instructions. Their method consisted of eye fixation with repeated suggestions for eye closure and sleep. They did not insist on sleep if the subject showed no such inclinations, but they manually pushed down the eyelids if the subject's eyes remained open more than a few minutes.* Any resistance was met by more forceful commands.

More than their predecessors, Liébault and Bernheim recognized individual differences in response to hypnotic suggestions. Hypnosis was not an all-or-none phenomenon but could be manifested at varying degrees of depth. The deepest level, somnambulism, and each of the lighter levels had characteristic features, although there were individual differences in response within each level as well as between levels. Once they made these advances toward greater scientific sophistication, the next step was to carry out normative studies on a large scale. According to Bramwell (1903/1956), Liébault compiled data from 755 subjects and found no differences in hypnotizability between males and females. The data were then restated in order to focus on age differences across the whole range from young children to the elderly. As shown in Table 2.1, the highest percentage of somnambules occurred in children 7 to 14 years of age. No subject in this age group or in the group of children younger than 7 years was entirely refractory.

---

*Although younger American children (e.g., under 7–8 years of age) today may sometimes opt not to follow suggestions for eye closure, we must remember that Liébault and Bernheim used more authoritarian methods than most clinicians now use and that their child subjects grew up in a more authoritarian culture than do most American children today. As such the differences in compliance are understandable.

TABLE 2.1. Norms of Hypnotizability

Age (years)	Somnambulism (percentage)	Less deep hypnotisim (percentage)	Refractory (percentage)
0–6	26.5	73.7	—
7–13	55.3	44.4	—
14–20	25.2	64.2	10.3
21–27	13.2	77.4	9.1
28–34	22.6	71.2	5.9
35–41	10.5	81.1	8.2
42–48	21.6	65.9	12.2
49–55	7.3	87.9	4.4
56–62	7.3	78.0	14.4
63 +	11.8	74.3	13.5

Note. Adapted from Bramwell (1903/1956).

J. MILNE BRAMWELL (1852–1925)

Bramwell was an English psychotherapist who began to use hypnosis in 1889. In 1903, he published *Hypnotism: Its History, Practice, and Theory,* a comprehensive review that was widely quoted as the major text in the field for many years. From vignettes of his own cases and those of his colleagues, we get a good idea of the range of childhood disorders treated with hypnotherapy at the turn of the century. These disorder included: behavior problems (e.g., stealing, lying, masturbation, insolence); chorea; eczema; enuresis; headaches; hyperhidrosis (excessive sweating); nailbiting; night terrors; seizures; and stammering (Bramwell, 1903/1956). The success rate was reportedly very high, but we are not sure whether all failures were reported. The children described ranged in age from 3 to 19 years.

THE BEGINNING OF CHILD HYPNOTHERAPY IN AMERICA

So far as we know, the first publication concerning child hypnosis in a major American journal was a paper in *Science* entitled "Suggestion in Infancy" (Baldwin, 1891). The author discussed the idea that the rise of interest in hypnosis had opened the way for increased understanding of infant behavior beyond mere physiological or reflex reactions. Such behavior could now be understood in terms of environmental influences, especially what he called *ideomotor suggestions.* For example, he described his use of reward and punishment to extinguish scratching behavior in a 3-month-old infant. He also discussed the child's development of imitative behavior, beginning at about 8 months. Baldwin did not use hypnosis per se but, rather, understood the possibility of understanding hypnotic phenomena as a point of departure for the study of consciousness, an idea that has only recently come back into sharp focus (E. R. Hilgard, 1977).

Lightner Witmer, who coined the term "clinical psychology" and opened the first American psychological clinic in 1896 at the University of Pennsylvania, published a sharply critical paper about hypnosis in the 1897 volume of *Pediatrics* (Witmer, 1897). He discussed his alarm that pedagogical uses of hypnosis were often considered a panacea. By his use of the term "pedagogical," he meant not only the use of hypnosis in formal education; he also included any hypnotic treatment in which suggestions were given chiefly for the purpose of educating the patient, for example, to expend constructive effort in work or to desist from objectionable habits. Like Charcot, Witmer thought that "the susceptibility to hypnotic influence is itself a stigma of neuroticism, perhaps of hysteria" (p. 26). He believed that hypnosis weakened the will and fostered impulsivity, adding that "mental tonic is what such persons need, not such mental perversion as hypnotism is" (p. 27).

R. O. Mason replied to Witmer's editorial in an earlier number of the same volume of *Pediatrics* (1897) with matching vehemence in support of pedagogical hypnosis, especially in the case of children. He described the beneficial effects of hypnosis for a wide variety of pediatric problems. He denied that he considered it a panacea, or that it weakened the patient's will or capacity for independent judgment. Countering Witmer's notion of hypnosis as a phenomenon seen chiefly in hysterics, Mason cited Bernheim's hypnotic research with large numbers of normal subjects.

Citing his own case records, Mason reported successful hypnotherapy with a 15-year-old girl suffering from lack of concentration and poor memory for schoolwork, a 7-year-old boy who was too frightened to cooperate with necessary medical treatment, a 5-year-old girl suffering frequent night terrors, and a 16-year-old boy referred because of masturbation and cigarette smoking. In each case "the treatment was essentially educational—the dismissal of the abnormal hurtful or evil ideas and tendencies and the restoration or introduction of new, normal and helpful ones in their place" (p. 104). Treatment time varied from one session to a long series of visits.

By 1900, both in America and in Europe, interest in child hypnosis was waning and would not revive again for nearly half a century. Then it got off to a slow start, not becoming a major research area until the late 1950s and early 1960s. During the two World Wars, interest in adult hypnosis increased briefly, as a result of pressure to get disabled soldiers back on the battlefield quickly. From the experiences of injured soldiers much was learned about how self-hypnotic anesthesia works. Injured soldiers would dissociate spontaneously and reduce discomfort. This was an important observation in the evolution of understanding about child hypnotic pain control. But, during these periods, little else was learned that was relevant to the treatment of children. When interest in child hypnosis increased again in the 1950s, researchers and clinicians began essentially where they had left off half a century before.

CONCLUSIONS

Early reports of hypnotherapy with children were primarily anecdotal, often in the context of emotional appeals to support or refute current theories and speculations about various aspects of human behavior. Nevertheless, by the end of the 19th century, those who had studied the field carefully already knew that children were suitable hypnotic subjects, that the peak of hypnotizability occurred in middle childhood, and that hypnotic techniques were applicable to a wide variety of childhood medical and psychological problems.

CHAPTER THREE

Norms of Hypnotizability in Children

The question of degrees of hypnotizability in children is not new. In the 1880s, Liébault (Tinterow, 1970), struggled with it in his studies of hypnotizability that included subjects from early childhood to over 60 years of age. In the 1930s, Hull (1933) and his students, especially Messerschmidt (1933a, 1933b), studied children's responses to waking suggestibility items. Although they did not equate suggestibility with hypnotizability, the two traits were positively correlated.

The results of the early studies were quite similar to more recent studies. That is, early research concluded that hypnotizability and suggestibility are quite limited in young children, increase markedly in the middle childhood years from about 7 to 14, and then decrease somewhat in adolescence, becoming quite stable throughout early and midadulthood, then tailing off again in the older population.

With all normative studies reaching essentially the same conclusion, one is tempted to review them rather briefly and then move on to other issues. The major problem is that these research findings are at variance with a growing body of clinical data indicating that children of preschool age, and perhaps even younger, do in fact respond positively to what is described as the therapeutic use of hypnosis. The issues involved in this controversy are complex. Thus, we choose to confront them head-on in order to leave the reader with some measure of the complexity of what appears on the surface to be an easy answer. We begin with a critical review of recent normative studies and then deal with the special problem of hypnotizability in young children.

NORMATIVE STUDIES

Stukát (1958) and Barber and Calverley (1963) administered tests of suggestibility to children at various ages. Since they did not claim to be using hypnotic techniques, we will not review their studies in detail. It should be noted that their findings for suggestibility are similar to studies measuring hypnotizability. This is seen in Figure 3.1, which compares their results with normative data for hypnotic susceptibility in children. One can conclude either that the traits measured by the three scales are highly correlated or that suggestibility, as measured by these tests, and hypnotic susceptibility are essentially the same trait.

Commenting on Tromater's (1961) review of early studies of childhood hypnotizability, London (1962) observed that early efforts to assess hypnotizability in children were in general agreement that children, as a group, are more susceptible than adults and that there is a curvilinear relationship between age and susceptibility, with a peak in the 8- to 12-year age range. London noted methodological problems in these early studies, especially the lack of an operational definition of susceptibility and imprecise measuring devices, and he set out to remedy these problems.

London developed a test called the Children's Hypnotic Susceptibility Scale (CHSS; 1963) that was based on the items in the Stanford Hypnotic Susceptibility Scale, Form A (SHSS, Form A; Weitzenhoffer & Hilgard, 1959). The CHSS contains 22 items in two parts, of which Part I is parallel in content to SHSS, Form A. Part II contains some more difficult items such

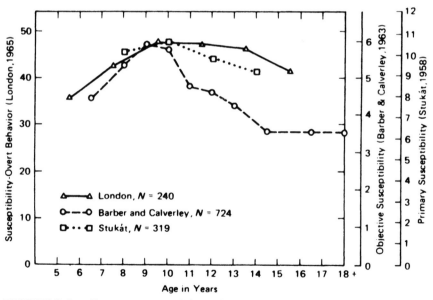

FIGURE 3.1.   Changes in suggestibility with age. Barber and Calverley's and Stukat's suggestibility scales (not involving hypnosis) correlate highly with hypnotic performances. London did use hypnotic techniques. Redrawn from E. R. Hilgard (1971). With permission.

as visual hallucinations and thirst and taste hallucinations. Administration of the scale requires 45 to 60 minutes for each child.

Because some children in the pilot studies (London, 1962) appeared to be faking or "playing along" with the instructions, the subjects received two scores for each item, one based on their overt behavioral response (OB) and the other based on the examiner's impression of the extent of the subjects' subjective involvement (SI), that is, whether they appeared to be (1) faking or role playing, (2) partially involved, or (3) deeply involved in the item. The product of these two scores yielded a total score (TOT). Usually, the score ultimately derived for each subject is the total for Part I and Part II combined. Sometimes the emphasis is on a part score. For example, if one wants to make comparisons with the SHSS, Form A, a 12-item test scored on the basis of the subject's overt behavior, then one would score the CHSS only for Part I, which contains the 12 parallel items, and only for overt behavior. Interscorer reliability, based on a pilot sample of 36 children retested after 1 week, was 92, indicating consistent performance in children similar to that found for adults.

Using data from 57 children, London (1962) found that children were more often successful on almost all CHSS items, as compared with adults on the SHSS, lending further credence to the notion that children are more susceptible. London was unable to establish a significant curvilinear relationship between age and susceptibility, although there was a trend in that direction. He predicted that the trend would become statistically meaningful when the sample size was increased, but he thought the curve would remain a shallow one, indicating that the relationship between susceptibility and age cannot be accounted for simply on the basis of age. He noted that "there is probably more variability among children at any given age than between children of any two successive ages" (p. 87).

To study the possibility that role playing might account for high scores among some children, London (1962) selected a new sample of 40 children, ages 5 to 11 years, the group in which role playing tended to occur. After performing six "playlets," each subject was engaged in a simulation task, following the motivation instructions for adults designed by Orne (1959). In his classic studies of hypnotic simulation, Orne compared nonhypnotizable subjects who were told to simulate hypnosis with highly hypnotizable subjects and found that even well-trained examiners could not tell which subjects belonged to which group. London's instructions to each child in his simulation study (1962) were as follows:

> We are going to be alone in this room for more minutes and then I am going to get Mrs. X. When she comes in, she will think that I have hypnotized you, and that you are in a deep hypnotic trance. Do you know what that means? Well, what I want you to do is make her think that you are

really hypnotized, and to do everything she tells you as if you were hypnotized. The things will be very easy for you, and the only thing you need to know is that, when she comes in, your eyes should be closed, and always keep them closed unless she tells you to open them.

Now, she may be a little bit suspicious that you aren't hypnotized because she knows that there will be one or two kids in here who are just faking, and she will wonder a little if it is you. If she thinks that you are faking, she will stop what she is doing right away—but as long as she keeps on going, you will know that you are fooling her into thinking you are hypnotized. (p. 87)

For children in this limited age range, there is a linear relationship between age and simulation ability. The simulation scores on the CHSS, Part II, were lower than those for hypnotic subjects below age 8 years but merged thereafter. In other words, simulation was obvious below age 8 years, but it was indistinguishable from hypnotic performance at higher ages. Noting that the youngest subjects were poor simulators and that older adolescents tend to be too honest to simulate on hypnotic susceptibility tests, London was left with the conclusion that "children in the middle group achieve peak scores because they can communicate simulated performances with the same effectiveness that they do real performances and we cannot tell them apart" (p. 90). This does not mean that all children in this group simulate, and those who do may do so only on selected items. Yet, when these children do simulate, it is not likely to be noticed, even by trained examiners. London concluded that the evidence for curvilinearity is weak and is even further weakened by the insensitivity of the CHSS to the simulation of individual items.

London noted that the subjects in these studies were chiefly from upper-middle-class backgrounds but did not speculate about the impact of social class distribution on his results.

London (1965) standardized his scale on a group of 240 children, ages 5 to 16 years, with 10 boys and 10 girls at each year level. These subjects came from a group of 303 children whose parents had responded to a form letter. Again the sample was markedly skewed toward the upper-middle-class professional and managerial level. For this new sample, interscorer reliability for the Full Scale CHSS ranged from .88 to .97 for the three obtained scores (overt behavior, subjective involvement, and total). Test–retest reliability ($N = 50$) after 1 week ranged from .75 to .84.

As in the pilot studies, there was a modest curvilinear relationship between age and susceptibility, with the peak in the 9- to 12-year range (Figure 3.2). And again the standard deviations were large at all ages. London (1965) noted that "the extent of susceptibility or the lack of it among different children within a single age group is more impressive than are changes across ages" (p. 195).

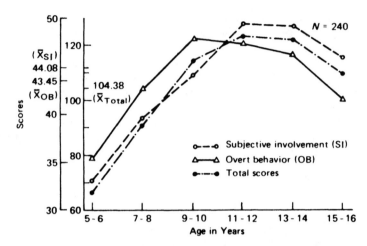

FIGURE 3.2. Mean Full Scale susceptibility scores, by age group, of the standardization sample ($N = 240$) for the CHSS. Redrawn from London (1965). With permission.

The mean score of the standardization sample of 240 children (8.16) was significantly larger than the mean score of college students (5.25) in the normative data for the SHSS, Form A. When scores were grouped into high, medium, and low categories for children, the largest group fell in the range of high susceptibility; for adults, the largest group fell in the range of low susceptibility. These data again support the notion that children are more responsive to hypnosis than adults (London & Cooper, 1969).

Cooper and London (1971) reported longitudinal data for a subset of the standardization sample. The intercorrelations across time periods, ranging from 1 week to 2 years, were significantly positive—but by no means perfect. Moreover, the correlations for younger children were lower than those for older children. These results are similar to those obtained in the measurement of intelligence, namely, that it is harder to predict from obtained scores to future scores for younger children than for older children. Results of this longitudinal study were similar to those of the cross-sectional studies, leading the authors to conclude that changes in susceptibility do occur with age and that these changes are extremely stable.

Morgan and Hilgard (1973) reported a massive study of age differences in hypnotic susceptibility for 1,232 subjects, ranging in age from 5 to 78 years. Again the subjects clustered in the middle socioeconomic class. The results for children, based on a slightly modified SHSS, Form A, were similar to those cited earlier, with a peak in the preadolescent years and a gradual decline thereafter. Morgan and Hilgard did not comment on the issue of simulation.

There were no significant sex differences in hypnotic susceptibility in any of these studies or in the report of Cooper and London (1966), which specifically addressed this issue.

The normative study of Morgan and Hilgard (1979) came to the same conclusions regarding age and hypnotizability as did the earlier studies. Its significance lies in the fact that the score is based on a short scale, The Stanford Hypnotic Clinical Scale for Children (SHCS-C) that can be administered in 20 minutes. This scale is presented in Appendix A. The brevity of the scale makes it feasible to use in a primarily therapeutic setting, although 20 minutes is a long time in most managed care settings.

Over the years, many clinicians have argued that the use of a scale to measure hypnotizability was, at best, irrelevant and at worst, improper. They argued that clinical and laboratory hypnosis are two different entities with little or no connection. Then they argued that, even if a scale could measure the kind of hypnotizability that is observed in a clinical setting, patients subjected to such a scale would experience frustration and failure that would both interfere with rapport and compromise therapeutic progress. Contrary to the assumptions of the first argument, E. R. Hilgard and Hilgard (1975) have found that adult subjects who score higher on a hypnotizability scale tend to respond more effectively to suggestions for pain control, both in experimental and in clinical settings. Contrary to the assumptions of the second argument, Morgan and Hilgard (1979) did not find any marked concerns about failure in the context of their permissive induction and suggestions. If a child began to apologize for a failed item, the examiner immediately countered with, "We are just as interested in what people don't experience as we are in what people do experience." Children in the clinical setting were told, "Not everybody does the same things. We have to find those things that are best for you, some you will find much more interesting than others. There will be some that we can build on" (Morgan & Hilgard, 1979, p. 154).

The Morgan and Hilgard (1979) study makes another major contribution to the field of hypnosis. Unfortunately, the authors make no mention of it, and we would like to take this opportunity to give them the credit they deserve. For the first time in the series of studies reported here, the term "susceptibility" has been omitted and the term "responsivity" used in its place. This shift reflects a growing awareness that the capacity to experience hypnosis is chiefly a skill or talent of the subject and not a phenomenon created by the hypnotist. The hypnotist is a teacher or coach rather than a controlling force. Thus, the term "hypnotic virtuoso" describes the behavior of the subject, not the hypnotist. The change in terminology reflects the change over the last few decades from an authoritarian to a permissive approach in hypnosis and hypnotherapy. We are in full agreement that the locus of control should be and is in the subject. Therefore, in this book, we use the term "responsiveness" or its equivalent except when referring to historical matters.

The SHCS-C includes one form for children 6 to 16 years old and another form for children 4 to 8 years old. The form for older children is based on an eye closure–relaxation induction followed by seven test items. The form for younger children is based on an active imagination induction, since young or immature children often respond negatively to suggestions for eye closure. This form contains six test items. In both forms, the items are intrinsically interesting to children, allow some success at all ages, and have direct relevance for choice of therapeutic techniques. The test correlated .67 with the longer SHSS, Form A, modified slightly for use with children.

In these early stages of its development, the SHCS-C consisted of only one form, utilizing an eye closure–relaxation induction. The second form (active imagination) was created when the authors discovered that the younger children failed most or all items in the relaxation condition but passed some of the same items in the imagination condition. At that time, exhibiting a degree of flexibility not seen in earlier studies, the authors modified the induction for younger children so that they could pass more items. The awareness of this need for flexibility now takes us into a new area, guaranteed to confuse more than to clarify what has already become a muddied field in the area of norms of hypnotizability in children.

HYPNOSIS AS A FUNCTION OF INDUCTION AND MEASUREMENT TECHNIQUES

Historically, the measurement of hypnotic susceptibility (responsivity) has consisted of a hypnotic induction emphasizing relaxation and eye closure followed by a number of test items reflecting various phenomena that most people agree typify hypnotic behavior. Subjects who score very low on these scales are said not to be hypnotizable. Moreover, some researchers (e.g., Barber, 1979) have taken the position that, if there is no formal hypnotic induction, the subject cannot be said to be in hypnosis at all.

We disagree with Barber's position. As yet, there is no absolute knowledge of the boundaries that define hypnosis. But we take the position that certain kinds of behavior can be described as hypnotic behavior. These behaviors include, but are not limited to, the behaviors elicited by standard scales of hypnotizability. And it is important to note that people vary in terms of their ability to experience different hypnotic phenomena. For example, two individuals with identical scores on a hypnotizability scale may have passed different kinds of items in order to obtain those scores.

We also believe that people vary in terms of the antecedent conditions that are necessary in order to experience hypnosis. In this regard, we find it refreshing that Morgan and Hilgard (1979) directed their research to show that some children respond positively to test items following one kind of induction but not another. Figure 3.3 shows the mean scores for their subjects following eye closure–relaxation and imagination inductions.

When children obtain different scores following different induction procedures, one might ask which scores are the "true" scores. We answer simply whichever scores are higher. That is, the purpose of a scale of hypnotic responsiveness is to allow the subjects to demonstrate their skills. But the findings of Morgan and Hilgard (1979) suggest that, in measuring hypnotizability, we have put some children in a position, through inappropriate induction techniques, where they do not do what they really can do. We then may come to the false conclusion that they are not responsive to hypnosis.

The situation is analogous to forcing a child into a sitting position and then measuring height by the distance of the child's head from the floor. Or, we could picture tying a child's hands behind his or her back and then concluding that he or she is not mature enough to tie his or her own shoes. We can only wonder what the normative data of London and Cooper and others would look like, particularly for younger children, if they modified the hypnotic induction in such a way as to maximize the child's ability to respond to the test items.

If the nature of hypnotic induction can affect scores on a responsivity scale, then the nature of the test items themselves will clearly also affect the scores. Logically, some items will be passed at virtually all ages, some at one

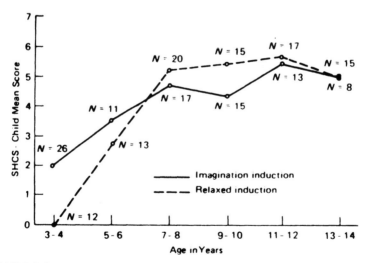

FIGURE 3.3.   Mean scores by age on seven items of the SHCS-C. Imagination induction is compared with relaxation induction. Redrawn from Morgan and Hilgard (1979). With permission.

age but not another, and some items might not be passed by children of any age. The test score will depend on which kinds of items and how many of each kind and which difficulty levels are included. As with intelligence, ultimately the meaning of hypnotizability is reduced to what precisely is tested by the test.

E. R. Hilgard and colleagues (E. R. Hilgard, Weitzenhoffer, Landes, & Moore, 1961) recognized the need for an operational definition when they wrote that "what we shall mean by hypnotic susceptibility for the purpose of our investigations is a relatively persistent tendency to yield the phenomena historically recognized as belonging to the hypnotic trance, *when the opportunity to yield these phenomena is given under standard conditions*" (p. 1). Adult scales of hypnotizability sample a variety of hypnotic phenomena, with items placed roughly in order of difficulty and high scores considered more "susceptible" than low ones.

In the case of children, degrees of item difficulty are not the same as those for adults or even for children of different ages. Therefore we must at least pause before we conclude that, on a particular scale of children's hypnotic responsiveness, a specific score necessarily means the same thing that it does on an adult scale. We must question whether the broad-sample-of-hypnotic-phenomena approach is as appropriate for children as it is for adults. That is, some so-called traditional hypnotic phenomena may be traditional for adults but not for children or for certain groups of children because of developmental issues. To use another analogy, we do not administer to young children the same types of intelligence test items we use for adults on the Stanford–Binet, recognizing that certain language and abstract reasoning skills are simply not developed in the young child. That is, we define intelligence somewhat differently for young children than for adults.

Moreover, if we want the concept "hypnosis" to mean roughly the same thing for children as for adults, then we should be reasonably confident that a given item is tapping the same quality in children as for adults as well as tapping the same quality in children of different ages. Such item equivalence is probably not the case in some instances, as evidenced by data relating age to item difficulty on scales of hypnotic responsiveness in children.

London and Cooper (1969) reported item difficulty for their standardization sample of 240 children for the CHSS, and they compared percent passing each item with the equivalent data for adults on the SHSS, Form A. In Table 3.1 we have adapted these data and rank ordered each item in terms of relative difficulty for children and for adults.

When these data are studied, the most striking finding is that eye closure is the most difficult item of all for children, whereas it is relatively easy for adults. We suspect that, in the case of children, suggestions for eye closure trigger negative attitudes and concerns about sleep and that these issues preclude the sort of detached interest in motor phenomena that most likely

TABLE 3.1. **Item Difficulty for Children on the CHSS and for Adults on the SHSS, Form A**

| | Rank order of difficulty[a] | |
Item	Children	Adults
Auditory hallucination	1.0	6.0
Postural sway	2.0	3.0
Hands together	3.0	2.0
Hands lowering	4.0	1.0
Finger lock	5.0	8.0
Posthypnotic suggestion	6.5	5.0
Amnesia	6.5	8.0
Arm rigidity	8.0	8.0
Verbal inhibition	9.0	11.0
Eye catalepsy	10.0	10.0
Arm immobilization	11.0	12.0
Eye closure	12.0	4.0

Note. Adapted from London and Cooper (1969).
[a]1 = easiest item; 12 = hardest item.

predominates for adults. If the item is tapping something in children that has little or nothing to do with hypnosis, then it really does not belong in the test.

R. K. Moore and Cooper (1966) commented on the difficulty with eye closure for children as compared to adults. They noted that the CHSS employs a Chevreul pendulum for this item with the instruction to hold the chain, look at the ball, and try to prevent it from moving. The parallel adult item (SHSS, Form B) requires the subject merely to look passively at a fixed target. They concluded that "for children, it may be that the interesting activity of trying to hold the attractive plastic ball stationary is less conducive to eye closure than focusing the gaze on a target some distance away" (p. 320). If this is true, then again, the two items are not measuring the same thing.

To give another example, children find the auditory hallucination item very easy (89% pass), whereas for adults, it is moderately difficult (35% pass). In this case, we have a notion that the item probably is measuring the same ability in children as in adults, with children simply being more skilled at this particular task.

R. K. Moore and Lauer (1963) studied item difficulty for a sample of 48 children, ages 6 to 12 years, and compared their data to adult scores, with essentially the same results as the sample of London and Cooper (1969).

Questions about the meaning of test items become even more interesting when we look at the data in Table 3.2, showing the relative difficulty of each item for children at different ages. Although we have not attempted any statistical analysis of these data, we are struck by several instances in which there are marked shifts in difficulty level from one age group to another. For example, it is astonishing that the amnesia item is the easiest of all for

TABLE 3.2. Relative Item Difficulty on the CHSS across Age Levels (N = 240)

Item	Age (years)[a]					
	5–6	7–8	9–10	11–12	13–14	15–16
Amnesia	1.0	11.5	13.0	10.0	16.0	12.0
Auditory hallucination	2.0	2.0	2.0	1.5	1.0	4.5
Hands together	3.5	6.0	5.0	12.5	4.5	3.0
Cold hallucination	3.5	4.0	5.0	7.0	8.0	6.0
Postural sway	5.0	9.0	8.5	3.5	2.5	1.5
Television	6.5	6.0	3.5	5.5	8.0	10.0
Visual hallucination	6.5	1.0	1.0	1.5	4.5	8.5
Finger lock	8.0	8.0	8.5	12.5	6.0	12.0
Hand lowering	9.0	3.0	11.5	10.0	8.0	4.5
Taste hallucination	10.0	6.0	5.0	3.5	10.0	15.5
Arm rigidity	11.0	11.5	10.0	16.0	19.0	19.5
Verbal inhibition	13.0	15.5	16.0	18.0	13.5	19.5
Smell hallucination	13.0	10.0	17.0	8.0	16.0	8.5
Dream	13.0	13.0	3.5	5.5	2.5	1.5
Post-hypnotic suggestion II	15.0	15.5	14.5	21.0	18.0	17.0
Arm immobilization	16.0	18.0	19.5	17.0	13.5	19.5
Eye closure	17.5	21.0	22.0	22.0	21.0	15.5
Post-hypnotic suggestion I	17.5	15.5	11.5	10.0	11.0	12.0
Eye catalepsy	19.5	15.5	14.5	20.0	16.0	22.0
Anesthesia	19.5	19.5	19.5	19.0	20.0	19.5
Regression	21.5	19.5	21.0	14.5	12.0	7.0
Post-hypnotic suggestion III	21.5	22.0	18.0	14.5	22.0	14.0

Note. Adapted from London and Cooper (1969).
[a]1 = easiest item; 22 = hardest item.

the 5- to 6-year-olds, whereas it is moderately difficult for children at all other ages and for adults. We strongly suspect that, although the item taps problems of memory retrieval for subjects beyond age 6, it taps problems of memory storage in the very young child. Since memory storage is not really what the item is designed to measure, it should probably not be in the test for this young age group.

Thus, we agree with E. R. Hilgard and colleagues (1961). If a scale purports to sample hypnotic phenomena, then it should do that and not something else. We would therefore anticipate some sort of revision of the CHSS in the same way and for the same reasons that intelligence tests or aptitude tests are subjected to item analysis and revised according to the data obtained.

After having dealt with some of the more formal problems involved in test construction, we now turn to the relevance of a hypnotic responsiveness scale of a therapeutic situation. Morgan (1974) and Morgan and Hilgard (1979) both address this issue. Morgan noted that the factor analytic studies on the SHSS, Form A, yielded three main factors: factor I included challenge items (e.g., arm immobilization, finger lock); factor II included direct suggestion items (e.g., hand lowering, eye closure); factor III included cognitive items (e.g., fly hallucination, post-hypnotic amnesia). Morgan noted that challenge items are relatively difficult for children and place the locus of control outside the child. Moreover, such items may encourage young children to balk because they have not yet resolved developmental issues in which oppositional behavior is a major response style. Morgan concluded that use of such items is probably undesirable in a treatment situation. On the other hand, direct suggestion items are easy for children, are readily converted to autosuggestions, and may therefore be especially appropriate in the context of treatment. Likewise, cognitive items are easy and also may provide information that is useful in treatment. Morgan and Hilgard (1979) applied these conclusions advantageously in the development of their short clinical scale for children. In other words, general hypnotic responsivity is not the same as the particular kind or kinds of responsivity that may be appropriate and relevant in a clinical situation. One should be able to predict something about treatment response from the latter but not necessarily from the former.

HYPNOSIS AND THE YOUNG CHILD

Available scales have indicated that 5- and 6-year-old children are not very responsive as compared with older children. And, it is generally assumed that children too young for the scales would score even lower than the 5-year-olds from whom data are available. However, several clinical reports have described the effectiveness of hypnotherapy with preschool children for such diverse problems as easing induction of anesthesia (Antitch, 1967; Cullen, 1958), alleviating distress and reducing pain (Gardner, 1978b; LaBaw, 1973; Olness, 1981b; Kuttner, 1991), controlling enuresis and encopresis (Olness, 1975, 1976), adjusting to contact lenses (Olness & Gardner, 1978), and asthma (Kohen & Wynne, 1988). The recent short clinical scale (Morgan & Hilgard, 1979) reaches down to age 4 years, and we have virtually no research information about children age 3 years and younger. Since we must assume that subjects who are not "hypnotizable" (as defined by the available scales) could not profitably utilize hypnosis in the course of treatment, we must either conclude that the claims for hypnotherapeutic efficacy are based on some aspect of the therapeutic relationship or process other than hypnosis, or we must revise our assumptions about the nature of hypnotizability.

Gardner (1977a) reviewed the question of hypnosis with infants and preschool children in some detail, noting that the primary problem lies in how one defines hypnosis:

> The tendency has been to look at a score on a scale, or to consider a response to some sort of formal hypnotic induction, or at least to assess the subject's verbal report of his own experiences. These criteria are not applicable to very young children; we have no scales below age 4, general-

ly recognized formal induction methods do not exist below about age 4, and the youngsters do not have adequate verbal fluency to describe their experiences in acceptable detail.

In the absence of the usual criteria for defining hypnosis, one must rely on observations of certain behaviors of the young child which are similar to behaviors associated with hypnosis in adults. These include (1) quiet, wakeful behavior, which may or may not lead to sleep, following soothing repetitive stimulation, which is a primary characteristic of most formal induction procedures, (2) involvement in vivid imagery during induction in children beyond infancy, (3) heightened attention to a narrow focus with concomitant alterations in awareness, (4) capacity to follow post-hypnotic suggestions as evidenced by behavior which deviates from what is known to be the child's usual behavior in a particular situation. (pp. 158–159)

Gardner (1977a) reviewed clinical evidence supporting the notion that small children develop reliable ways of soothing themselves, such as rocking or talking rhythmically. She noted that parents also find reliable ways of calming their young children. Specific examples include stroking some part of the body, playing music, turning on a vacuum cleaner, and putting an electric shaver near the child. She found that the sound of a small hair dryer has the same quieting effect on a fretful infant. She described young patients who responded positively on rhythmic stimulation. She noted studies of hypnosis (Morgan, 1973; Ruch, 1975) in which the authors suggest that hypnotic talent may be present from a very young age or even from birth, and she also reported pertinent studies in child development that show children as young as 2 years having the capacity for fantasy and rapport and the desire for mastery intrinsic to the hypnotic situation. Bowers and LeBaron (1986) have noted the importance of developmental factors in assessing hypnotic responsivity. They note that most 7-year-old children have the cognitive ability to experience most aspects of hypnosis reported by adults. They also note that many children find hypnotic suggestions to be as natural as play. LeBaron (1983) found a significant relationship between the occurrence of fantasy-oriented activities in children's family environment and their hypnotic susceptibility. One can also speculate on the possibility that neurobiological differences produce some parents who are fantasy-oriented and are able to provide their children with both the genetic and environmental resources for enjoyment of fantasy. Furthermore, preschoolers are often in states equivalent to if not hypnosis, when they are in fact active, noisy, moving about, especially when they are "play acting" or "role playing."

Gardner (1977a) suggested developing a scale that might tap hypnotic potentialities in very young children, adding that hypnotherapy might be more appropriate for this age group than hitherto recognized. A test of hypnotic responsiveness may be conceptualized as a work sample; for any subject, one must be sure that the work sample is relevant to available behavior and abilities. Rather than insisting that hypnotic responsiveness is present only if a large number of hypnotic phenomena can be elicited, it might be more useful in the case of very young children to start from a position closer to Bartlett's (1968) definition of hypnosis as "a control of the normal control of input (information) for the purpose of controlling output (behavior)" (p. 69). Some hypnosis researchers seem to be moving in this general direction. For example, Hilgard and Morgan (1978) noted the following:

> First, for the young child, approximately the age group of four to six, with as always a few exceptions, it is inappropriate to rely upon formal hypnotic procedures. These procedures involve two major elements: (a) the implied difference between voluntary and involuntary action, and (b) the expectation of distraction through self-controlled fantasy. Instead, this group is more responsive to a kind of protohypnosis, in which the distraction has at first been set up in the external situation. That is, the very young child is better able to be distracted by listening to a story or by participating in a verbal game with a friendly adult than by removing himself from the scene through his own fantasy or through reliving an earlier game or experience on his own. Gradually the content of the external stimulation can be altered in such a way that the child achieves the control. From the beginning, the primary goal is to give the control to the child. This technique of distraction works with children who are unable to use formal hypnosis; such a group also includes some of the older children. (p. 286)

In a later paper (Morgan & Hilgard, 1979), the same authors concluded that "the child under 6 is hypnotizable, but not according to the sample practices commonly used with older children" (p. 154).

In the 1979 paper, Morgan and Hilgard noted the rather poor response of youngest children to hypnotic suggestions for pain and anxiety control during such major medical procedures as spinal taps and bone marrow aspirates. We would add that, even if these results follow from the use of fully appropriate induction techniques and suggestions, the fact that the young subjects did not respond much to hypnosis for this purpose does not mean they might not respond positively in some less threatening situation. General hypnotic responsiveness and responsiveness in a particular laboratory or clinical setting may be two very different things.

In the case of young children, the field is wide open for advances in the study of hypnotic responsivity and its clinical applications.

CONCLUSIONS

We have strayed far from the simple curvilinear relationship, with its peak in the middle childhood years that is often assumed to describe accurately the norms of hypnotizability in children. Major problems include the difficulty in identifying instances in which subjects in middle childhood simulate hypnosis, use of samples limited to the middle socioeconomic class, very large standard deviations, weaknesses in test construction, frequent use of induction techniques that may interfere with hypnotic responsiveness, use of items to measure hypnotizability that may actually be measuring something quite different, and lack of data and methods of assessing hypnotizability in very young children.

The truth is that we really cannot say very much with confidence concerning hypnotic responsiveness in children. Although there is obviously a tremendous need for more research, we believe we can conclude two things. First, most studies err on the side of underestimating children's hypnotic talent. Second—and this conclusion derives from the first—the lack of solid evidence concerning children's hypnotic responsiveness does not imply that we should abandon our clinical efforts to help children through hypnotherapy. On the contrary, in a context of proper modesty, we should continue to expand both research and clinical efforts and thereby enlarge the data bank. Many children do respond to hypnotherapy, and many reports conclude that the crucial element in treatment is hypnosis and not something else. In a field where the state of the art is not as primitive as it is in child hypnosis, such an argument would, at best, be considered very weak. In this field, however, it seems to be the only reasonable place to stand for the time being.

CHAPTER FOUR

Correlates of Childhood Hypnotic Responsiveness

Researchers and clinicians have wrestled with the problem of determining why children, as a group, are more responsive to hypnosis than adults. Some suggested answers are based on research; others are derived from theories of child development; still others are derived from informal observations of children. In this chapter, we discuss a wide variety of possible correlates, evaluating the available data. A few correlates have already been discussed, and we mention them briefly for the sake of completion.

VARIABLES

Age

The relationship between age and hypnotic responsivity is very complex. The repeated finding of a modest curvilinear relationship, with its peak in middle childhood, may or may not be entirely accurate. Some of the correlates postulated below derived from the assumption that the results of the normative studies are truly a reflection of reality.

Sex

We have noted that there are no significant differences in hypnotic responsiveness between boys and girls at any age. Therefore, it is reasonable to combine data for both sexes in discussing research and clinical findings.

Nature of the Induction
and of the Suggestion Item

Children of different ages respond best to different kinds of inductions, and specific items may measure different dimensions at one age than at another. The reader will have to bear this in mind in evaluating clinical findings presented in later chapters.

Genetics

Morgan, Hilgard, and Davert (1970) studied hypnotic responsiveness of 76 pairs of twins, together with their parents and siblings close in age, using the SHSS, Form A (Weitzenhoffer & Hilgard, 1959). Morgan (1973) later increased the twin sample to 140 pairs, including the original 76. Since larger samples yield more reliable data, we report data only from the more recent study. The twins' age range was 5 to 22 years. Zygosity of the twin pairs was based primarily on the mothers' reports, this method having been found to correlate very highly with serological methods. Both members of a twin pair were hypnotized simultaneously, in separate rooms, in order to avoid experimenter bias or communication between the twins. Parents also completed a questionnaire, rating each child for similarity to father and to mother on 11 personality and temperamental variables.

The correlations for monozygotic twins were statistically significant both for males ($r = .54$) and for females ($r = .49$). Correlations for dizygotic twins and for sibling nontwin pairs were not different from zero ($r = .08-.25$). Moreover, the correlation for monozygotic pairs ($r = .52$) was significantly higher than the correlation for like-sexed dizygotic pairs ($r = .18$). These data, together with a computed heritability index of .64 and a low but significant correlation between midparent and mean child susceptibility, were consistent with the interpretation of a genetic contribution.

Personality resemblance, as rated by the parents, was positively related to hypnotizability scores for either sexed child and the like-sexed parent. No such interaction existed for either sexed child and the opposite-sexed parent. Morgan (1973) interpreted these results as suggesting an environmental contribution to hypnotizability, based mainly on identification with the liked-sexed parent and modeling of that parent's behavior. She concluded that "hypnotizability thus appears to be the product of both a genetic predisposition and subsequent environmental influences, as well as their interaction" (p. 61).

The capacity for eidetic imagery ("photographic mind") is known to exist in approximately 6% of children in the Western world but is also known to be nearly universal in certain tribal groups in Africa. This may be a genetic trait that would relate to the capacity for hypnotic responsiveness. However, this phenomenon has not been studied. It has been our clinical experience that children who have eidetic imagery learn and apply self-hypnosis very easily.

Cognitive Development

London (1965) correlated hypnotizability scores on the CHSS (London, 1963) with intelligence test scores for a group of 42 children, ages 8 to 12 years, taken from his standardization sample and for a group of 54 children, ages 6 to 12 years, participating in the Fels Institute Longitudinal Study. For the first group, IQ scores were extrapolated from scores on the Vocabulary subtest of the Wechsler Intelligence Scale for Children (WISC; Wechsler, 1949). For the Fels group, complete WISC scores were available. The relationship between hypnotizability and intelligence was positive but modest. Comparing the difference in the correlation coefficients for the two samples, London concluded that standardization sample ($r = .43$).

L. Jacobs and Jacobs (1966) studied hypnotizability of 64 school children, ages 4 to 17 years, who were referred because of poor school achievement associated with a variety of factors including manifest brain injury, mental retardation, delinquency, behavior disorders, and psychoses. No standardized scale of hypnotizability was utilized. The subjects were considered to be in hypnosis "when eye closure with rhythmic eyeball movements, increased and forceful swallowing, masked facies, regular slow respiration and muscular relaxation were obtained, followed by a catalepsy of the eyelids or extremities" (p. 270).

Sixty of the children were given one or more of several individual intelligence tests, either privately or by a school psychologist. The IQ distribution was skewed toward the lower end, with five subjects scoring from 50 to 70 and five subjects below 50. Only three subjects scored above 130. Visual inspection of the data indicated that those with the highest IQs achieved a trance state more often than those rated below average or retarded. No tests of statistical significance were performed. The large incidence of severe neurological and emotional disorders and the likelihood that the children came from a wide range of social class backgrounds make it impossible to compare these data meaningfully with the London (1965) data.

At this time, therapists are not trained to adapt hypnotherapeutic or other forms of communication to the specific learning capabilities of each child. It is possible that some children would respond better to visual or nonverbal teaching strategies than to talk strategies. It is hoped that research will provide screening assessments to guide therapists in their choice of teaching strategies.

Child Behavior

Although child hypnotherapists generally agree that usual teaching strategies are ineffective with children who have an attention-deficit or attention-
deficit/hyperactivity disorder, such children may focus very well on hypnotic inductions that include physical movement or provide appealing biofeedback.

A study by Kohen and colleagues (Kohen & Ondich, 1992) found no
correlation between the SHCS-C and the Achenbach Child Behavior Checklist and its subscales with 100 children.

For the present, we cannot predict hypnotic responsiveness based on
specific behaviors of children.

Electroencephalographic Patterns

Children's electroencephalographic (EEG) patterns have been studied in hopes
of finding some relationship to hypnotizability. Cooper and London (1976)
and London (1976) studied a sample of 35 normal children, ages 7 to 16
years. Hypnotic susceptibility was significantly correlated with alpha duration ($r = .29$) when the children's eyes were open. Although the alpha duration increased as expected when the children were told to close their eyes,
the relationship between alpha and hypnotizability vanished ($r = -.09$).
The authors (Cooper & London, 1976) noted that alpha represents a relatively alert state of consciousness in children, and they surmised that

> since it is well known also that young children do not like to keep their
> eyes shut for long, the relatively higher incidence of alpha duration in the
> Eyes Closed condition of this study may represent exactly the opposite of
> what it would represent in an adult study; namely, that the children are
> more alerted when their eyes are closed than when they are open. (p. 146)

They concluded that it might have been more appropriate to study theta
waves. The data were further confused by the finding that the magnitude
of the correlations varied markedly from one experimenter to another.

L. Jacobs and Jacobs (1966) found, in a group of children with poor
school achievement, that children with markedly abnormal EEGs showed
poor responsiveness to hypnotic induction. As noted in the section on intelligence, many of their subjects manifested mental retardation and frank brain
damage, thus making the data even more difficult to interpret.

Walters, E. Green, and A. Green at the Menninger Clinic have developed an EEG biofeedback unit that produces alpha, beta, and theta feedback
concurrently and also provides a quantitative measure of various brain wave

percentages. In piloting these units, we have noted that the brain wave measures vary rapidly and directly according to the type of thinking that a child is asked to do. Children are also able to develop skill in changing brain wave pattern voluntarily. These units have been used therapeutically in working with children who have attention-deficit disorders and seizures (D. Walters, E. Green, & A. Green, personal communication, 1986). Camp and Ledbetter at the University of Colorado are currently developing EEG standards for such training, and they will implement a controlled trial of EEG feedback for children with attention deficits.

Response to Thermal Biofeedback Training

Several studies of adults have found no relationship between scores on various hypnotizability scales and response to biofeedback training for control of peripheral skin temperature (Engstrom, 1976; Frischholz & Tryon, 1980; Roberts, Schuler, Bacon, Zimmerman, & Patterson, 1975). Engstrom (1976), however, found that when subjects attempted to change skin temperature using hypnosis alone, with no biofeedback, low-hypnotizable subjects failed while highly hypnotizable subjects succeeded.

Children respond to thermal biofeedback training (Hunter, Russel, Russell, & Zimmerman, 1976; Lynch, Hama, Kohn, & Miller, 1976). We know of no studies of children in which success in such training has been correlated with hypnotic responsiveness. Dikel and Olness (1980) studied control of peripheral skin temperature in children ages 5 to 15 years. Most children succeeded at this task. There were no differences in temperature control between children who used hypnotic imagery alone and those who combined hypnosis with biofeedback training. Moreover, neither of these two groups differed from a third group, with no previous hypnosis training, that achieved temperature control using biofeedback alone. Since some children in the third group reported using spontaneous thermal imagery (e.g., putting their hands into snow) similar to the imagery offered to the first two groups by the experimenters, it seemed possible that the third group had actually used hypnotic techniques in spite of the effort to control for this variable. A few children who achieved little temperature change using hypnosis alone were much more successful when biofeedback was added. Although the authors did not measure hypnotic responsiveness, it is possible that these subjects were at the lower end of that continuum. Subjects who responded minimally to biofeedback alone were not offered the opportunity to see whether they might do better with hypnosis training.

We attempted to correlate skill in peripheral temperature control in two clinical studies (Olness & Singher, 1989; Olness, MacDonald, & Uden, 1987). These involved training in self-regulation of pain in children with cancer and with juvenile migraine. There were no correlations between ability to control peripheral temperature and ability to demonstrate pain control in a clinically useful manner. This was because the majority of children demonstrated rapid, significant changes in peripheral temperature, as has been described in other studies. The variation in this ability was not sensitive enough to provide a predictor with respect to application of skills in self-hypnosis.

King and Montgomery (1980) discussed complex methodological problems in evaluating the results of thermal biofeedback training. Given the additional complexities of measuring hypnotic responsiveness in children, we anticipate that it will be some time before there is clarification of the relationship between the two skills. Our hunch is that the two skills are unrelated in children as well as in adults. We wonder whether children whose locus of control is external may respond better to biofeedback training, whereas those who tend more toward internal locus of control may be able to change skin temperature more easily with hypnosis. As cyberphysiological (self-regulatory) skills, however, biofeedback training may be applied clinically in a variety of complementary ways (Culbert, Reaney, & Kohen, 1994).

Control of Tissue Oxygen

A pilot study by Olness and Conroy (1985) did show that some children were able to control tissue oxygen using self-hypnosis techniques, but it did not conclude that self-hypnosis was a causative factor or essential to success in such control.

Achievement Motivation

In 1966, London despaired of ever finding personality variables that would correlate with hypnotizability in children. Later reports (Cooper & London, 1976) were somewhat more optimistic with respect to achievement motivation. In the study of 35 children, in which EEG data were also reported, the subjects were asked to solve puzzles 1 week after the CHSS was administered. They were asked to try to get the solution independently, although they could request parental help if they wished. Children with the highest hypnotic susceptibility scores tended to wait the longest before requesting help, indicating higher achievement motivation. London suggested that these findings reflected variations in child-rearing practices, especially with respect to independence training.

The research on hypnotizability and achievement motivation is consistent with clinical impressions that children's natural desire for mastery of skills and for understanding of, and participation in, their environment is directly related to their responsiveness to hypnosis (M. H. Erickson, 1958b; Gardner, 1974a). Clinicians capitalize on these qualities when they introduce hypnosis to a child as "something new you can learn how to do — not everybody knows how to do it, just as not everybody knows how to ride a bike."

Role Playing

London (1962) observed that some subjects seemed to be faking on the CHSS, especially those in the 8- to 12-year age group. This observation was supported by the ability of children in this age group to simulate hypnosis when instructed to do so.

In further examination of these findings, especially in the context of Sarbin's (1950) role theory of hypnotic susceptibility, Bowers and London (1965) compared the abilities of 40 children, ages 5 to 11 years, on two role-playing tasks. One was a measure of dramatic acting skill; the other was a hypnotic simulation test. When age and intelligence were held statistically constant, there was no correlation between the two measures.

Madsen and London (1966) then explored the relationship of these two skills to hypnotic susceptibility scores on the CHSS. The subjects were 42 middle-class children ages 7 to 11 years. The dramatic acting test measured the extent to which the children could portray the cultural stereotype of such familiar roles as mother, bully, teacher, and sheriff. The hypnotic simulation test was the one described in the earlier London (1962) studies. All subjects were given the CHSS, followed 1 week later by the two role-playing tests. Hypnotizability scores were significantly correlated with scores on the simulation test, but there was no relationship between CHSS scores and dramatic acting ability. Thus, role playing is a complex behavior, made up of several skills that may or may not be related to each other and to other variables.

Madsen and London (1966) noted that children who scored low on the CHSS scored about five points higher on the simulation test given 1 week later. For high scores on the CHSS, the later simulation score was essentially unchanged. The authors postulated a possible rehearsal effect for the low susceptible children and designed another study to test that hypothesis.

In the second study (London & Madsen, 1968), 34 children, ages 7 to 11 years, were given the same tests as in the first study, but this time the order was reversed, with the CHSS following the role-playing tests. Unlike the earlier (1966) study of these authors, there was no significant correlation between hypnotic simulation and hypnotic susceptibility. In other words, if the subjects were familiarized with the various phenomena on the CHSS, they could role play the part of a hypnotized person with some proficiency.

But they could not simulate a set of behaviors about which they knew very little. With respect to overt behavior scores, prior simulation experience had virtually no effect on the later CHSS scores. However, to the surprise of the experimenters, prior simulation experience led to a significant decrease on CHSS subjective involvement scores measuring the degree to which the experimenters thought the subjects were really involved in the items.

The experimenters concluded that attempting deliberately to act like a hypnotized person inhibits ability to become deeply involved in a similar task. To put it in another framework (Fromm, 1977), approaching a task in the context of ego activity may interfere with later ability to perform the task in a more ego-receptive mode.

Imaginative Involvement

Several studies of child development have clearly established that children in the 2- to 5-year age range not only are capable of imagery and fantasy but spend a great deal of their time in various types of imaginative behavior (Gould, 1972; L. Murphy, 1962; Singer, 1973, 1974).

Kosslyn, Margolis, Barrett, Goldknopf, and Daly (1990) conducted a study in which they compared mental processing of visual images by 5-year-olds, 8-year-olds, 14-year-olds, and adults on four imagery tasks. These included image generation, image maintenance, image scanning, and image rotation, for example, to decide which pieces can be loaded into a car's trunk. All tasks were computer administered, and subjects generally responded by pressing the appropriate key on the keyboard. Adults and 14-year-olds were tested in a single session, but younger childen were tested in two separate sessions. Subjects were asked to memorize upper case block letters as they appeared drawn in 4 × 5 grids, and later they were asked to look at two X marks in an empty grid. They were to decide whether a specified upper case letter would cover both marks if it were present in the grid as previously seen. Ten letters were used; five were relatively simple (L, C, U, F, H). Five (P, J, O, S, G) were relatively complex. Twenty trials were used. Response times were slower with younger children. Male children took relatively more time to generate images of complex letters than did female children. In an image maintenance task, younger children were as adept at holding images as the older children. For a scanning task, the 5- and 8-year-olds were slower than the 14-year-olds and adults, but 8-year-olds were very adept at accurately generating images of simple letters.

This is one of the first studies of mental processing of images in children and is important. However, whether or not it is relevant to spontaneous use of imagination in children is not known. The researchers defined a visual image. Letters may not be familiar to all 5-year-olds; this may have given an advantage to older children. Letter reversals are also frequent in many 5-year-olds, and this may have impacted on the results. However, the finding that the female children were superior in generating and maintaining images as defined in this study is worth noting. No studies have been done relating sex to image preferences in children or to hypnosis teaching strategies for children.

The idea that imagination is an important factor in hypnotic responsiveness is at least as old as the commission that investigated Mesmer's theories in 1784. The positive relationship between various kinds of imaginative involvement and hypnotizability in adults is now well established, particularly as a result of careful investigations by J. R. Hilgard (1970). In her elaborate study of young adults, she not only found that highly hypnotizable subjects engaged in a variety of imaginative involvements as adults, but also that these subjects—in contrast to those who were low on susceptibility tests—more frequently had engaged in imaginative experiences in childhood, according to their own reports. In the highly hypnotizable subjects, imagination was typically related to stimuli outside the person rather than autistic or inner-stimulated imagination. Parents either reinforced fantasy or at least did not interfere with it. LeBaron's study (1983) showed a significant relationship between fantasy-oriented activities in the family environment and children's hypnotic responsiveness.

Many child clinicians are convinced that the readiness with which children respond to hypnosis is related to their imaginative skills and involvements (Ambrose, 1961; Boswell, 1962; Erickson, 1958b; Gardner, 1974a; L. Jacobs, 1962; Kohen & Olness, 1993; Kuttner, 1988, 1991; Olness & Gardner, 1978). Gardner (1974a) has described several aspects of cognitive and emotional development in children that are probably related both to imaginative involvement and to hypnotizability. These include (1) capacity for intense concentration, immersion, focused attention on a limited stimulus field, and full absorption in the immediate present; (2) a tendency toward concrete, literal thinking; (3) limited reality testing, love of magic, and readiness to shift back and forth between reality and fantasy; (4) intensity of feeling states, often in an all-or-nothing way; and (5) openness to new ideas and delight with new experiences in a context of felt safety and trust.

Some writers have offered explanations of changes in hypnotic responsiveness with age largely in terms of development and decline of imaginative skills. E. R. Hilgard (1971) made the following interpretation:

> Hypnosis reaches its height in the preadolescent period because by that time language and experience have stimulated imagination and given it content, so that those characteristics described as child-likeness have had a full opportunity to bloom. . . . [In late adolescence] reality-orientations conflict with the free enjoyment of a life of fantasy and adventure, and for many people this means a reduction in their hypnotizability. (p. 38)

J. R. Hilgard (1970) commented similarly on declining hypnotizability with age:

> One may hazard the guess that the conditions of increasing rational sophistication and the needs for competency and achievement bring with them a decline in wonderment; these changes with age somehow counteract the imaginative involvements so important in hypnosis and substitute for them interactions on a reality level that make hypnosis increasingly difficult. (p. 189)

Whether this is true, or whether the change in imaginative involvement with age makes hypnosis *different* with increasing age, rather than more difficult, is unclear.

In London's (1966) study of a large number of personality variables in relation to childhood hypnotizability, he included information about the children's tendency to be imaginative and to engage in an active fantasy life, obtaining his data through interviews with parents of 111 children. Specific questions concerned imaginary playmates, extent of dreaming, whether the child talked to him- or herself much, and whether the child played imaginative games either alone or with other children. None of these items—alone or in combination—correlated with CHSS scores, although they correlated positively with each other. There was, however, a certain moderating effect of imagination on age and susceptibility. That is, there was a significant correlation between age and susceptibility for children low in imagination, but there was no age–susceptibility relationship for children whose imagination scores were high. Considering the very large number of variables studied, London was hesitant to make very much of these findings.

LeBaron, Zeltzer, and Fanurik (1988) conducted two pilot studies to assess the relationship between hypnotizability in children and the extent of involvement in fantasy-related activities during early childhood. They developed a structured interview questionnaire regarding fantasy activities that occurred between ages 4 and 7 years. These included questions such as: "What were your favorite games and activities?"; "What games or activities did you like best when you were all alone?"; and "Did your parents ever read to you or tell you stories?" They administered the SHCS-C and the fantasy questionnaire to 30 children with medical problems, ages 6 to 18 years, and to 37 healthy children, ages 6 to 12, years from a school population. They found that the distribution of fantasy scores was approximately normal, but, as has been true in many other studies, the hypnotizability scores were strongly skewed toward the high end of the scale. They found that there was a correlation of .42 ($p < .03$) between fantasy and SHCS-C scores in the children with medical problems and .39 ($p < .02$) for the healthy children. They recognized a confounding variable that the older subjects might have had difficulty in recalling imaginative involvement from childhood or be more reluctant to reveal childhood interests to the interviewer. Authors note a problem in the SHCS-C is that criteria allow for passing the "fantasy" items such as dream with a minimum of detail, so that the total score does not distinguish between children who are able to experience richly detailed fantasies and those who report only a few images.

In 1991, Plotnick, Payne, and O'Grady reported a study using the fantasy questionnaire used in the LeBaron study, the Children's Social Desirability Questionnaire (CSDQ), the Zeltzer and LeBaron (1984) revision of the Stanford Hypnotic Clinical Scale for Children (SHCS-C-R), and the Children's Fantasy Inventory: Absorption and Vividness Scales (CFI: A&V). This study had recruiting difficulties, and investigators ultimately studied 42 children from 26 families and sent the script of the SHCS-C to the parents before they brought their children in for the study. This could have resulted in contamination of results. Authors found that absorption in imaginary involvements in children (CFI:A) related significantly to the hypnotizability scores for Observed Behavior ($r = .42$, $p < .01$). Scores on the vividness of imagery scale (CFI:V) and involvement in fantasy play also correlated positively with hypnotizability scales for Observed Behavior, Realness, and SHCS-C-R ($p < .01$). Social desirability scores did not relate to hypnotizability scores for Observed Behavior, Realness, or SHCS-C-R. Authors noted that several children appeared to be somewhat wary of the procedures, and they suspected that some of the children did not consider it socially desirable to respond. They suggest that the Attitude-Toward-Hypnosis-Scale of Spanos, Lush, Smith, and deGroh (1986) should be adapted to children and used in future similar studies.

A weakness of the reported studies is that the terms "fantasy" and "imagery" are interpreted to refer to visual mental constructions. It would be important to determine whether or not subjects prefer auditory imagery to visual or kinesthetic to visual images. Some children enjoy olfactory imagery. We use a simple imagery questionnaire that is useful clinically in developing hypnotic inductions for children (see Appendix B). We welcome the use of this questionnaire or a modification in future clinical studies.

Attitudes toward Adults

Gardner (1974a) has hypothesized that children may be especially responsive to hypnotic suggestions because they are generally predisposed to trust adults, responsive to social influence and authority, and comfortable about engaging in help-seeking behavior. Most children feel safe when they experience regressive aspects of hypnosis in the presence of a presumably competent adult. In most cases they do not experience the degree of anxiety about control that often interferes with hypnotic responsiveness in adults. There has been no research to test these hypotheses.

Parent-Child Interaction

Several psychoanalytic writers (Ambrose, 1963, 1968; Boswell, 1962; Call, 1976; Krojanker, 1969) focus on transferential and regression aspects of the hypnotic relationship. In this context, it becomes possible to specify the kinds of parent–child relationships most conducive to hypnotic responsiveness in the child. For example, Call (1976) theorized that, while in hypnosis, the child subjectively experiences a relationship with the powerful, internalized parent image. Therefore, the child who has had a past experience with a well-defined, powerful, omnipotent parent would be more responsive to hypnosis than a child who had less well-defined parental influences.

Results of two retrospective studies of young adults (J. R. Hilgard & Hilgard, 1962; J. R. Hilgard, 1970), found that subjects who identified with work habits and attitudes of neither parent were low in hypnotizability. The same was true for identification with parental temperament. In both studies, highly hypnotizable subjects identified most strongly with the opposite-sexed parent. The families of highly hypnotizable subjects were characterized by a combination of warmth and strict discipline, a setting in which the likelihood of clear identifications and strong ego development was optimized. J. R. Hilgard (1970) hypothesized that the hypnotizable subject may later incorporate the hypnotherapist in the same way that the parents were incorporated, with a certain readiness to conform to authority even if it seems rather illogical.

In a longitudinal study, children who had initially been studied in kindergarten were tested for hypnotizability and related behaviors when they reached their senior year in high school (Nowlis, 1969). The results indicated that "a rather stern, restrictive, and punitive home environment at the time the children were in kindergarten was related to higher susceptibility to hypnotic-like experience when the children reached the twelfth grade in high school" (p. 114). In these comparisons, "hypnotic-like experience" was measured by Shor's Personal Experiences Questionnaire, Form L (Shor, 1960; Shor, Orne, & O'Connell, 1962), an inventory of trance-like experiences in everyday life that predicts hypnotizability but is not itself a test of hypnotizability. On an actual hypnotizability scale, the Harvard Group Scale of Hypnotic Susceptibility, Form A (Shor & Orne, 1962), only antecedent child-rearing variable was significantly related to hypnotizability, namely, pressure for conformity with table standards. In view of the many variables studied, the author concluded this one finding should probably be attributed to chance.

In the only study in which parent–child relationships and childhood hypnotizability have been studied concurrently, L. M. Cooper and London (1976) found that parents of highly hypnotizable subjects tended to rate themselves as more strict, anxious, and impatient than parents of low-hypnotizable subjects. When these parents offered help to their children on a puzzle task, the suggestions given by parents of highly susceptible children were more abstract and constructive than the suggestions given by parents of low-susceptible children. Cooper and London suggested caution in interpreting these results because of the large number of variables studied.

Despite methodological differences and difficulties in the studies of J. R. Hilgard (1970), Nowlis (1969), and L. M. Cooper and London (1976), the results of all three point in the same direction, leading to a position of greater credence than would have been possible from any of the studies taken alone.

FACTORS THAT MAY COMPROMISE HYPNOTIC RESPONSIVENESS

In an extensive review of correlates of hypnotic responsiveness in childhood, it is necessary to go beyond the developmental issues that have concerned us so far. We will discuss several variables not directly related to hypnotic talent but that may enhance or impede hypnotic responsiveness.

Misconceptions about Hypnosis

We have found that may children (as well perhaps as their parents) approach hypnotherapy with a great deal of misinformation. Often they may believe that they will somehow be put to sleep or, as commonly depicted in cartoons, be "put into a trance" and then be under the absolute control of the "hypnotist," and not remember anything that transpires during the hypnotic session. While sometimes children get these notions from parents and other adults, more often the "information" comes from television. For example, one children's program portrayed a mad scientist who used a shiny ring to bring various people under his spell. When his victims wore the ring, they walked around in an obvious trance-like state, followed his instructions including engaging in embarrassing and antisocial behavior while muttering "Yes, master," and had no memory of their behavior when the trance was lifted by removal of the scientist's ring. The currently popular film "Aladdin" also portrays hypnosis in such a fashion, that is, as a controlling "power" by the sinister "bad guy" used to further his cause of evil.

Fortunately the effect of such programs is usually more positive than negative with respect to children's willingness to experience hypnosis. They are more intrigued by the "magic" portrayed than they are concerned about being controlled or made to engage in unacceptable behavior. However, for therapeutic as well as for educational reasons, we strongly advise that any first hypnotic induction or experience be preceded by a didactic session in which children's (and parents) prior ideas (and fears or worries) about hypnosis are solicited and understood, misconceptions are clarified, and myths put to rest. We are aware of one 12-year-old boy who initially refused hypnosis on religious grounds because he thought it involved some sort of demonology or witchcraft. Only after being assured that neither he nor the therapist were possessed by demons did he consent to hypnotic induction.

Some children refuse therapeutic hypnosis despite all efforts at clarification. In a few cases, the children have even demonstrated that they are hypnotizable but still refuse to apply their skills to a particular problem. Reasons for these examples of apparent resistance are not always clear, but they may include (1) being unwilling to give up a symptom because of secondary gains; (2) equating hypnosis with loss of autonomy and choice; (3) equating freedom from pain and anxiety with death, in severe illness; (4) being unwilling to give up a symptom that serves a major defensive function against debilitating depression or psychosis; (5) experiencing anxiety with certain induction techniques that compromise coping mechanisms, for example, resisting dissociative imagery because of a need or cognitive mastering during medical procedures; and (6) having had a previous negative experience with another hypnotherapist. When the therapist understands the resistance, sometimes further clarification or modification of technique will be helpful; at times the therapist will decide that hypnotherapy is contraindicated. Occasionally the therapist will be unable to understand the apparent reluctance, and the child will remain (seemingly) refractory to hypnosis. And, sometimes what seems like "resistance" may simply represent a mismatch between therapist and child patient. In such cases rather than abandon the (potential) use and value of hypnosis, the therapist may opt to refer the child to a colleague who also uses hypnotherapeutic strategies and with whom the child may well "connect" more easily or positively. This of course remains a matter of personal judgment by each clinician.

Attitudes of Significant Adults

Some clinicians treating children despair of attempting hypnotherapy with children because of presumed negative attitudes on the part of patients' parents, teachers, clergy, and other adults from whom children get their concept of reality and of appropriate behavior.

Attitudes in Institutional Settings

Misconceptions, negative attitudes, and a lack of information about hypnosis among child health professionals not only limit the number of children who might be referred for hypnotherapy; they also can sabotage ongoing hypnotherapy done by a qualified professional with a motivated and capable child. It is disheartening to give a post-surgical child patient hypnotic suggestions for increased and comfortable food intake only to discover that someone else has put the emesis basin closer to the child than the dinner tray! Another common problem in hospitals is that colleagues may consider using hypnotherapy but only as a last resort when a child has developed severe conditioned fear and anxiety about procedures in general. Although such children can benefit greatly from hypnotherapy and overcome their conditioned negative responses, this usually takes multiple therapy sessions. When the hypnotherapist is called 30 minutes prior to the procedure and cannot "deliver" a calm child to the treatment room, the naive colleague will say, "It doesn't work." Although this has the logic of complaining that a child's throat still hurts after one dose of penicillin, the scenario occurs all too frequently.

It is important that the child health professional who uses hypnotherapy take time to educate colleagues. This must be an ongoing process such as our program to provide inservice education programs about hypnotherapy at a children's hospital (Olness, 1977c). These programs were available not only to the pediatricians, nurses, house officers, and medical students, but also to administrative, secretarial, and housekeeping personnel. House officers rotate frequently, but they are often the first physicians to make decisions about pain and anxiety management for children. It is important to teach them about hypnotherapy not only for their patients but for themselves. The inherent stresses of being a houseofficer can be reduced by self-hypnosis practice. Sokel, Lansdown, and Kent (1990) developed a Pain and Symptom Management Team for the pediatric services on Great Ormond Street in London. They found a dramatic increase in referrals. Of the first 51 cases referred, 36 were taken on for hypnotherapy. They note that "it is essential to demystify hypnotherapy in a hospital context, to convey to children and their parents, and often to colleagues, that we are harnessing a normal power" (Sokel et al., 1990).

In recent years nurses in children's hospitals have become very active in promoting hypnotherapeutic techniques especially on post-surgical or chronic illness units. Valente (1990) and Hobbie (1989) have both described how nurses can apply hypnotherapy. Valente (1991) has also detailed the myths, research, and effectiveness of hypnotherapy as a strategy for managing cancer pain of school-age children.

Regardless of whether a treatment is pharmacological or nonpharmacological, it benefits the child patient and increases efficiency if all members of the treatment team know something about that treatment.

Parents

Traphagen (1959) found a preponderance of positive attitudes toward hypnosis among parents (65%), higher than she expected. We find positive attitudes among most parents of our prospective child hypnotherapy patients.

Some parents are interested to discover that they have unwittingly been using hypnotic-like techniques with their children. For example, Katie, age 12
years, frequently gagged or vomited when taking oral medication. Her mother
spontaneously developed the idea of helping her child by describing in detail
her favorite foods while the child swallowed her pills. When we pointed out
the similarity to hypnosis, Katie quickly learned to use the favorite food imagery independently and easily resolved her problem with taking medication.
Even when parents are at first reluctant, it is usually possible to help them
shift to a more positive stance toward hypnosis. Gardner (1974b) described
techniques designed to help parents who are reluctant about hypnosis to move
from being obstacles to becoming allies in their children's treatment. The
approach includes three basic steps: educational, observational, and experiential. Details of each of these steps follow:

> It is usually best to begin with a relatively didactic discussion with the
> parents, especially eliciting and responding to their specific questions and
> concerns. Hypnosis can be defined as basically a state of mind, usually com-
> bining relaxation with concentration on a desired point of focus so that other
> undesired thoughts or feelings then fade into the background. Such shifts
> of attention are easily demonstrated by asking the parents to focus on sounds
> which were not previously noticed, such as the typing in the reception area
> or the soft hum of the air conditioner. The heightened attention which
> characterizes hypnosis is then described in the context of everyday events
> such as a mother's ability to waken to her infant's cry while sleeping through
> other louder but insignificant noises. [In answering other questions con-
> cerning hypnosis generally, brochures available from the American Society
> of Clinical Hypnosis may be helpful.]
>
> This general discussion easily leads to the specific issue of why hypno-
> sis may be appropriate for a particular child. Thus, the mother may be told
> that the goal is to help the child focus on comfort so that pain will ease,
> on feelings of well-being so that anxiety will diminish, or on pleasant hun-
> ger in order to counteract nausea and vomiting. A few basic principles of
> induction techniques, such as relaxation training and guided imagery, can
> then be explained, emphasizing the need to tailor the induction to the needs
> of each child, and providing some understanding of simple physiological
> and psychological principles that account for the success of the techniques.
> Throughout, the parents' specific questions are answered, and misconcep-
> tions are clarified including such things as the distinction between hypno-
> sis and sleep and concerns about spontaneous hypnosis or greater
> susceptibility to charlatans. The goals are (a) to teach the parents that hyp-
> nosis can be described in simple, everyday terms without resorting to con-
> cepts suggesting magic or witchcraft and (b) to help the parents understand
> that hypnosis may be a specifically useful treatment modality for their child.
> This writer finds that, after this discussion, almost all parents are willing
> to let their children have a trial of hypnotherapy. For those who are not,
> the issue is not pushed any further.

If the parents become enthusiastic about the possible value of hypnotherapy for the child, they have already accomplished a major step toward becoming a hypnotherapeutic ally. Usually children look to their parents for guidance and assurance when facing new situations, and if the parents communicate a confident attitude toward hypnosis, the child is much more likely to be trusting and cooperative.

For those parents who permit hypnotherapy for their children, the second phase of parent training consists of having them observe their children in hypnosis. Observation is usually postponed, however — and especially in older children — until after the initial induction, since this is often the point of maximum concern for both the child and the hypnotherapist regarding whether a state of hypnosis can be achieved and whether it will be effective for the problem at hand. This writer finds that having any third party present, e.g., parent, doctor, or nurse, increases the likelihood of anxiety about successful performance. This anxiety may then seriously interfere with success, since it draws attention away from the task and replaces desired relaxation with tension. However, occasionally the parents may be invited to observe the first session if the child is particularly anxious and wants his parents to stay with him.

When rapport is established between the therapist and the child, and when it is clear to both that the child can use hypnosis to alleviate his problem, the parent is then invited to observe a hypnotic session. Ideally this is done after the child has been taught self-hypnosis (easily mastered by most children eight years of age or older), because then the parents see that the child can be in control both of induction (usually simple techniques such as eye-fixation, visual imagery, or reverse hand-levitation) and dehypnotization. . . .

An important part of the observation session is to have the parent watch the therapist communicate with the child in hypnosis, requiring the child to give both nonverbal and verbal responses and then to transfer hypnotic rapport to the parents and have them also communicate verbally and nonverbally with the child. This exercise helps assure the parent that the child is in contact with his surroundings and in control of the hypnotic state as much as necessary. Parents who initially went along with the idea because of desperation or "blind faith" now have keener understanding and are able to be even more supportive, both in sessions with the therapist and when the child is asked to practice self-hypnosis for use with a chronic condition or for repeated painful procedures or unpleasant experiences where the therapist may not always be available. With a little further training, they are also now in a position to help their child deepen or maintain a hypnotic state or achieve the initial induction when the child may be too anxious or in too much discomfort to concentrate effectively alone.

The parents' effectiveness as hypnotherapists is usually enhanced by the third phase of parent training, namely, having them experience hypnosis themselves. This step further dispels the idea of hypnosis as magic, removes any remaining doubts and fears, and allows review of details not previously discussed. Often this occurs informally as a natural consequence of the observational phase. That is, the parents spontaneously report feelings of relaxation compatible with light hypnosis while watching their child in hypnosis. The dynamics of this phenomenon are not clear, though this writer has seen it with adults watching other adults as well as with adults watching children. Usually the observer is a "participant observer" in the sense of having warm, tender feelings for and/or identifications with the subject. There may also be an element of contagion of the trusting relationship between the subject and therapist. Once, when both parents observed a hypnotic session with a six-year-old nauseated girl, suggestions were given that she could feel quiet and a bit sleepy and that soon she would experience nice hungry feelings so that it would feel good to take fluids and medicine. Not only did the suggestions prove effective for the child, but mother later reported that she became pleasantly sleepy, while father said he developed marked hunger and went out for a snack! Both parents describe their experience with amusement, commenting also that they were glad to know something of what their child experienced. Another parent, after experiencing a formal induction, reported that experiencing hypnosis herself really convinced her that a person in hypnosis is "awake and aware" and that this allowed her to feel more secure when she helped her son use self-hypnosis.

For parents who experience a formal induction, there is usually only one hypnotic session, focusing mainly on aspects of induction, deepening, and dehypnotization, often in the presence of the child so as to maximize mutual trust and confidence. The experiential phase of training may be omitted, if it is not anticipated that the parents will actually assume the role of hypnotherapist . . . or if the parents resist the idea of experiencing hypnosis themselves, even though they accept it for their child. In most cases, only one parent goes through this phase, and this writer uses formal parent induction in less than half the cases of child hypnotherapy. (pp. 45–47)*

Since publishing the 1974 paper on parental attitudes, Gardner (1974b) continued the educational and observational steps of parent training but decreased the frequency of having parents actually experience formal hypnotic induction. Moreover, when parents did request formal hypnotic induction for themselves, Gardner asked that the child not be present, at least initially. This change developed when it became clear that some parents — even in brief hypnosis — might use the opportunity to experience grief or other feelings whose full expression might be inappropriate in front of the child.

Situational Variables

Sometimes a child's physical or psychological condition may temporarily preclude the use of hypnosis. Such conditions include: unconsciousness, anxi-

---

*From Gardner (1974b). With permission.

ety, or pain to such an extreme degree that the child is unable to focus any attention on the hypnotherapist, or at least in any way that we are able to detect; and extreme debilitation with inability to move from a passive to an active posture in a hypnotherapeutic relationship. Only rarely do time limitations preclude the effective use of hypnosis. Although concerns about time limitations often seem to be a preliminary or theoretical deterrent for therapists new to the use of hypnosis, we have been impressed repeatedly with how much can be accomplished in a very short period when circumstances seem suboptimal, for example, in an emergency situation when everyone, including the patient and perhaps the clinician, is markedly anxious.

CONCLUSIONS

Gardner and Hinton (1980) reviewed correlates of hypnotic responsiveness in children. Considering the great diversity of possible correlates, they noted the lack of any serious attempt to ground the findings in the context of a cohesive theory. Even the comments of psychoanalytic writers have been limited in scope. In light of advances in theoretical conceptualizations of hypnosis (e.g., Fromm, 1977; Fromm & Gardner, 1979; Fromm & Hurt, 1980), we anticipate that future research will more clearly identify correlates of childhood hypnotic responsiveness and evaluate their relative significance in a more orderly way.

CHAPTER FIVE

Hypnotic Induction
for Children
Techniques, Strategies,
and Approaches

Children respond to a large number of hypnotic induction techniques, strategies, and approaches, each with countless variations. Any induction method may also be used as a method of deepening, or intensification of the hypnotic experience; and methods may be combined in almost any order. The choice of an appropriate induction for any given child depends on the needs and preferences of the child and on the experience and creativity of the therapist. Success is certain to be limited if a therapist is competent only in the use and application of one or two induction techniques for children or attempts to utilize techniques suited for adults without providing or integrating modifications that may be necessary for child patients.

Any health specialist who undertakes hypnotic induction with children must first have considerable knowledge of child development and expertise in working with children in the context of his or her primary profession (pediatric, child psychology, psychiatry, dentistry, etc.). One must also know something about the social and cultural backgrounds of child patients, their general likes and dislikes, themes of interest related to books, television programs, current movies, music, and video and computer games. For individual patients, successful hypnotic inductions are those that are often based on knowledge of the patient's particular likes and dislikes, comfort areas, language preferences, past experiences, and aspirations about the future. Sometimes unexpected "resistance" to one technique demands a rapid shift to another. In short, a child hypnotherapist must first be a competent child therapist/clinician. The same requirements apply to researchers studying hypnotic phenomena in children.

Compared with adults, children are more likely to squirm and move about, open their eyes or refuse to close them, and make spontaneous comments during hypnotic inductions and, perhaps, through the hypnotic procedure as well. Although these behaviors may seem at first experience to represent resistance, this is not usually or necessarily the case. In moving about or opening his or her eyes, most often the child is simply adapting the induction strategy to his or her own behavioral style, and the thoughtful hypnotherapist also adapts accordingly, reinforcing positively whatever behavior the child has reflected, thus creating a "win–win" experience, rather than an adversarial or problematic interaction. Many children have negative attitudes about going to sleep or, having been told that a favorite pet has been "put to sleep," equate being put to sleep with being put to death. Therefore, we usually avoid such words as "sleepy," "drowsy," and "tired" both in our inductions and in our hypnotic language in general. Likewise, since some children—especially 4- and 5-year-olds—resist closing their eyes and may even be frightened by the idea itself, we do not stress eye closure as important to induction, although we sometimes tell children that they may be able to concentrate better *when* they close their eyes. In all instances, of course, the choice is theirs. We aim to be ever alert to adapting our language to the children's level of understanding, neither talking down to them nor using overly complex language.

The induction techniques that we will describe share characteristics of being permissive in nature, emphasizing children's involvement and control and encouraging their active participation in the process of experiencing and utilizing the hypnotic state. We avoid authoritarian methods widely used in the past, including avoiding phrases such as "You will . . . ," or "I want you to do this now . . . ," or "You won't be able to. . . . " Such methods, in which the hypnotherapist uses a controlling or commanding manner, may indeed result in successful induction and initiation of hypnosis in some children, although much less so now than in earlier times or in cultures in which children expect adults to be very strict and authoritarian.

When hypnotic induction is employed in the context of medical or psychological therapy, we believe that authoritarian methods and approaches are contraindicated, as they risk interfering with the evolution of a child's sense of mastery over the medical and/or psychological problem(s) with which he or she is dealing or struggling. The use of challenges (e.g., "You will not be able to open your eyes no matter how hard you try") is especially to be avoided for these reasons, as such challenges risk the emergence of helplessness as opposed to the quality of empowerment that hypnotherapy offers: The purpose of therapy is always to increase the child's control of a desired feeling or behavior, and any induction that emphasizes loss of control can only inhibit therapeutic progress. We do not mean to imply that the therapist avoids any structuring of the situation or dilutes the patient's perception of him or her as a competent, helping person. We do, however, emphasize the distinction between being appropriately authoritative (as the clinician, guide, teacher, coach) and being authoritarian.

Although we shall describe several specific hypnotic induction techniques, our list is by no means a complete or exhaustive compendium. Nor is this chapter intended as a substitute for direct training with experts in the field. We suspect that many professionals who give up hypnotherapy do so because they never acquired a solid base of personal, experiential training. Appropriate avenues of training are discussed in the Introduction and in Chapter 17.

Although some children expect and benefit from relatively formalized induction techniques, many respond equally well or better to a more simple, casual approach. For example, in some cases it may be sufficient to say, "Just think about how you feel when you are building a house with Legos at home; just let yourself feel that way now." Or, it may be very effective to say, "Just pretend you're not here and that instead you're somewhere where you are very happy."

M. H. Erickson (1958b) was particularly aware that children frequently go into hypnosis without any formal induction, and he taught that careful and sensitive observation by the hypnotherapist would allow him or her to know what would best facilitate effective hypnosis and to "go with the child." This phenomenon can present problems to researchers who define hypnosis as whatever occurs following a hypnotic induction. However, the criteria for determining the presence or absence of hypnosis can only be based on patient or subject behaviors known to be characteristic of the state of hypnosis and not on behaviors of the person doing the induction.

The choice of induction techniques depends not only on patient variables but also on the style and preferences of the therapist. A hypnotherapist is not likely to be successful using a method with which he or she is uncomfortable. Moreover, hypnotherapists should always be alert to the possible value of new methods along with inevitable changes in cultural trends such as norms for social behavior, child-rearing methods, and educational approaches.

New developments in science and the arts that shape children's interests and attitudes will also have relevance for hypnotic induction approaches. It may turn out that some methods currently in general use will be outdated or inappropriate for children of future generations. We emphasize here as well as in application sections that follow, the importance of recognizing childhood as an ongoing, fluid, and dynamic state. In this context we must be mindful, therefore, that the maturing child patient who finds one or several hypnotic induction strategies effective and pertinent to him- or herself now may have no use at all for those techniques 6–12 months from now as he or she moves into a new phase of development. Careful attention to our patients' developmental needs, therefore, will allow us to work closely with them to tailor hypnotherapeutic inductions (and suggestions) that fit with their developmental as well as social–emotional needs.

Some of the techniques we describe have been invented by our child patients or by children in our families or their friends. For techniques in use for a long time, and with several variations, we have been unable to trace their originators, and we apologize to these unsung heroes.

In the course of any hypnotic induction, we give positive feedback to the child's responses, and we communicate expectations of and for success by focusing on possibilities, and by avoiding words such as "try," which imply that failure may be the outcome. Since we believe our patients will benefit most from hypnotherapy if they enjoy the induction, we work in ways that are enjoyable to us as well, using humor liberally where appropriate, and never taking ourselves too seriously.

THE PRE-INDUCTION INTERVIEW

Depending on the needs of the child, the pre-induction interview may be quite brief or very extensive. In emergency situations, it may be deferred entirely. The interview usually includes discussion of the reasons for utilizing hypnosis in relation to a particular problem, review of the child's ideas about hypnosis, clarification of misconceptions, and full reply to questions. If details of the child's likes and dislikes, significant experiences, fears, hopes, and comfort areas have not already been ascertained, these areas are also discussed at this time.

A SAMPLE OF HYPNOTIC INDUCTION TECHNIQUES FOR CHILDREN

The following descriptions of these techniques consist of the actual words we might say to a child. Obviously our own phrasing varies from child to child, as it does (and must) vary from one therapist to another. We emphasize again that these are samples and that variations are inevitable, as well as necessary and appropriate. We find that a questionnaire for families (see Appendices B and E) is helpful in learning about a child's interests, fears, and wishes, and as such is helpful in guiding our selections of suggested imagery during the hypnotherapeutic process.

Visual (Multisensory) Imagery Techniques

Favorite Place. "Think about a favorite place where you have been and where you like to be. It might be easier if you close your eyes, but you can leave them open if you like or leave them open until you close them, or until they close by themselves." For children who cannot think of a real favorite place, ask them to think of an imaginary one, such as "one you have always wanted to go to and will probably visit some day."

It sometimes helps to ask children to tell the therapist their favorite place and several of their favorite or valued activities. The therapist can then enhance the imagery by adding specific details. Important information about the child is sometimes obtained, similar to the information obtained, for example, from psychological projective tests that elicit fantasy. When children offer more than one favorite place and indicate no preference, the therapist may enhance rapport by suggesting the one with which he or she is most familiar, and thus able to talk most easily and comfortably about, thereby conveying a sense of comfort and confidence in turn to the child patient. The therapist may also suggest the situation involving the patient most actively, especially if the goals of treatment include enhanced competence and active mastery of a problem. The imagery utilized in induction need not be related at all to the problem: "See yourself, feel yourself in that favorite place which you have chosen, or which has popped into your imagination. Look around and see the shapes and colors, hear the sounds there. Let yourself really be there now . . . because you really are there in your imagining (or daydreaming, or pretending). It's good for everybody to be in a favorite place sometimes, a place where you like to be, a place where you like how you feel. You can feel those good feelings now. Take some time to enjoy it. When you feel as if you are really there—even part way there in your mind—let me know by lifting one finger to say yes." If the child looks troubled, the therapist should inquire directly as to the difficulty. A comment that not everyone likes to go to a favorite place will be reassuring, and then one can suggest a different method. Occasionally a child who successfully imagines a favorite place may then have an unexpected negative reaction—for example, sadness because a grandparent who also enjoyed that place has died. Depending on the goals of treatment, the therapist may choose either to shift to another method or to help the child explore the emotional reaction, in or out of the hypnotic state, depending upon the individual circumstances. Prior to the beginning of the induction, the child can be told that he or she can talk in hypnosis, especially if a hypnotic interview is part of the treatment plan. This can be presented easily as part of the clinician's demystification and education about hypnosis and is often a great relief to children (and parents) who, like many, had misconceptions about an all-powerful, controlling "hypnotist." It may be useful to tell a child before and/or during hypnosis that "even hearing yourself talking can help you help yourself be even more comfortable and to see things in your imagination more clearly." This kind of gentle "challenge" encourages and eases the child's ability, desire, and willingness to talk. One can add additional simple motivational suggestions to this, such as "When you talk and tell me what you are imagining about, then I can be an even better coach to help you help yourself." Such statements reinforce the cooperative nature of the hypnotherapeutic relationship and as such are easily accepted and experienced by patients as facilitative.

Multiple Animals. "Do you like animals? Good. Which do you like best? Fine. Just imagine that you can see yourself sitting in a very nice place with a puppy [or whatever animal the child has chosen]. It might help to close your eyes. Feel that puppy's soft fur [kinesthetic imagery] and see its color [visual imagery]. Now, just for fun, pretend it is another color or striped or polka-dotted. Let it be any way you like, and the puppy is happy too. You can change the color anytime you choose *because* [this is the motivating portion of the suggestion] it's *your* imagination, and you are the boss of your imagination. And you can imagine a second puppy just like the first, the same colors, the same soft fur. Two puppies, and you can see yourself playing with them. Now, you may choose to make three puppies and change their color back to the first color or to another color. You can tell me about the puppies if you like."

Flower Garden. "You said you like flowers. Just let yourself imagine being in a beautiful big flower garden with all your favorite flowers. You may have your favorite toy or stuffed animal with you. See the bright colors [visual imagery]. Smell the sweet smells [olfactory imagery]. If you like, you can touch the petals and feel how soft they are [kinesthetic imagery]. Imagine that it's all right for you to pick as many flowers as you want from this big flower garden. You can keep them for yourself. Or you can pick some for someone special. Feel your arms widening around a bigger and bigger bouquet until you have all you want. If you take them to a special person, you can see how happy that person looks when you give the flowers. And, you can feel happy too!"

Favorite Activity. "Tell me something you like to do." [The child answers.] Or, one might begin by saying, "It says on this paper your Mom and Dad wrote on the questionnaire that you like to do [name three or four things from questionnaire]; I wonder which is your very favorite?" And then, "Good, just imagine that you can see yourself doing that. Let yourself really enjoy it, and do it better than ever before." This method emphasizes the active participation mentioned in the favorite place technique. Some children actually engage in physical activity appropriate to the imagery, such as strumming their fingers as if playing a piano, or pretending they are throwing a ball or holding ski poles or bicycle handlebars.

Cloud Gazing. "What are some colors you like? Good. Let yourself imagine some beautiful clouds in the sky and see them change into one of your favorite colors. Good. Now let them change into another color. Or perhaps several nice colors. The clouds may change shape too, as you continue to watch them. It will be interesting to see what they become. You can be part of those clouds, if you like, feeling very comfortable, very good." This technique may not be appropriate for a child who has been told that death means "going up to heaven to live with God." Use special caution if there has been a recent death of a family member, friend, or pet, or if the child has an illness that may result in death.

Letter Watching. "You have told me that you like to write. Let yourself see a blackboard, or a piece of paper with an *A* on it. Now watch the *A* turn into a *B*. Then, let the *B* turn into a *C*. See as many letters as you like. When you are feeling very comfortable, very good, let me know by lifting one finger." One can do the same with numbers. If the child looks troubled, consider the possibility that letters and numbers may have symbolic meaning, for example, letters as grades or numbers as ages. One may notice the occurrence of spontaneous age regression or age progression with the number method, and this may or may not be desirable, depending upon the purpose and therapeutic goals of the hypnotic experience.

Television [or Movie] Fantasy. "You told me you like to watch TV and that your favorite program is _____." For children who name a particularly violent program as their favorite, some therapists prefer to inquire about other interests and use a different method. It is probably better to inquire casually for other interests than to ask the child for a less violent program, since the child may interpret the latter as a rejection or as a controlling statement. "Just imagine yourself getting ready to watch your favorite TV program. Where is the TV set you are watching? Good. Just get comfortable, and when you are ready turn on the set, either on the set or on the remote controller. Feel yourself push the button of the controller and get to the right channel. Now you can see your favorite program. When the sound and the picture are just right for you, let me know by lifting one finger. Good. Just continue watching and listening, and feeling very comfortable, very good!" If the child is undergoing a medical treatment procedure, the therapist may give repeated suggestions for continued watching. If the therapist intends to give hypnotic or post-hypnotic suggestions, these may often be interspersed in the context of the program. For example, if the child has "resisted" (refused?) taking oral medication, the therapist can suggest that the TV hero or heroine is happy to take medicine that will cure illness. Or, the child can be asked to name a favorite food, then given the suggestion that the TV character is eating that food and wants to share it with the child. The medication is then hallucinated as the favorite food. Most children have no problem merging and immersing themselves into a TV program or a video.

The advent of "controllers" and awareness of multiple channels allows the clinician to use this TV or videotape imagery to move easily from induction into utilization and to "solve problems." Thus, in going from induction to utilization (or working on some specific area of your life), one could simply say, "Now switch to the *Bobby [child's name] channel* where you see yourself in your mind—how you are now **OR** how you want to be." This imagery also allows for a kind of "safety valve" in the event of an unpleasant experience in trance. As noted, the clinician may decide in some cases to focus on the sadness or some other unsuspected feeling that may appear abruptly; or he or she could simply invite the child to "just change the channel; you are the boss of your imagination."

We have seen desperately ill children accept oral medications in the context of these suggestions. In psychotherapeutic treatment, the therapist may use the TV technique to explore problem areas or to help the child toward constructive resolution. Similarly, this imagery may be used constructively to help a patient with changes he or she may wish to make as part of the therapeutic agreement. In such an approach of the "split-screen technique" one can visualize the "old way" or "the problem" on one video screen or on one-half of the video screen; and on the other half, the patient can be instructed to "let the way you want it to be [i.e., the desired outcome] now come into view on the other screen [or other half of the screen]." Multiple variations can then be explored, such as inviting the child to visualize one image (the old one) getting smaller while the other gets bigger. Or, one might suggest one image gets dimmer and the other brighter, or one blows a fuse and the other is made out of invincible parts from outer space, and so forth.

As reflected in this example, in this and virtually all other hypnotic induction techniques, there is really no sharp distinction between induction and therapeutic work. Even when an induction technique is used without any therapeutic suggestions, the child's experience of the induction itself will be either therapeutic or countertherapeutic. The same is true, of course, for all aspects of the clinician–patient interaction in hypnotherapy as well as in other forms of treatment.

Auditory Imagery

Favorite Song. "You said that you like to sing. Where do you like to do that best? Good. Imagine that you are there now, singing your favorite song. Sing the song through in your mind. Enjoy doing it very well, making just the sounds you like. When you have come to the end of the song, let me know by lifting one finger. Or you can sing it again if you like, and *then* let your finger lift." [Note: "Lifting one finger" is a conscious act, whereas "let your finger lift" is a hypnotic suggestion/request for dissociation and *in*voluntary (*ideomotor*) movement.] The patient may be asked to tap out the beat with one or more fingers. When the tapping ceases, the therapist knows the patient has ended the song.

Playing a Musical Instrument. If the patient enjoys playing a musical instrument, the therapist can adapt the *Favorite Song* technique accordingly.

Listening to Music. "You said you liked music. What kind of music do you like to listen to? Exactly what piece of music would you like to hear now? Good. Just imagine yourself hearing that very clearly now, as loud or soft as you like. You might want to turn it up . . . and then down. . . . You may imagine watching the musicians too. You can let me know when the music has ended." For some children actually listening to a tape recording may be better than imagining it. We occasionally ask children to bring in taped music, or have brought in a tape ourselves of a patient's favorite music (Gardner & Tarnow, 1980).

Movement Imagery

Flying Blanket. This method, invented by one of Karen Olness's children, should not be used if the patient is afraid of flying or of heights. "Imagine that you are going on a picnic, going with your favorite people to a special place for a picnic. You have your favorite things to eat and drink. You can see and smell and taste them. You can enjoy playing games with your family and friends. Then when you are finished eating and drinking and playing games, you may see a blanket spread out there on the ground. It's your favorite color, smooth and soft. You may sit on it or lie on it. Pretend it's a flying blanket, and you are the pilot. You are in control. You can fly just a few inches above the ground, just above the grass or higher, even above the trees if you want. You're the pilot. You can go where you want and as fast or as slowly as you wish, just by thinking about it. You can land and visit your friends or you can land at the zoo or anywhere you like. You're the pilot, and you're in charge. You might fly by a tree and see birds in a nest. You can speed up and slow down. Enjoy going where you want. Take all the time you need to feel very comfortable. When you are ready, you can find a nice comfortable landing spot and land your flying blanket. When you have landed, let me know by lifting one finger." Therapeutically one might also say, "When you are ready to learn more about how your inside mind can help your body or the way it can help with those problems that have been bothering you, then land your blanket."

Movement Imagery. "Do you like to do things like ride a bicycle or ride a horse? Good. Which do you like best? Fine. Just get comfortable and imagine that you are doing that now. You are just where you want to be, and it's a perfect day. Imagine going exactly where you wish at the speed you wish. You are in control, and you can go wherever you like. Enjoy what you see. Enjoy the feeling. Enjoy being able to go at any speed you like. And each time you change speed or direction, let that be a signal to get even more comfortable than you were before. When you are very, very comfortable, you can gradually slow down. Find a good stopping or resting place and rest, very comfortably." For children who are frightened of passivity, it may be best to omit the suggestion to slow down and stop. Therapeutic suggestions may be given, of course, while the trip is in progress. Or, the end of the movement can be the signal for the therapeutic suggestions; for example, "When you are ready for me to tell you about the suggestion for dry beds [or control of that tic], you can gradually slow down and stop in a favorite place. When you are there, just let your yes finger lift. Then I'll know you're ready." This has the added advantage of emphasizing the child is in control.

Sports Activity. "You told me that you like to play football. Imagine yourself at the age you are now, or maybe older, playing on your favorite football team, wearing its uniform, playing the position you like. Let yourself get very comfortable as you imagine a game with your team winning. You are helping your team win. Feel your control as your muscles move the way you tell them, running, or throwing, or catching or kicking. Enjoy being with the winning team, and continue until the game is won. Perhaps you'll hear the crowd cheering for you and your team. Let me know when the game is over by lifting one finger." This method may be especially suited for children for whom enhanced muscular control is a therapeutic goal, provided they do not have excessively negative attitudes about their sports ability.

Bouncing Ball. "Sometimes it's fun to think of going wherever you want. Pretend you're a bouncing ball, maybe a big one, and you can be any color you want, even striped or with polka dots. It might be easier if you shut your eyes. Be that bouncing ball, and bounce wherever you want. Bounce, bounce, bounce. You can go wherever you wish. You can bounce up a tree and along a branch. You can bounce over your house or over the hospital. You can bounce along a path in the woods or on a sidewalk. If you like to swim, you can bounce and float, bounce and float. If anything is bothering you, you can let it bounce right off. Keep bouncing until you find the right place for you to stop and when you've stopped, let me know."

Playground Activity. "I know you like to go to the playground and play on the swing and the slide. You can pretend you are there now. Imagine yourself getting on the swing and starting to swing back and forth. Just a little at first, then more, back and forth, just as fast or as slow you like, back and forth. Back and forth. Feeling very good. So easy. And when you are ready to go to the slide, just let the swing slow down and imagine yourself at the top of a nice, long, smooth slide, a slide that is just right for you. As you go down that slide, you can feel more and more comfortable. Feel your body going gently down and down. So smooth. So easy. Down and down. When you reach the bottom, you may find something you like very much. So comfortable. When you reach the bottom, you can just enjoy what you find there. Lift one finger when you get to the bottom. If you like, you can tell me what you find there, or you can tell me later, or you can keep it private."

Be a Snowman (Snowgirl) > > *Be a Tree.* "Just be a beautiful frozen snowman (snowgirl). That's great, what a nice-looking snowman (snowgirl). Now Mr. Snowman, it's the end of winter, and the sun is going to come out, and it's getting quite warm. [Note: Most children will start to 'melt' from the top down without any help. Most of the time it may help to have them do it 'in slow motion.'] That's right, so melty until you get all the way to the ground and become a beautiful puddle in Springtime, and now with the new spring, the seeds in the ground are going to use that water and start to grow now into a tree [Note: Most children do not need any further verbal or physical cue to start getting up.], a beautiful, big, strong tree with roots deep into the ground, big, beautiful branches this way and that, with beautiful leaves and maybe even lots of fruit. Now the winds of Spring come and begin to blow, and the tree sways this way and that but is so strong and the roots are so deep that the tree stays up and strong, and comfortable, and safe."

Storytelling Techniques

With young children or those who are too anxious to participate much in other imagery techniques, the therapist may decide to make up a story suited to the child's needs and interests. This technique may be especially useful with small children who are undergoing painful or frightening medical procedures. The story may be an entirely new fantasy production or it may be a variation of a TV program or other theme with which the child is familiar. The therapist may take full responsibility for the story or may ask the child to contribute ideas to the extent that he or she is able. This method provides an opportunity for the therapist to engage the child in humorous fantasy, a good antidote for anxiety. For example, the clinician might begin by telling a familiar story and then substitute doctors, nurses, or family members for the original characters. Most young children delight in these antics, although a few will of course insist that the story be told "the right way." Although some might consider storytelling a distraction technique rather than a storytelling technique, we do not see these as mutually exclusive; and we have seen narrowed focus of attention and altered sensation, which typically characterize the hypnotic state. Of course the therapist can also intersperse into the story suggestions for comfort, analgesia, and calm. Just as these techniques may function as inductions for younger children, so storytelling may play an important role in the formulation of hypnotic therapeutic suggestions for all age groups and for a wide variety of problems as described in later chapters. We do not offer any examples here, since this method is almost entirely a function of the therapist's own creativity and ingenuity in the context of individual child patients and their own personal lives and stories.

Ideomotor Techniques

These methods are distinguished from movement imagery techniques because the latter do not necessarily involve any actual movement by the child, though movement may occur. Ideomotor techniques ask the child to focus mentally on the *idea* of a particular movement and then to *let* the movement occur without conscious muscle activity. Such methods are especially valuable when the therapist wishes to communicate the idea that the child can gain increased control over pain and other physical responses that previously seemed beyond control. They may also facilitate the idea that one's attitudes can affect the healing process and that willingness or openness to change can replace complete passivity in treatment. These methods are most often suited for children of at least school age, but sometimes younger children may benefit.

Hands Moving Together. "Hold your arms straight out in front of you, your palms facing each other, about a foot apart [Figure 5.1, left]. Good.

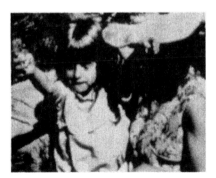 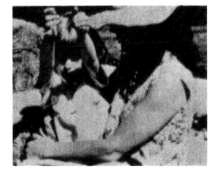

FIGURE 5.1. Hands-moving-together technique. Left: Initial position. Right: Progressive movement of hands toward each other.

Now imagine two powerful magnets, one in each palm. You know how magnets attract each other. Just think about those two very strong magnets, and you may notice that your hands begin to move closer together *all by themselves,* without you doing anything [Figure 5.1, right]. Don't help your hands . . . just notice. Good. Notice that the closer the magnets are together, the stronger they pull. And the stronger they pull, the closer your hands move together. Don't help your hands; see what they'll do all by themselves. Soon they will touch. When that happens, just let go of those imaginary magnets, let your hands and arms drift down to a comfortable position, take one deep breath and let yourself relax all over."

Hand Levitation. "Let your hand and arm just rest comfortably on the arm of the chair. Notice and feel the texture of the fabric beneath your fingers. Now imagine that there is a string tied around your wrist and that big, bright helium-filled balloons are tied to the other end of the string, the kind of balloons that float up all by themselves. Lots of balloons, your favorite colors, just floating, so light, so easy. Effortless. As you focus on the lightness of those balloons, you may notice how that hand begins to feel light too" [Figure 5.2]. Note the shift from "your hand" to "that hand" in order to facilitate dissociation. "Soon one of the fingers may begin to feel especially light. One of the fingers may begin to lift up." Notice carefully which finger moves and comment accordingly, for example, "Good, I see that finger moving, I wonder what will move next. Yes. Good. Now another finger is moving. Now the whole hand. Just focus on the balloons and on the feeling of light-

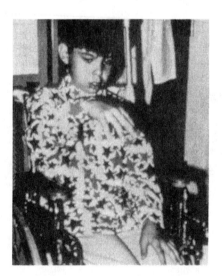

FIGURE 5.2. Hand levitation technique.

ness in that hand. And the higher it goes, the lighter it can feel, and the lighter it feels, the higher it goes. Just floating up all by itself. Drifting higher and lighter and higher and lighter. Now imagine a soft breeze. That hand may float over toward your lap, or it may float even higher, or it may just stay where it is now. Very comfortable, very relaxed all over. You can just let that hand [or arm] float, or, if you choose, you can let the string loosen and the balloons float away and let that hand slowly drift back down to a comfortable resting place, *because* it's fun and because it feels good to do. . . . So easy. Just effortless." If the child seems to be having difficulty, the therapist can first induce a hand or an arm catalepsy and then suggest further movement.

Arm Lowering. "Stretch one arm out straight in front of you with the palm of your hand facing up." Assist the child as necessary. "Good. Now imagine that I am putting a dictionary on that hand." For young children the image of a large rock might be preferable. "You may notice that it begins to feel pretty heavy. Now, imagine a second dictionary [rock] on top of the first one. That arm can feel even heavier. Soon it will want to drift down. When it feels heavy, just let it drift down. Heavier and heavier, down and down. I can see it moving down now. Good. Just let that happen." As with most inductions, timing and especially pacing and leading are essential to success. The therapist can add dictionaries as needed but should be careful to comment on actual movement that occurs. For the few children who seem to resist this technique, the therapist can shift to another kinesthetic strategy, such as arm rigidity or arm catalepsy.

Finger Lowering. This method appeals to young children and may also be used with older children for whom arm lowering may be difficult, as perhaps because of physical debilitation. The therapist helps the child rest the little finger on the bed or arm of the chair, leaving the other fingers extended in the air. "Pretend that this little finger is having a nice rest or nap on the arm of the chair. The other fingers would like to rest or nap too, watch them. Soon they will want to drift down and down . . . until they are resting too. I wonder which finger will drift down first. Look, that one is resting now. When they are all resting, you can feel very comfortable and rested all over too. You can close your eyes if you like, or leave them open until they close all by themselves, rested. More and more comfortable."

Arm Rigidity. "Stretch one arm straight out to the side and make a tight fist. Imagine that the arm is very strong, just like the straight strong branch on a tree. Stronger and stronger. So strong that I cannot push it down. I cannot bend it. That arm is very powerful. It can be as strong and powerful as it wants, even as powerful as a superhero [Fill in the name of the child's

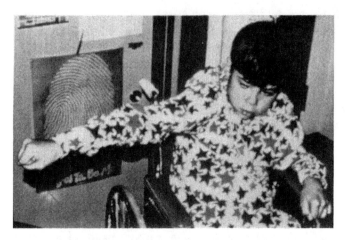

FIGURE 5.3. Arm rigidity technique.

favorite female or male superhero.]" (Figure 5.3). Note how easily this method can lead into ego-strengthening suggestions.

Mighty Oak Tree. This method is especially useful in groups but is also appealing to young children who do not naturally or easily sit still. It also serves as a wonderful method for modeling and/or teaching parents that children can experience and learn to utilize hypnosis without having to insist that they "sit still." "Stand up, tall and straight as a strong oak tree. That's good. Let your arms be branches and stretch toward the sky. Your feet are roots that go down through the floor. Feel how strong you are! Very strong. You can't be moved. Feel the sun and air and rain come in through your branches to make you even stronger. Feel those strong tough roots hold you even while the wind blows through your leaves. When you're ready, when you feel like a powerful oak tree, I'll try to lift you."

Arm Catalepsy. "Is it okay with you if I pick up this hand? Good. Just let it relax. Let me do the work." If the child cooperates by raising the hand and arm, indicate that such conscious cooperation is not necessary and repeat until there is no conscious cooperation. This is usually accomplished easily by saying something like "Thank-you, but just let your arm do it by itself, you don't have to help your arm. . . . Good. Just let the hand rest. Let me do the work of lifting it. Fine. Now look at that hand as though it were part of a sculpture, just floating there by itself. Just imagine it floating there all by itself." The therapist gradually loosens hold of the hand, sensing when the catalepsy has been achieved. "Good. That hand is floating by itself now. Now just raise the other hand and notice the difference. Now you can begin to understand how your strong unconscious, inside mind can help you do what you want."

Progressive Relaxation Techniques

These methods are essentially the same for children as for adults. They are often used as inductions with adolescents and sometimes with younger children who have medical problems that can benefit by deliberate programming of physiological relaxation [e.g., the child with quadriceps (leg muscle) spasm associated with a fractured femur]. The main difference in response between children and adults is that children often respond very quickly with total body relaxation. The therapist must observe the rate of response and through careful pacing and leading be ready to terminate the induction with a simple suggestion for complete relaxation. Lengthy details about specific muscle groups may be necessary for some children, whereas others will experience boredom that can then interfere with response to further suggestions.

Following Breathing. "Focus your eyes easily on some point on your lap or anywhere you like, and pay attention to each time you breathe out. Notice what happens to your shoulders *automatically* while you breathe out . . . they go down, don't they? Good. That's the mind and body working together all the time; even without thinking about it, every time we breathe out we relax some automatically. That feeling is relaxation. When you breathe out you loosen your chest muscles. Each of does that about 10 or 12 times each minute. Pay attention to breathing out, and each time extend your own relaxation feeling a little further. Past your chest and into your tummy muscles. Next time you breathe out, let the comfortable feeling move down into your hips and your upper leg muscles. Relax your lower leg muscles now and feel a flow of comfort, loosening relaxation feeling from your chest muscles down to your ankles, your feet, and your toes. Go at your own pace and your own speed. When you're ready, focus on your lower back muscles, and let them feel very comfortable. Loosen your upper back muscles. And now let a flow of relaxation spread past those shoulders that were already relaxing, down into your upper arms, gradually past your elbows and into your lower arm muscles, into the small muscles of your wrists, hands, and even the little muscles of the fingers. When you're ready, allow your neck muscles to become comfortable more than they were already. Loosen them but just the right amount to keep your head very comfortable. Let the flow of relaxation move into your cheek muscles, your forehead, around your eyes, even to the tiny muscles of your head and scalp, and even into your hair muscles. When you're nice and comfortable all over, please give me a signal by nodding your head or raising a finger. You can tell me if there is any part of your body that doesn't seem ready to be comfortable yet, and we can do some other things so that you can be even more comfortable all over."

Teddy Bear. This method is especially useful for young children for whom sleep is desirable, as in pre- or post-operative situations, but for whom direct suggestion for sleep might produce resistance. A doll or stuffed animal might be substituted according to the child's preference. "What does your teddy bear do when he is sleepy? Hold him the way he likes to be held. Let his head get very comfortable. Maybe you should pat him gently . . . so gently. That's good. Is he getting sleepy? Let his arms get cozy and comfortable. Don't forget his tummy . . . comfortable and sleepy. Let his feet get comfortable. Pretty soon the whole teddy bear is sleepy. Comfortable, drowsy, dozy and cozy. You can rock him if you like . . . maybe even sing him a nice quiet song. So comfortable. So nice. Such a good feeling. So easy. So quiet. So nice of you to help him (her) this way."

Balancing Muscles. "Sit forward, drop hands to your sides, and move your feet out and spread them a little apart from each other on the floor. Move your body forward until you feel your abdominal muscles pull, then move back until your back pulls. Do this until you find a balanced, neutral position for your trunk. Do the same with your head. Move a little forward, a little back until it feels right. Imagine a thread from the ceiling to your head. Think of your head stretched up a little, hold the position easily for as long as you wish, then think of the thread being cut, and your head bending forward, very relaxed and comfortable throughout."

Floppy Raggedy Ann or Andy. "Pretend that you are Raggedy Ann (Andy), floppy all over, so loose and comfortable. Let's be like Raggedy Ann and feel floppy. Let me check this arm. Good. See how it flops down when I pick it up. Just like Raggedy Ann. Now let me check the other arm. Good. That's floppy too. Now let yourself feel floppy all over, loose all over, and very comfortable all over; you can be floppy Raggedy [name]."

Eye Fixation Techniques

Coin Technique. Present a coin and ask the child to hold it between the thumb and first finger (Figure 5.4). For some children, attention is heightened by first drawing a smiling face with a colored marking pen on their thumbnail. Younger children often prefer to have their favorite stuffed animal hold the coin, sometimes in a "paw," sometimes under a nose. Whether they fix their eyes on the coin held by themselves or by the stuffed animal is immaterial. "Just look at that smiling face on the thumb that's holding the coin

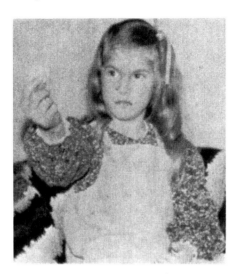

FIGURE 5.4. Coin technique.

[or just look at that coin] real easy. That's good. After a while the fingers [or paws] begin to get a little tired of holding it, and after a while the coin can slip down to the floor [or sofa or bed.] It will be safe there. You can get it later. When it falls, that is your signal to yourself to just let those eyes close by themselves. That's right."

Looking at Point on Hand. "Move around until you have a comfortable position and let your eyes look down, easily, at a point on your hands or fingers, on your ring, or on a painted nail or some other spot. Just hold your eyes there easily while you take five . . . long . . . deep . . . comfortable breaths. After the fifth breath, or even sooner if you choose, let your eyes close easily and comfortably."

Stereoscopic Viewer. The photo chosen for the viewer should, of course, be of something which the patient is known to enjoy. "Hold this viewer easily in front of your eyes. I'll turn the light on. Can you see the kitty walking in the leaves? Maybe she's looking for someone to play with. See the colors. What else do you see?"

Biofeedback. Children as young as 3 or 4 years are intrigued by watching changing numbers on a thermal biofeedback monitor and have a remarkably long attention span for the machine (Figure 5.5). Some children may simply be asked just to watch the numbers change. This induction strategy combines simple eye fixation with absorption and fascination with the chang-

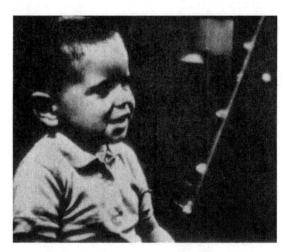

FIGURE 5.5. Biofeedback technique.

ing colors and numbers. In addition, some children may be encouraged to change finger temperature by specifically thinking about hot or cold. This process emphasizes bodily control and may be a good introduction to related therapeutic suggestions; for example, "This machine tells you how warm or cold your fingers are. Look at the numbers [invitation for eye fixation]. When they go up, that means your fingers are warmer. When they go down, that means your fingers are cooler [education]. Sometimes you can *make* the numbers change by just *thinking* about your fingers being warm or cool [hypnotic suggestion about mind–body connections]. I wonder which way the numbers will go for you. Good. The number went up. Your fingers are warm and comfortable. Look. The number has changed again. Just watch the numbers and feel more and more comfortable [definitive link between visual biofeedback—'Look'—and the hypnotic suggestion to feel more comfortable]."

Computer game biofeedback, used in our programs, is very appealing to many children and is becoming increasingly useful in the therapeutic approach to a variety of pediatric and adolescent biobehavioral problems. Computer-based biofeedback technology now permits easy access to recording and displaying a wide variety of physiological parameters [e.g., blood pressure, pulse, respiratory rate, electrodermal activity (galvanic skin response), muscle tension (EMG), (peripheral) temperature], which are "fed back" to the child patient/client through visual and/or auditory displays. The liberal use of colors and the implementation of increasingly creative, attractive games and scenarios tap into the child and adolescent's sense of adventure, challenge, and desire for active participation. Linked to either direct or indirect measurement of their "problem," such biofeedback opportunities provide a natural connection to hypnotic inductions and hypnotherapeutic strategies. Culbert et al. note (1994) that individual patient problems suggest a need for varying degrees of integration of biofeedback and hypnosis; and as discussed in detail in Chapter 14 our belief is that there is a hypnotic induction component for all biofeedback. These two cyberphysiologic (self-regulatory) methodologies may thus be combined creatively in the best interest of the patient and his or her individual problem(s). Computer games for these purposes are now being displayed prominently in museums around the United States and varying forms may soon be available for home use. Many children continue to be delighted and intrigued with watching simple biobands or biodots applied to their fingers; these change color as temperature changes, and children can use these at home to reinforce their learning.

Distraction and Utilization Techniques

These methods, based on techniques developed by M. H. Erickson (1959), are especially helpful with children who are frightened or in severe pain. They attract attention often by a seeming lack of logic, shifting focus from a negative to a positive aspect of the situation. Once the therapist can get the child's attention, trance often may occur spontaneously, and therapeutic suggestions may be easily accepted. The success of these techniques is chiefly a function of the therapist's creativity. We give only a few examples.

> "It hurts, and it's going to hurt a while longer. It will probably keep right on hurting until it stops. [The child hears 'it stops.'] I wonder if it will stop hurting in 5 minutes or 7 minutes or 30 seconds or right now?"
> "Your right hand is hurt. Let's be sure the left hand is not also injured. Does it hurt here . . . or here . . . or here?"
> "Those are pretty sparkling tears. Can you cry some more of them? I wonder which eye will have more tears."
> "What's that dog in the corner doing?"
> "What color is the air today?"
> "Listen to that scream. You certainly have strong lungs. Now scream a few more times, and then we'll count in a whisper. One, two, three . . . You're good at whispering. We'll count when you scream, and we'll count when you whisper . . . four . . . five. . . ."

Using Modern Technology: Technology-Aided Induction Techniques

Videotape. Young children who are shy or hesitant may benefit by watching a videotape of a child of similar age responding to hypnotic induction. These often are very valuable in pre-hypnotic conversations with children and families to demystify the forthcoming hypnotic experience expected to be of help for the child. They also serve to remove misconceptions as well as to clarify modern mythology about what hypnosis is and is not. With the increased prevalence of home and school videocameras, many children are camera-eager rather than camera-shy; and videotaping of a given hypnotic experience sometimes serves to facilitate a child's interest, concentration, and absorption. Such a videotape might also be used as a form of personal — video and audio — biofeedback in later, ongoing therapeutic work with a child, for example, to show the child through a previous video how he or she looked, how well he or she was relaxing, how pain-free he or she was during hypnosis.

Audiotape. For some children who have difficulty learning to go into hypnosis without the therapist present, inductions may be recorded on cassette tapes for use at home, in a hospital room, or even in the nurse's office at school. We have a strong preference, however, that children achieve full independence in using hypnosis for their own benefit, rather than becoming dependent on our audiotaped induction/therapeutic suggestions. Although we acknowledge and wish to promote the value of audiocassettes for rehearsal reinforcement and review, in the interest of avoiding dependence, we most often prefer to wait until a child has demonstrated comfort and facility with self-hypnosis before offering to prepare an audiotape. Once a child has learned hypnosis and upon one or more return visits has demonstrated through discussion and self-induction of hypnosis that he or she has begun to integrate self-hypnosis into his or her life, then we may offer to prepare a tape for home use. A typical approach might be: "Now that you know how to do this for yourself, I know that some times there must be days/nights when one part of you knows that you probably should practice your RMI [relaxation/mental imagery, self-hypnosis], while another part of you is too tired, or bored, or just doesn't feel like it. So, I was thinking that maybe what we could do is today, when we practice in a couple of minutes, maybe I'll just record what I say, and then if it comes out good, you can have the tape, and it will be like having the coach at home. Then, sometimes if you know you should practice and don't feel like it, that would be a good time to put the tape on, and it will be easier to just listen the way you do when you're here. What do you think?" The vast majority of children and teenagers like this idea and are eager and thrilled to have the audiotape that they then use in widely disparate ways. Occasionally, however, the child experiences the offer of a tape as something of an insult to his or her ability to do this for him- or herself and refuses, saying "Naw, I don't need it, thanks anyway."

The availability of portable, personal Walkman-type playback units has been a boon, especially for chronically ill children. Their use during procedures may allow for and promote rapid induction of hypnosis when the child's favorite music is played or a specific tape is used with instructions for entering and maintaining the hypnotic state.

When a tape is requested by a child or family, the therapist should ask for recommendations from the child regarding what should be placed on the tape. Each tape should be tailored to the child's particular needs. Some children like to dictate their own induction onto the tape, thus taking a major step toward mastery. The child should be told that this tape is for his or her use only and is not to be played for other children. We have not seen children abuse taped inductions when the therapist explains that the tape would probably not be helpful to other children. In the interest of promoting mastery and autonomy, we usually urge parents to not listen to the child's tape unless and until the child invites them to share the experience. We often present this to the parent(s) by pointing out in the child's presence that although we don't mind if the child shares the tape with the parents, that the parents don't mind (we hope!) if the child decides to keep it private (at least for "a while").

Telephone. We have found that children respond easily to hypnotic induction rehearsal, review, and reinforcement by telephone so long as patient and therapist are well known to one another. Sometimes distance precludes a face-to-face visit or the therapist is not immediately available when some unexpected special circumstance arises in which immediate reinforcement of hypnotic suggestions is advisable. For example, a burned child may suddenly be faced with an unexpected procedure or may otherwise experience intense pain and be unable to use techniques of self-hypnosis. Although privacy and quiet are desirable, we have used telephone inductions in a busy intensive care unit where as many as a dozen adults were working with our patient and others. In long-term follow-up of children with habit problems, Olness (1976) has children telephone the office on a regular basis. Many selected children also call us with follow-up reports after frequent office visits are no longer necessary. In addition to updating progress, during these conversations the patient also verbally reviews self-hypnosis exercises, and the therapist reinforces suggestions. Obviously it is important that the patient be able to use inductions that do not require the therapist's actual presence. After the patient has told the therapist about the current situation, the therapist can begin the induction. In selected situations, especially with preschool children and hospitalized/immobilized patients, parents may help by holding the telephone receiver near the child's ear and mouth.

Group Inductions

Simultaneous induction of several children in a group has been reported to be successful, particularly with children who have chronic illnesses such as hemophilia (LaBaw, 1975) or asthma (Kohen & Wynne, 1988), or leukemia or other cancers (Olness & Singher, 1989). This method may be especially useful with very young children, who often feel more comfortable in groups and can capitalize on their natural tendencies to imitate their peers. Sometimes parents also enjoy desired relaxation and confidence when they are given the opportunity to participate with their children in group exercises. They may also enjoy sharing the benefits of learning self-hypnosis to reinforce these general goals. The therapist may choose to have all participants use the same induction, such as favorite place imagery or the coin technique, or storytelling, a particular favorite with preschool children. At other times, and especially if the children in the group differ widely in age, the therapist may use a patient's-choice induction in which each patient uses a self-hypnotic technique most beneficial (for themselves) in the past. During this time the therapist may choose to purposely remain silent, may play music, may address general comments to the group, or may intersperse particular statements directed to specific individuals or to the whole group. When the therapist makes hypnotherapeutic suggestions, these may be addressed to the group as a whole or to individual members. Rivalry can be eliminated or minimized in such a setting when each member receives a brief personalized comment or suggestion during the group hypnosis.

In group inductions, some children—especially the younger ones—may choose to have their eyes open, at least at the beginning, so that they can observe and imitate their peers. For most children, the therapist may comment that distraction will be lessened and concentration heightened if they close their eyes at the outset, perhaps opening them briefly from time to time as needed.

Arousal: Ending the Hypnotic Experience

When choosing a method of terminating a trance, the therapist takes into account the child patient's need for structure and (normal) tendency to resist finishing the experience for the moment. Compared with adults, children usually need less formality and ritual. If structure appears to be helpful or important for a particular child, the therapist may count or ask patients to count to a certain number. Or, children may count silently, using suggestions that they will open their eyes at some point in the counting and feel fully alert, aware, and refreshed by the end of the count.

If a less structured approach seems best, as it commonly does, the therapist might say, "Enjoy that experience [or scene or place or game] for a little while longer, and then, when you're ready, slowly, comfortably, easily open your eyes and return to your usual way of being, and your usual regular self." For an older child or teen-ager, one might address him or her as one might an adult, noting, "When you're ready, slowly, comfortably, easily open your eyes and return to your usual state of consciousness and alertness. . . . " For a younger child, "Do that a little longer, and when you're ready, go back [or return] to what you were doing before we began this practice." For all age groups, it is useful to combine the invitation to complete the experience with acknowledgment of the difference and value of the hypnotic state as compared to the nonhypnotic state by saying, ". . . and be sure to bring your good and relaxed feelings with you when you come back here." If the child is in pain or distress before the induction, the therapist needs to add some clarification such as "We can do this with you lying in your bed with your teddy bear, and you can keep all the comfortable nice feelings you have now." Some children may be told to enjoy the hypnotic state "for as long as you like," but this phrase should be avoided with children who might use it to extend the session beyond appropriate limits or otherwise seek to manipulate the therapist. Occasionally a child in a group hypnotherapy session may compete with peers by resisting arousal from the trance. The therapist can usually solve the problem with a casual remark such as "I wonder who will be the first one to be able to get fully alert again." Rarely, a direct comment to the child may be in order.

Consistent with our usual avoidance of the terms "asleep, sleepy, tired, drowsy," we also avoid the terms "wake up" from the trance experience. However, when doing an induction with a child for whom it would be appropriate to drift from the state of hypnosis to the state of sleep without intermediate arousal, we would say, "Now, if you wish, you can just drift off to sleep. When you wake up, you can feel fully refreshed and alert. When you wake up, you will no longer be in hypnosis; you can be in your usual state of awareness and give yourself an inside message to enjoy the rest of the day."

Self-Reinforcement Using Patient-Recorded Audiotapes

It is helpful to some children to make recordings of themselves dictating the self-hypnosis exercise. This is done after several sessions with the hypnotherapist. When they are practicing at home, some children do far better when they actually hear themselves speaking on the tape recorder than when they try to concentrate on the exercise by memory. It is important that the therapist also hear the tape at some point in order to make sure that appropriate suggestions are recalled and given. Aronson (1986) has reported the use of the technique with a 15-year-old adolescent. Sometimes older children and teen-agers may benefit from writing a "script" of what they want their tape to say, occasionally brainstorming and reviewing it with the clinician and then preparing a tape for themselves.

INDUCTION TECHNIQUES
FOR DIFFERENT AGES

Children of different ages often prefer different induction techniques. Although we can group techniques roughly according to the age groups for which they are most often appropriate, there are no hard and fast rules, especially in cases where levels of cognitive or social–emotional development are at variance with expectations based on chronological age. Immature adolescents may do well with techniques that normally would appeal to younger children. Likewise, some young children succeed best with methods that appeal to older age groups, especially techniques they know are used by older siblings or parents. As usual, we remain flexible and let the patient be the guide, tailoring techniques to the individual and developmental needs of a given child.

In Table 5.1, we have included methods that need no description and therefore have not been discussed previously.

MODIFICATIONS FOR CHILDREN
WITH SPECIAL PROBLEMS

It is especially important that the therapist working with children who have various disabilities be familiar with a variety of induction strategies and techniques and be capable of creative modification to suit and accommodate to special circumstances and needs.

Physical Disabilities

Hypnotherapeutic induction can be successful with children who are at bedrest or who have motor limitations, verbal dysfluencies, blindness, or deafness. Even delirious or comatose children may respond (D. M. Markowitz, personal communication, 1980). In general, the therapist chooses a method in which the disability itself is not involved or appropriately modifies a method while taking account of the problem. For example, in the case of a child who is deaf, it may be necessary to agree on written suggestions and/or enlist the aid of someone fluent in sign language. In so doing it is obviously critical to provide education about hypnosis for, and spend time developing rapport with, the individual(s) who will be doing the signing in order to maximize hypnotherapeutic communication and success.

Korn and Johnson (1978) reported using hypnotherapy to facilitate rehabilitation of a 16-year-old girl with significant brain damage. The patient

TABLE 5.1. Induction Techniques by Age

Preverbal (0–2 years)	Middle childhood (7–11 years)
Tactile stimulation, stroking patting	Favorite place
Kinesthetic stimulation: rocking, moving an arm back and forth	Favorite activity
	Cloud gazing
Auditory stimulation: music or any whirring sound such as a hairdryer, electric shaver, vacuum cleaner placed out of reach of the child	Flying blanket
	Videogames (actual or imagined)
	Riding a bike
	Arm lowering
Visual stimulation: mobiles or other objects that change shape, color, or position	Blowing breath out
	Favorite music
	Listening to self on tape
Holding a doll or stuffed animal	Coin watching
	Fixation at point on hand
	Hands (fingers) moving together
Early verbal (2–4 years)	Arm rigidity
Blowing bubbles	
Pop-up books	**Adolescence (12–18 years)**
Storytelling	
Stereoscopic viewer	Favorite place/activity
Favorite activity	Sports activity
Speaking to the child through a doll or stuffed animal	Arm catalepsy
	Following breathing
Floppy Raggedy Ann or Andy	Videogames (actual or imagined)
Teddy bear	Computer games (actual or imagined)
Watching induction or self on videotape	Eye fixation on hand
	Driving a car
	Playing or hearing music
Preschool and early school (4–6 years)	Hand levitation
	Fingers/hands together as magnets
Blowing breath out	Fantasy games (e.g., Dungeons and Dragons)
Favorite place	
Multiple animals	
Flower garden	
Storytelling (alone or in a group)	
Mighty oak tree	
Coin watching	
Letter watching	
Pop-up books	
Television fantasy	
Stereoscopic viewer	
Videotape	
Bouncing ball	
Thermal (and other) biofeedback	
Finger lowering	
Playground activity	

was comatose when the therapists first began making suggestions for induction of hypnosis. She responded to specific imagery designed to help her recapture her ability to swallow, to move extremities, to dress herself ("Imagine yourself dressing a life-sized doll"), and to speak. Over a period of weeks, this patient became alert and regained autonomic reflex responses, motor skills, and speech.

Mental Retardation and/or Developmental Delay

Hypnotic induction with developmentally delayed children and adolescents must take into account the mental age of the patient. The therapist can then proceed to some extent as if the child's chronological age were the same as his or her mental age. As development in children with delays may be very uneven, and social skills may sometimes be far more advanced than cognitive skills, it will be particularly important for the clinician to have not only developed a careful rapport with the child, but also to have a clear understanding of the child's level of ability and disability. We have had successful experiences with relatively mildly retarded children (e.g., IQs 50–70), and with young adults who are developmentally child-like.

Children with more severe delays or retardation usually respond poorly or not at all to hypnotic induction. Such patients do not seem capable of necessary levels of ability to relate to the therapist, of focusing attention selectively, and of following instructions. Even if they do respond to induction, they usually do not benefit from hypnotherapeutic suggestions, probably because of limited conceptualization, memory, and language skills.

Learning Disabilities

As much as possible, the therapist must understand the specific areas of disability in order to modify induction and hypnotherapy accordingly. Many children with learning differences and difficulties may also have difficulties with associated inattention, impulsivity, distractibility, and a variety of behavioral problems, some of which may be secondary to their learning problems, and some of which may be part of an overall problem such as attention-deficit disorder (with or without hyperactivity). Increasingly, clinicians and educators who work with children with learning difficulties are utilizing creative approaches such as various forms of hypnotherapeutic-like self-regulation (e.g., imagery or biofeedback) to maximizing learning.

Abused Children

Prior to the consideration of hypnotherapy for a child or teen-ager who has been abused, the clinician must assure that the young person is safe; and that thorough medical, psychological, and family assessment have been conducted, and care for all involved is ongoing. Recognition of the powerful and potentially far-reaching impact of physical and/or sexual abuse will remind clinicians to think carefully about the principles of forming relationships, and the critical aspects of developing rapport with abuse victims. In so doing, we will recognize the (potential) vulnerability of abuse victims and will be more effective in becoming part of the solution rather than part of the problem.

Children and adolescents who have been the victims of physical or sexual abuse may be best understood to have experienced some degree of post-traumatic stress disorder (PTSD). Friedrich (1991) suggests that a hypnotic state is induced/occurs at the time of abuse [similar, perhaps, to the "negative" trance phenomena experienced by children or adults in emergency situations (Chapters 7 and 12), during natural disasters such as floods, tornadoes, earthquakes; or to victims/refugees of wars]. Because of our awareness of this vulnerability, we encourage clinicians to proceed with caution even in initial history-taking and rapport-development and to be alert to the reappearance of spontaneous hypnotic states for their potential diagnostic and therapeutic value. In his work with abused children, Friedrich (1991) emphasizes that hypnotherapy may be used therapeutically for symptom stabilization and removal, for controlled uncovering of the traumatic events through regression, and toward integration with the goal of facilitating mastery and a return to optimal pre-trauma functioning. As we have noted for many clinical situations, Friedrich (1991) emphasizes "joining" with the child victim and notes that by listening carefully and through the use of his or her own language the clinician can more easily help the child victim hypnotically to begin to understand and reframe his or her traumatic experience to facilitate positive rather than maladaptation.

Rhue and Lynn (1991, 1993) describe the application and value of storytelling as a hypnotherapeutic strategy for treatment of sexually abused children. They, too, emphasize the importance of therapeutic rapport and describe collaborative storytelling (1993) with a major beginning focus being the identification of a "safe context" and "building a safe haven, a favorite place," in which ongoing hypnotherapy can proceed.

Clinicians who work with victims of abuse and/or other trauma are encouraged to review Friederich's (1991) and Rhue and Lynn's (1991, 1993) detailed case reports for more specific information and the description of various thoughtful, creative, and successful hypnotic strategies.

Autistic and Severely Disturbed Children

There is one case report (Gardner & Tarnow, 1980) of the use of hypnotic induction with a mildly autistic adolescent. Efforts to use traditional approaches to induction were met with minimal responses. Listening to a favorite piece of music proved to be a successful induction, during which this patient responded with spontaneous eye closure, neck and jaw relaxation, and hand catalepsy. Severely autistic children who have little capacity for interpersonal relationships are not likely to respond to hypnotic induction.

Olness has found use of eye fixation on a biofeedback monitor to be a successful induction method for some severely disturbed children. As they watch the shapes, lines, or numbers change, appropriate suggestions are made regarding their ability to concentrate, to control their body, and to do positive things for themselves. As with other children, such approaches must be individualized to the unique needs, likes and dislikes, and style of each child.

It seems reasonable that children with severe ego deficits might respond best to induction techniques that are adaptations of soothing, comforting, nonverbal methods similar to those recommended for use with young children.

Terminally Ill Children and Adolescents

It is very important that induction of hypnosis with terminally ill children and adolescents enhances their sense of mastery. It should be clear to such patients (and their families) that they are involved in treatment planning from the beginning and that the methods chosen are their own. Whenever possible, clinical consultation for possible hypnotherapy with young people who are dying should take place well before their "final hours." Unfortunately, that does not commonly happen, and many of these patients are weak, and sometimes affected by sedatives and pain medications when we meet them. If possible, the timing of initial hypnotic induction should be the maximum possible number of hours after the last sedative or pain medication. Sometimes, however, even a heavily sedated child will respond. For these patients, reinforcement via cassette tapes may be helpful so that they may choose to listen both whenever and as often as they choose and are able. Parental assistance and telephone reinforcement from the therapist are necessary more often than in those with self-limited or non-life-threatening problems (see also Chapter 13).

TEACHING SELF-HYPNOSIS

It is almost always useful and important to teach children self-hypnosis, particularly when problems relate to recurrent difficulties or discomfort, or to undesirable habits. This subject has been discussed in the literature both separately (Gardner, 1981) and in the context of treatment of specific pediatric problems such as hemophilia (LaBaw, 1975) or functional megacolon (Olness, 1976), or habits (Kohen, 1991). For children who practice self-hypnosis, the advantages are (1) their sense of control and mastery is acknowledged, and (2) desired behavior is more frequently reinforced by repetition of appropriate imagery exercises.

Gardner (1981) noted that brief didactic teaching concerning abuse of self-hypnosis is usually sufficient to prevent children from giving demonstrations to their friends or acting as well-meaning but untrained hypnotherapists. The risk of abuse is higher in children with poor judgment or poor impulse control or children with sociopathic tendencies; teaching self-hypnosis as such is usually contraindicated in such cases. Using these guidelines, we have not known any of our patients to abuse their self-hypnotic skills.

We find that the major problem with teaching children self-hypnosis is ensuring that they actually do practice the exercises on a prescribed daily basis. In one study (Kohen, Colwell, Heimel, & Olness, 1984), some children reported becoming bored with the prescribed practice, or "forgot" to do it. Even with cooperative parents, an excellent response to hypnotherapy, and office or telephone reinforcement from the therapist, relatively few children will continue self-hypnosis practice beyond a few months. This is particularly so if they've had success in resolving their problem.

Some children resist the recommendation of using self-hypnosis. Factors producing this sort of "resistance" include inadequate motivation to solve the problem, the age and developmental level of the child, transference to the therapist, and fear that therapy visits will cease if the child uses hypnosis independently, and parental interference.

It is usually possible to deal successfully with resistance to using self-hypnosis. In the case of very young children, we prepare a cassette tape for the child or involve a parent in the practice, striving and encouraging the process to be both creative and fun as well as, hopefully, successful. The involvement of the parent serves a dual purpose, as the parents of children with chronic illness benefit from acknowledgment by health care providers that they are able to contribute in some way to the therapeutic process.

Children who resist self-hypnosis because of fear that therapy visits will cease can be specifically reassured that this will not occur. The therapist can also make phone calls for a time in order to effect a smooth termination in cases where cessation of therapy is, in fact, appropriate and desirable. We have also found that writing letters to the patient after or as part of the ongoing termination / separation process can have a positive effect in encouraging regular self-hypnosis practice.

Some children resist self-hypnosis as a reaction against parental interference, sometimes well-intentioned and sometimes not. The problem is especially likely to arise in the case of children with enuresis (Kohen et al., 1984), probably because wet beds can be especially vexing to parents and can trigger their anger and frustration more easily than other problems such as pain or anxiety.

L. Jacobs (1962) reported a case history of a 6-year-old girl suffering from enuresis. The child believed that her parents didn't love her. When the child was in trance, suggestions were given that she would learn a "signal" when her bladder was full, and also that her parents loved her whether or not she was wet. At first, she did very well. The mother was instructed that each night she put the child to bed she should hold her and kiss her, tell her what a good girl she was, tell her how much the family loved her, and how easy it would be to remember the signal, thus reinforcing the therapist's suggestions. After family financial setbacks, the mother subsequently became distraught, shouted at the child, spanked her, and the patient experienced a relapse. After discussion with the therapist, the previous suggestions were reinforced, and the patient had no further problems. It is important to remember that unpleasant habits and behavior patterns in children commonly induce unpleasant habit reaction patterns in family members, and therapists must consider those patterns in developing a treatment plan that is tailored to that particular child in the context of his or her family.

We specifically request that parents not remind children who have habit problems to practice self-hypnosis, often suggesting more positive ways for them to give attention. We tell children in the presence of the parent that their parents are not to remind them. We then focus in detail with the child concerning how best to remember to practice. Possibilities include putting a sign on the door, tying a string around the toothbrush, having a placecard beside the dinner plate, and tying a sign around the neck of a favorite stuffed animal. The goals, of course, are to engage the parent to agree with and acknowledge the child's decision and to shift a negative frame of mind (about this problem) to a positive one for child and family alike. Following this, the parent is asked to leave, and the therapist works with the child alone.

It also seems useful to agree on the place where the child will practice self-hypnosis and to allow for trips out of town or overnight visits to friends. In general, we ask that the child practice, in a sitting position (because it is too easy to fall asleep if one practices imagery and relaxation in the recumbent position!), in his or her room. Occasionally, and in consultation with the parent, the therapist and child might decide on a particular chair in the study or living room. The chosen place should be quiet. The child should usually practice alone, although we know of children who successfully practice during rest periods or other breaks during their school day.

When desired therapeutic objectives are being accomplished and frequent office visits are not necessary, we recommend that the child call and/or write to the therapist on a regularly scheduled basis. The child is then asked to verbalize the self-hypnosis exercise over the phone, and the therapist reinforces where necessary. It is also essential to arrange for a time to terminate self-hypnosis exercises, for example, 1 month after all beds are dry. This implies that the therapist expects success and that the patient is motivated to continue. Occasionally a child will be bored or tired of a certain image in the induction, and suggestions can be provided for change.

Gardner (1981) described a three-step method for teaching children self-hypnosis, easily accomplished in one session:

Step 1. The therapist uses various induction and deepening methods, usually emphasizing imagery and ideomotor techniques. The latter are especially useful for children who want some outward and visible sign that hypnosis has been achieved. After allowing time for enjoyment of the imagery, the therapist asks the child to count silently up to five, eyes opening at three, fully alert at five. The therapist comments that the child now knows how to come out of hypnosis and return to the alert state without help. Rapid alerting in emergencies may also be discussed.

Step 2. Therapist and patient discuss which of the induction techniques employed in step 1 were most helpful and agree to discard the rest. The child is then asked to describe to the therapist in detail the techniques chosen for induction, to feel the same good feelings, and to go into hypnosis easily and naturally as the description proceeds. The therapist may add details if the child's wording is too general. After another pause and a reassuring comment, the therapist asks the child to return to the normal alert state. Problems are discussed as necessary.

Step 3. This is the same as step 2 except that the child is asked to recall and to decide to experience the induction silently. Neither child nor therapist speaks. The child nods when trance is achieved. After another pause, the child returns again to the usual state of alertness. Any remain problems or questions are then discussed. The child is then ready for full independent use of self-hypnosis.

Alternatively, one of us (DPK) invariably teaches self-hypnosis during each patient's first hypnotic experience, with incorporation of Ericksonian-like expectancy suggestions and liberal use of ego-strengthening and future-oriented suggestions. Following induction and intensification (deepening) of hypnosis, and whatever therapeutic utilization suggestions may be offered during the first hypnotic experience, suggestions for and training in self-hypnosis are provided along with post-hypnotic suggestions before the end of the experience:

> "Before you come to the end of what you have learned so well today, be sure to congratulate yourself for how well you've done; and be proud of how your brain and body are learning to talk to each other so well. It's nice before you finish to remind yourself of what you did to help give yourself the good feelings you have now, so that *when* you practice this one or two or three times each day for 10 or 15 minutes, you'll know exactly how to do it. So, just picture in your mind where you might sit at home when you practice, and then see yourself doing the fingers-together game [or whatever induction was used] to start off your self-hypnosis [or self-relaxation and imagination or whatever words are being used]. Great . . . now notice that as your eyes close and you start to get comfortable that you can imagine about anything you want . . . perhaps it will be about playing soccer or [add choices of several of child's favorite activi-

ties] . . . and you can notice everything about it . . . and when you practice this at home in this same way, you'll be able to notice just as you have
today and now the way your muscles relax as you breathe out. And you
can allow the relaxation feeling to move down your body all the
way . . . that's right . . . and then, just like today, as soon as the relaxation has gotten all the way to your head [or toes], then you can let your
head nod [or your finger lift], and that will be the signal to yourself that
you are as comfortable as you want to be for that practice time. And then,
before you finish practicing, make sure you give your mind and body any
directions or new ideas you want them to have [substitute here any hypnotherapeutic suggestions specific to the child and his or her problem(s)].
And the last thing that you need to know when you practice at home and
here, is that if you happen to be practicing at bedtime, you don't have to
even finish, you can just let your self-hypnosis practice finish by falling
asleep. And if you happen to be practicing at some other time, then when
you're finished, you'll be done, and you can open your eyes and bring your
good feelings back with you."

CONCLUSIONS

Hypnotic induction is usually a pleasant and creative experience both for
child patients and for their therapists. Techniques can be modified to suit
children of different ages or with special problems such as physical disability. Most children readily learn self-hypnosis and can benefit from this additional skill. It is important to consider learning styles and family and cultural
differences of an individual child before deciding which hypnotic technique
is most apt to be suitable for that child. The choice of specific induction techniques is based on the therapist's ingenuity as well as on the child's needs,
preferences, and abilities. Although such choices are now based on clinical
judgment, future research may show that some problems or some children
respond better to one technique than to another. To date, such studies have
not been reported.

PART TWO

HYPNOTHERAPY WITH CHILDREN

CHAPTER SIX

General Principles
of Child Hypnotherapy

We will now review techniques and results of hypnotherapy for a wide range of childhood problems. Most published accounts of hypnotherapy for specific childhood problems include some general comments concerning principles, indications, contraindications, and pitfalls of this therapeutic modality. A few papers (Call, 1976; Kaffman, 1968; Olness & Kohen, 1984; Williams & Singh, 1976; Wright, 1960, 1987) focus directly on basic issues.

In order to avoid excessive repetition in succeeding chapters, we devote this chapter to a discussion of general principles of child hypnotherapy. Some of our thoughts are shared by most people in the field, whereas others will provoke varying degrees of controversy.

DEFINITION AND BOUNDARIES
OF HYPNOTHERAPY

Hypnosis and hypnotherapy are two different entities. *Hypnosis is an altered state of consciousness* that may have certain temporary beneficial effects, such as tension reduction but is not in itself designed for that purpose. *Hypnotherapy is a treatment modality* with specific therapeutic goals and specific techniques utilized while the patient is in the state of hypnosis.

We also distinguish between a hypnotist and a hypnotherapist, for these terms are often confused in the context of clinical work.* A hypnotist—

---

*We do not mean to imply that the term "hypnotist" always has a negative connotation. For instance, in research on various hypnotic phenomena, the scientist who does a hypnotic induction and explores the subject's hypnotic behavior is a hypnotist, not a hypnotherapist. Use of the term "coach" or "instructor" may be preferable to use of "hypnotist."

often found listed in the classified advertisements of newspapers or in the yellow pages of the telephone directory under "hypnotists"—may be a person with limited education whose only skill is the use of hypnosis and who accepts virtually everyone for treatment. Although such people often get good results—otherwise they could not stay in business—they may engage in indiscriminate use of their one skill, sometimes with unfortunate results.

A hypnotherapist is, first of all, a *therapist*. A child hypnotherapist has advanced training in one of the child health professions and uses hypnotherapeutic techniques as part of a comprehensive approach to the diagnosis and treatment of certain disorders. In this context, it is a good rule of thumb that one should not attempt to treat a problem with hypnotherapy unless one is also competent to assess the problem and recommend other therapists if appropriate. When parents ask us about hypnotists, we do our best to educate them with regard to these distinctions.

We believe that the practice of hypnotherapy with children should be limited to health professionals who typically assume primary responsibility for treating children's problems, for example, child psychologists and psychiatrists, dentists, pediatricians, and other physicians and surgeons who work with children. Furthermore, these professionals limit hypnotherapeutic work to their own areas of competence. This does not mean, for instance, that a psychologist should never treat organic pain with hypnotherapy. It does mean that the psychologist who does so is also competent to treat organic pain with other methods (e.g., supportive psychotherapy or biofeedback).

In selected cases, it is appropriate for nurses, physical therapists, speech pathologists, and other child health specialists to use hypnotherapy. If their specialized treatment of a child is performed under the supervision and/or responsibility of a physician, dentist or psychologist, then their use of hypnotherapy should also be conducted under the direct supervision of a health professional who assumes responsibility for the patient and who is competent in the use of hypnotherapy.

To give an example, a surgeon might have primary responsibility for the care of a burned child and may have ordered extensive physical therapy as part of the total treatment regimen. The surgeon—if he or she is not trained in hypnotherapy and is not also a psychotherapist—might request that a psychologist, who is trained in hypnotherapy assume primary responsibility for the child's emotional well-being and for helping to maximize the child's cooperation with treatment, including painful physical therapy sessions. The psychologist consults with the surgeon and the physical therapist and evaluates the child in order to design specific hypnotherapeutic strategies to maximize the child's opportunity for physical and emotional recovery. The psychologist might then train the physical therapist in some of these methods for the purpose of facilitating cooperation with necessary procedures in physical therapy and remain available for continuing consultation and supervision.

GOALS OF HYPNOTHERAPY

People who come to us requesting hypnotherapy begin by saying, "I have a problem." Often they really mean to say, "A problem has me." That is, they perceive themselves as having been rendered passive and helpless, the victim of a situation over which they have virtually no control. Previous therapeutic efforts either have been of limited value or have contributed to the patient's passive–dependent stance by forcing continued reliance on external powers such as machines and medication.

The goal of hypnotherapy is always to teach the patient an attitude of hope in the context of mastery. The patient learns to be an active participant in his or her own behalf, to focus on creating a solution rather than on enduring a problem, and to discover and use resources for inner control as much as possible.

The goal of mastery does not mean that the patient necessarily turns away from external aid, although this may sometimes be possible. An anxious child may no longer need tranquilizers; a child with asthma may no longer need a nebulizer. Often, however, the child successfully using hypnotherapy continues to require external help, albeit now in a different psychological context. Thus, a child in renal failure continues regular dialysis, but has less anxiety and depression, is more motivated to participate in treatment, and is more cooperative with necessary dietary restrictions. Such a child keeps the need for dialysis to a minimum and may perceive the machine as a useful aid rather than as an external imposition.

The so-called First Law of Hypnosis emphasizes that the patient must be able to define or perceive a desired therapeutic outcome. It is essential that the therapist also keep this in mind. Sometimes, the outcome desired by the parents or therapist is not the same as that desired by the child. This can be explored in various ways with children; for example, "We've been talking for a while. Am I right in understanding that what you want is to have all of your beds dry?" Or, during the first hypnotic induction the therapist can ask the child to indicate which finger represents "Yes," which represents "No," and which represents "I don't know." Then, when the child appears very comfortable, the therapist can say, "I'll ask some questions that you can answer with your fingers. Do you like chocolate ice cream? Do you like to go to bed at night? Do you like the color blue? Would you like to have dry beds at night? Do you like to eat pizza?" Occasionally, the ideomotor response will be "No," and this is an indication that further work must be done before teaching the child self-hypnosis. It is also important in structuring suggestions to include "future programming." An example is, "Think of something you're looking forward to next summer. You needn't tell me what it is. Imagine that it's next summer, and you are enjoying what you're doing, just as if you were really there. And, while you are enjoying it, you can also enjoy thinking how nice that your beds are all dry because of your work, because you have become the boss of your bladder—and then you can continue to imagine you're enjoying what you are looking forward to next summer."

RECOGNIZING DEVELOPMENTAL ISSUES

That a child is not an adult seems obvious, but it is a fact sometimes overlooked in hypnotherapy. If a child patient is to achieve the goal of mastery through successful response to hypnotic induction and treatment techniques, language must be adapted to the level and interests of that child, being neither too complex nor too simple and patronizing. As in any therapy, the hypnotherapist must take into account the child's perceptual and conceptual skills with respect to problems and possible solutions. For this reason, it is often best to let the child select some of the details of imagery used in hypnotherapeutic suggestions. The therapists might say, "Think of a way you can feel safe" and then follow the child's lead instead of suggesting a particular plan.

If the child patient is seen at different points over a period of time, it is important to remember that techniques that were appealing and helpful at one age may have no value or even be aversive at a later age.

The degree to which children mix reality and fantasy is often a cause of fears and other problems. But this developmental tendency can become an advantage in hypnotherapy. For example, the child may respond particularly well to imagery techniques such as rehearsal in fantasy, experiencing a new behavior first in hypnotic imagery and then quickly becoming able to make the transition to incorporating that behavior in reality situations.

PARENTAL INVOLVEMENT

In some instances, particularly when the parent has been overprotective or when the child needs greater autonomy, it is best to minimize the parental role in hypnotherapy. The parents may be asked specifically to refrain from reminding the child to practice self-hypnosis and to allow the child privacy during practice sessions. The therapist gives the parent a general explanation of the treatment program. The following vignette is an example of this approach.

Hugh N., age 7 years, suffered from severe asthma. Finding self-hypnosis very helpful, he became able to participate more fully in school and in sports and was especially proud of being able to help himself and not always have to rely on his parents for medication. Soon after hypnotherapy began, his mother said to the therapist, "When Hugh begins to wheeze, he goes to his room and closes the door. After about 5 minutes, he comes out, and he's not wheezing, and I don't know what he does in there!" The therapist answered, "I know what I asked him to do, but I don't know what he really does in there either. What is important is that Hugh is better." The mother continued to allow her son the privacy and independence he needed.

In some cases, the child may need the parent's presence either in the therapist's office or during use of self-hypnosis in order to help focus on hypnotic suggestions or to provide reassurance. For example, Ellen L., an adolescent girl, had difficulty sleeping because of chronic, progressive organic pain with associated anxiety. Although she learned self-hypnosis, the severity of her pain sometimes interfered with her ability to concentrate on hypnotic suggestions. Her mother willingly served as a surrogate therapist when needed, with the results that both mother and Ellen got more sleep and felt more hopeful about Ellen's condition.

Most parents abide by the therapist's recommendations concerning the degree of their involvement. A few parents consciously or unconsciously sabotage the therapy. In a particularly unfortunate case, Billy R., a 6-year-old, was brought for hypnotherapy to seek relief from the itching of severe eczema. He responded well in the first few sessions, easily controlling the itching as he sat in the therapist's lap. He learned self-hypnosis and was asked to practice twice daily for 5 to 10 minutes at home. He said he needed his mother to help him, and the therapist agreed that mother's presence would be useful. But the mother refused, saying she already spent too much of her time with his expensive skin care. She also refused to seek help for her own resentment and related problems. Billy's itching continued unabated.

Sometimes careful assessment points to the need for the parents or other family members to be involved, not just to support the child but as full participants in family therapy, with or without hypnotherapy. Just as in child psychotherapy, parents of children presenting for hypnotherapy may focus the pathology on the child when they also need help. If the parents absolutely refuse to participate in therapy, sometimes it is possible to make at least partial gains with the child alone. In such cases, the parents may be willing to be seen every few weeks for counseling or for a review of the current home situation. We prefer this "half-measure" approach to that of no therapy for the child. Sometimes the parents' trust will eventually increase to the point that they enter therapy. At the least, it may be possible to teach the child more effective ways of coping in the family situation. We realize, however, that this therapeutic strategy may reinforce the parents' conviction that the locus of the problem is in the child, making the parents even more resistant to treatment for themselves. There is the added risk, if hypnotherapy with the child is successful, that the parents may then find another target for the pathology, perhaps another child or even the marital relationship itself.

TYPES OF HYPNOTHERAPY

To say that a child is using hypnotherapy really tells us very little except that hypnosis is being employed somehow in the treatment program. Hypnotherapy refers to the use of a variety of hypnotic techniques in the context of some form of psychotherapy, using that term in its broadest sense. Thus, hypnotherapeutic methods may be employed in the context of relationship or supportive therapy, behavior modification, psychoanalysis and dynamic therapies, gestalt therapy, or rational–emotive therapy. Some hypnotherapeutic methods are common across several psychotherapeutic approaches, whereas others have more limited application. For example, hypnotic relaxation is used to facilitate progress both in analytically oriented therapy and in behavior modification. Hypnotically induced dreaming, on the other hand, might be employed in the analytic approach but probably not in a behavior modification program.

The specific hypnotherapeutic techniques used with a particular patient are derived from the nature of the presenting problem, the patient's goal, other patient characteristics, the therapist's theoretical orientation, and certain situational factors such as the amount of time available for treatment. There are a large number of possible hypnotherapeutic techniques, each with many variations. Specific examples will be described in Chapters 7 through 15. At this point, we simply divide hypnotherapeutic methods into three broad categories.

Supportive, Ego-Enhancing Methods

The chief goal here is to help the patient feel more worthy, more capable of dealing effectively with problems and challenges, more able to contribute to his or her own well-being, and be in control of circumstances both internal and external. Patients who fear necessary surgery, who experience pervasive anxiety, or who manifest borderline or psychotic behavior often derive special benefit from supportive techniques. These methods may also be used prospectively in the course of routine pediatric care; for example, "I will look forward to your telling me about the fun things you do in kindergarten." "Your muscles feel strong. I think you can use them to learn to ride your new bike." Such supportive phrases may be applied appropriately in emergency situations, such as when a child arrives in the emergency room with a laceration.

Symptom-Oriented Methods

Here the therapeutic effort is directed at removing, altering, or alleviating specific symptoms, either physical or emotional in nature. Difficulties associated with phobias, pain control, and habit control, among many others, often respond to symptom-oriented approaches, especially if the patient is highly motivated to be rid of the symptom. These symptom-oriented approaches are contraindicated if the symptom serves as a major defensive purpose such as to protect the patient from severe underlying depression or the outbreak of psychosis.

Dynamic, Insight-Oriented Methods

Again the goals are symptom relief and ego strengthening, but now special methods are employed to help the patient understand issues that create and maintain problems, gain insight into and work through underlying conflicts, and achieve a more extensive shift toward personality maturation in broad cognitive, affective, and social spheres.

Generally speaking, supportive and symptom-oriented methods are most often used with children, and dynamic methods are used to a somewhat lesser extent. For many child patients, hypnotherapy includes a combination of all three methods.

INDICATIONS FOR HYPNOTHERAPY

Since the rest of this book is devoted to a detailed review of situations in which children can benefit from hypnotherapy, we limit this section to a few general comments. It is generally accepted that hypnotherapy is underutilized in the treatment of children. Moreover, hypnotherapy is too often considered as a last resort, despite the fact that it might have several advantages over other treatment modalities. These advantages include frequent appeal to and acceptance by the child patient, few risks and side effects, frequent rapid response to treatment, and the fact that hypnotherapy fosters attitudes of independence and mastery in coping with problems.

A child can be considered a suitable candidate for hypnotherapy if (1) the child is responsive to hypnotic induction methods, (2) the problem is treatable by hypnotherapy, (3) the child can relate positively to the therapists, (4) the child has at least minimal motivation to solve the problem, (5) the parents or other responsible adults agree to the treatment plan, and (6) the use of hypnotherapy for the problem at hand would not harm the patient.

CONTRAINDICATIONS

As child hypnotherapy achieves greater acceptance by health professionals and the general public, the problem of underutilization gives way to excessive enthusiasm and inappropriate utilization. Parents and other well-meaning adults sometimes put great pressure on us to use hypnotherapy as rapidly and forcefully as possible with child patients so as to eliminate troublesome symptoms. Children, too, sometimes make inappropriate demands for hypnotherapy. It is encumbent on us to resist this pressure. A few parents and children will then threaten to seek the help of a "hypnotist." At this juncture, sometimes we are successful in offering guidance and sometimes not.

We also see excessive enthusiasm about hypnotherapy in some health professionals who have just begun training in this subspecialty and have been exposed to accounts of dramatic cures such as those one often hears about in hypnosis workshops or reads about in hypnosis journals. Sometimes these professionals think of their most difficult patients and conclude that hypnotherapy is bound to be the answer to their unsolved problems. Occasionally this is true; more often it is not. In detailed discussion of such cases, we tend to find either that the therapist has underestimated the patient's degree of pathology or that the therapist has problems with a countertransferential need "to be all things to all people." In such cases, we try to educate professionals toward more rational use of hypnotherapy.

The situations in which we believe hypnotherapy is absolutely contraindicated may be subsumed in the following categories of patient requests: (1) granting the request could lead to physical endangerment for the patient; (2) granting the request could aggravate existing emotional problems or create new ones; (3) the request is simply to "have fun" experimenting with hypnosis; (4) the problem is more effectively treated by some method other than hypnotherapy; and (5) the diagnosis is incorrect, and the real problem should be treated some other way.

There are also some relative contraindications for hypnotherapy, usually based on inappropriate timing of the referral. In these situations, granting the request for immediate hypnotherapeutic treatment would involve overlooking a significant medical problem, overwhelming the patient's ego, or trying to impose change on an unmotivated child. In such situations, hypnotherapy may be appropriate if utilized at a later time or in a manner different from what the patient or parent demands.

Absolute Contraindication:
Risking Physical Endangerment

Eddie Y., a 15-year-old, admitted with some embarrassment that although he enjoyed playing football he became frightened when he was rushed by larger players. Convinced that anxiety impaired his running and passing skills, he said, "Could you hypnotize me so that I couldn't see those big guys, and then I wouldn't be afraid?" Eddie was told that it might be possible for him to experience such a hypnotic negative hallucination, but that it was most inadvisable since he couldn't dodge players if he couldn't see them. He quickly understood that he would not only endanger himself by such use of hypnosis but would also quickly become a detriment to the team. He also agreed with the idea that a mild degree of anxiety can be appropriate and even beneficial to his performance. Reconsidering, he concluded that his anxiety was within normal limits. He felt assured that he could seek more appropriate kinds of treatment, with or without hypnotherapy, if ever his anxiety truly reached irrational and maladaptive proportions. He continued playing football without further difficulty.

Absolute Contraindication: Risking Aggravation of Emotional Problems

Cynthia N., an angry and depressed adolescent girl, telephoned the therapist to report a very unhappy experience with a boyfriend and requested one or two sessions of hypnotherapy for the sole purpose of developing amnesia for her entire relationship with him. The therapist explained that it was unlikely that she could achieve and maintain such an extensive amnesia; hypnotherapy could not produce such "magic cures." Even if she could accomplish this goal, however, it was inadvisable since she might then develop much more serious emotional difficulties. For example, instead of learning skills for coping with this circumscribed problem, she might achieve only partial repression and then develop a maladaptive reaction such as general depression or anxiety, perhaps leading to deeper problems in relating to men. The therapist suggested a longer course of psychotherapy that might include hypnotherapy, but not for the purpose of creating amnesia. Cynthia refused and insisted that she would continue her search until she found someone who would grant her request. We have no follow-up on this girl.

Absolute Contraindication: Hypnosis for Fun

Walter B., an adolescent boy who had recently met the therapist socially, asked to be hypnotized "just for fun." The therapist denied the request and explained why hypnosis should be limited to research and therapeutic situations. Walter agreed with the decision after he understood that hypnosis is an altered state of consciousness in which he might have unexpected emotional reactions that could not and should not be treated in a brief social encounter. He was impressed by a few vignettes of professionals participating in hypnotic inductions as part of hypnosis workshops. Although the hypnotic suggestion was simply to recall and enjoy a pleasant experience, two persons developed unexpected grief reactions, and a third developed a mild paranoid reaction. Though such reactions are rare, they are unfortunate. Walter saw that one might choose to risk such a reaction as a participant in a hypnosis workshop, or as a subject in a research study, but that there was no sense in taking such a risk when the only goal was "to have fun."

Absolute Contraindication: Hypnotherapy Considered Not the Most Effective Treatment

Bobby A.'s mother sought hypnotherapy for her 5-year-old son to help him overcome an extreme fear of dogs. He refused to play outdoors for fear of meeting a dog, and his little sister was now beginning to share his fear. In an initial interview, Bobby demonstrated little fear when talking about dogs and cheerfully joined the therapist in playing with toy dogs. Further discussion with the mother soon revealed that it was really she who had a moderate fear of dogs and that Bobby was basically doing what she expected him to do, although he did have a mild degree of fear. The therapist counseled with the mother, who achieved rapid fear reduction. As a further means of helping her family move from inappropriate fear to adaptive enjoyment of dogs, she agreed to buy a puppy. A week later, the dog joined with the therapist, the mother, and her two children in a playful visit on the lawn outside the therapist's office. Bobby and his little sister easily resolved their fear, and the boy proudly took charge of feeding his new pet.

Absolute Contraindication: Request for Hypnotherapy Based on Misdiagnosis

Tim, R., a 6-year-old, had trouble paying attention in school and failed to follow the teacher's instructions, although he had at least average intelligence. When his mother requested that Tim have hypnotherapy for his "behavior problem," the therapist insisted on taking a careful history. It turned out that Tim had had recurring middle-ear infections and that his failure to pay attention was chiefly related to a previously undetected hearing loss. When Tim was treated for his medical problem, his "behavior problem" disappeared.

Relative Contraindication: Immediate Medical or Surgical Treatment Takes Precedence over Hypnotherapy

Anne C., a 10-year-old, had a long history of complaints of vague abdominal pain associated with reluctance to go to school. One day, when the complaints became particularly severe, the mother requested hypnotherapy for Anne. The therapist insisted on a physical examination that resulted in a diagnosis of acute appendicitis and immediate surgery. Following Anne's recovery from surgery, the therapist reevaluated her, and she successfully used hypnotherapy to resolve a relatively mild school phobia.

The frequency of occurrence of such cases, in which the children referred for hypnotherapy were proved later to have biological bases for their symptoms, inspired a survey by Olness and Libbey (1987). Of the 200 children surveyed, 39 had unrecognized biological bases for their symptoms; within this overall group, 80 had been referred specifically for hypnotherapy, and 20 of these had previously unrecognized organic conditions that explained their symptoms. Within this group of 20 patients, the average duration of symptoms prior to diagnosis was 18 months. All had been seen by physicians within 1 year before their referral to the clinic. Eleven had been in psychotherapy for periods ranging from 3 to 30 months; of these, 2 had been hospitalized for 6 to 12 months in inpatient units.

Each child had a complete remission of the presenting symptoms with treatment of the underlying disease.

Although it is important to recognize the psychological or behavioral aspects of most illnesses (LeBaron & Zeltzer, 1985a; Leventhal, 1984; Starfield, 1982), it is also important to recognize a biological base for certain behavioral symptoms.

Relative Contraindication: Another Form of Psychotherapeutic Management Takes Precedence

Larry W., age 14 years, was hospitalized because of total body weakness and rapidly developing inability to walk. Finding no organic basis for the problem, the physician made a diagnosis of conversion reaction and requested hypnotherapy. In psychodiagnostic interviews, it became clear that Larry's symptoms served as defense against psychosis. After consulting with the physician, the therapist refused hypnotherapy for symptom relief and urged the parents to admit their son to an inpatient psychiatric program for intensive treatment. The parents denied that their son could have such a serious psychological problem, and they took him home. Follow-up about 1 year later revealed that the patient had indeed developed a frank psychosis. It is possible that, at some point in the course of intensive inpatient psychotherapy, hypnotherapy might have been a useful adjunct, but its use for abrupt symptom removal was clearly contraindicated.

Relative Contraindication: The Symptom Provides Significant Secondary Gain for the Child

C. J. Erickson (1991) described a teen-age girl who was able to use hypnosis quite well to control the pain of her sickle-cell disease. However, after several months, when she was hospitalized for crisis pain and the therapist came to see her, she would refuse hypnoanalgesia on the first day although she was in pain. The therapist would stay with her for half an hour, talking with her. On the second hospital day, she was willing to use her self-hypnosis skills. After several hospitalizations during which she demonstrated the same pattern, she was able to explain that everyone avoided her when she was in pain. Her therapist was the only person who was willing to be with her when she was in pain; therefore she rejected helping herself because the presence of a sympathetic human being was more important than pain reduction.

CONCLUSIONS

This brief review of general principles is intended to provide a framework in which to consider the disparate problems presented in succeeding chapters.

The following clinical material includes techniques that were utilized and why, what suggestions were given, and how the results were interpreted. We have done this in spite of the fact that there is little conclusive evidence bearing on the efficacy of any of the hypnotherapeutic programs. We take the position that as long as a given hypnotherapeutic endeavor has not been shown clearly to be ineffective there may be at least some features of it useful to child hypnotherapists and their patients. We maintain this position even when we are critical of the claims made for positive results, departing from it only when it appears obvious that the use of hypnotherapy had no relationship to the results obtained.

Given the scope and complexity of problems to be discussed, we have sometimes had to be arbitrary about including a particular problem in one chapter rather than another.

CHAPTER SEVEN

Hypnotherapy for Psychological Disorders

Hypnosis is not a therapy in itself. When it is combined with various forms of medical and psychological treatment, it becomes hypnotherapy. Some authors express this clarification by avoiding the term "hypnotherapy" and utilizing the phrase "hypnosis as a therapeutic adjunct," but these efforts often result in a return to semantic confusion with the use of such phrases as "the patient was treated with hypnosis" or "hypnosis produced no substitute symptoms." Therefore we maintain the distinction between "hypnosis" as an altered state of consciousness or awareness and "hypnotherapy" as a treatment modality in which the patient is in hypnosis at least part of the time. Our departure from this distinction is in our use of the term "self-hypnosis." Technically we refer to "self-hypnotherapy," but we will avoid that term since it is not yet in general use. Related to this is the emerging discipline of cyberphysiology, with emphasis on self-regulation via strategies such as self-hypnosis (see Chapter 15) or biofeedback (see Chapter 14).

In this chapter, our discussion of hypnotherapy refers to the use of hypnosis in the context of psychotherapy, omitting treatment of habit disorders and learning problems. There are fewer reports of child hypnotherapy for primary psychological problems than for medical and surgical problems. The difference may be related to the greater frequency of positive attitudes toward hypnotherapy expressed by pediatricians and pediatric nurses as compared with child psychologists and psychiatrists (Gardner, 1976a). Yet interest and acceptance of hypnosis in psychotherapy is growing as evidenced by Division 30 of the American Psychological Association, the hypnotherapy section. We hope that our review of this area will stimulate further use of psychological hypnotherapy by pointing out some of its advantages and applications. Cautions and contraindications have been discussed in Chapter 6 and are also reviewed well in a recent major text, *Handbook of Clinical Hypnosis* (Rhue, Lynn, & Kirsch, 1993).

ADVANTAGES OF
PSYCHOLOGICAL HYPNOTHERAPY

Williams (1979) commented on the essential value of psychological hypnotherapy: "Hypnosis can accelerate and augment the impact of psychotherapeutic intervention. . . . The increased therapeutic leverage afforded by hypnosis can often facilitate both the conversion of insight into action and the more rapid relief of disabling symptoms" (p. 108).

We believe that children in hypnotherapy are more able to accept the therapist's interpretations and to utilize their own capacities for achieving insight into conflicts and other dynamic issues. Increased readiness for insight follows from the combination of heightened ego receptivity and ego activity, intensified transference, and focused attention that characterize the hypnotic state. Moreover, the emphasis on mastery that underlies contemporary permissive hypnotherapy further enhances children's motivation to solve their problems, for they are taught that the solution truly belongs to them and not to anyone else (Fromm & Gardner, 1979).

The chief difference between hypnotherapy for children and for adults is that child therapists are less likely to use hypnotic techniques for the purpose of eliciting intense emotional abreactions (Williams, 1979). Specific hypnotherapeutic techniques vary with the age of the child, the nature of the problem, and the therapist's theoretical orientation. The techniques described below are not an exhaustive inventory, but rather a sample based on available clinical material.

In presenting clinical data, we are aware of the problem of diagnostic nomenclature, an area in which the very nature of child development makes for greater disagreement among child therapists than among those working with adults. Changing trends in the meaning and use of diagnostic labels further complicate the issue. In general, we have retained diagnostic labels contained in published reports or as they were used when we treated those patients described. In grouping cases, we have usually followed the guidelines of the American Psychiatric Association's (1994) *Diagnostic and Statistical Manual of Mental Disorders* (DSM-IV). During the past 5 years, a collaborative task force composed of pediatricians, psychologists, and psychiatrists has been developing a *Diagnostic and Statistical Manual for Primary Care* (DSM-PC) in conjunction with the American Academy of Pediatrics' Task Force on Coding for Mental Health Disorders in Children. The DSM-PC, to be published in 1996, is likely to become a practical standard for diagnosis by primary care providers.

RISKS OF PSYCHOLOGICAL HYPNOTHERAPY

With respect to subsequent discussion of behavior disorders, anxiety disorders, sleep disorders, or somatoform disorders, we strongly emphasize the importance of careful diagnostic procedures. In a retrospective review of 200 children referred to a behavioral pediatrics clinic, a subset of 80 patients had been referred specifically for hypnotherapy. Overall, 39 of the 200 children (19.5%) had unrecognized biological bases for their symptoms; within the subset, 20 (25%) had previously unrecognized organic conditions that explained their symptoms. Each of these children had a complete remission of presenting symptoms with treatment of the underlying disease. Examples included children with a presenting symptom of anxiety who proved to have hyperthyroidism or those with cyclic vomiting who had a genetic enzymatic defect. It is essential that child hypnotherapists keep in mind the possibility of such biological bases for presenting symptoms (Olness & Libbey, 1987).

BEHAVIOR DISORDERS

The problems in this group are manifested by children of all ages and are essentially characterized by impulsive and/or aggressive infringement on the basic rights of others or violation of major societal rules. Examples include delinquent behavior, rebellion at home or at school, poor self-control, and tantrum behavior. Hypnotherapy is rarely utilized early in the treatment of such problems. Psychotherapists often use behavior modification as a first approach, although insight therapy may also be employed.

Although hypnotherapy has often been a last resort in treating primary behavior disorders, reports describing its value tend to be positive provided both that the patient experiences distress and therefore is motivated to achieve change and that the parents are willing to cooperate in the treatment program. Younger children often respond better than older ones. By the time the behavior problem has crystallized into character pathology, manifested by ego syntonicity and minimal anxiety, then treatment by any method becomes exceedingly difficult if not impossible (Crasilneck & Hall, 1985; Mellor, 1960; Solovey de Milechnin, 1955).

Much recent research has elucidated the neurochemistry and neurophysiology of neurotransmitters and how they are involved in the regulation of major behavioral systems. For example, norepinephrine, dopamine, and serotonin are significant in the regulation of an individual's behavior with the external environment (Rogeness, Javors, & Pliszka, 1992). A behavioral facilitatory system (BFS) and a behavioral inhibitory system (BIS) have been described (Gray, 1987). The BFS, controlled by the mesolimbic dopaminergic system, is activated primarily by environmental stimuli that are appealing such as a plate of cookies on the table, and it is unrestrained by internal systems. The BIS, controlled by the septohippocampal system, can inhibit the BFS. Children with a strong BFS relative to the BIS would internalize poorly and be much more dependent on environmental controls (such as a parent in the vicinity), have less insight into reasons for punishment, and be more likely to blame others for their behavior. Several behavioral disorders of children may be secondary to dysregulation of neurotransmitter systems that impact the BFS or BIS. Kagan (1994) has noted that children with behavioral inhibition had increased urinary norepinephrine and increased heart rate. He has also noted a striking persistence of personality types in following children from 2 to 13 years. Although the intrinsic personality types and behavior were modified somewhat by parenting styles, Kagan also noted evidence that differences in behavior and physiology reflect differences in thresholds of responsiveness in the limbic system. We also know that the limbic system is a mediator of short-term memory, that is, mental images to be stored, and connects many different systems involved in perceiving threats and responding to stress. One can speculate also that deliberate changes in mental images, as occurs in hypnosis, may be mediated in the limbic system. Behavioral inhibition in children has been associated with major depression and panic disorders. Children with conduct disorders have been found to have decreased noradrenergic activity and decreased serotonergic function. Although there is much research in progress to develop medications to normalize these neurotransmitters, we speculate that, with increased precision in understanding the neurotransmitter abnormalities' relationship to chronobiological or nutritional or activity factors, it may be possible to combine hypnotherapy with biofeedback of relevant physiological responses for more predictable treatment of conduct disorders.

Assessment of Learning Styles

It is important that the hypnotherapist consider the possibility of learning disabilities as contributing to the presenting symptom and to modify therapeutic approaches accordingly. A study by Gualtieri, Koriath, Van Bourgondien, and Saleeby (1983) reported a survey of 40 consecutive admissions to a child psychiatry inpatient service, in which at least half of the patients had moderate to severe language disorders. Routine intelligence testing did not discern most of the disorders. This was especially true in the areas of auditory analysis, memory, or integration, rather than in the more general test areas covering expressive or receptive language. Children with the former types of disorders demonstrated peculiar responses to instructions, compensatory talkativeness, and tantrums. They often did not understand or respond to verbal instructions. Awareness of their limitations led therapists to simplify language and use pictorial charts, drawings, and other nonverbal approaches. There were marked improvements in the progress of these children when therapy was adapted to their language disorders. Studies also note that learning disabilities are more apt to be missed in high-IQ children (Faigel, 1983). Although learning deficits are obvious with respect to some conditions such as pervasive developmental disorders, they may not be obvious in bright children who present with a variety of behavioral problems. Grynkewich (1994) has documented that mental imagery strategies, including hypnotherapy, may be adapted to improved school performance in children with significant learning disabilities.

Behavior Disorders in Young Children

Behavior problems in preadolescent children are sometimes described as tension discharge disorders, commonly a reaction against inconsistent parenting, family strife, or inability to adjust at school. Genetic or physical problems such as the fragile X syndrome can lead to disruptive behavior. Very often the behavior disorder represents an immature and maladaptive defense against anxiety and low self-esteem. The therapeutic task is to provide a context in which the child can cope more adaptively. Hypnotic relaxation and the intensity of the transference to a benign therapist may provide such a context when other methods fail, or even provide a primary therapeutic modality.

Williams and Singh (1976) reported briefly on the case of a 10-year-old boy who presented a 3-year history of temper tantrums. He had not responded to previous therapeutic efforts including medication, psychotherapy, and behavior modification. After three sessions of weekly hypnotherapy, there was marked abatement of temper tantrums. Specific hypnotherapeutic techniques with this child were not described. Over the next 19 months, he maintained his gains in individual and family therapy, together with medication and special class placement. He also used self-hypnosis successfully at times of stress. We can assume that the parents willingly involved themselves in the treatment and that negative reactions to the tantrums from peers and family enhanced the child's motivation. This case is an example of the way in which hypnotherapy seems to provide the added impetus necessary for change to occur.

Two single case reports (M. H. Erickson, 1962; Lazar & Jedliczka, 1979) describe hypnotherapeutic treatment without any formal hypnotic induction, emphasizing utilization techniques, especially "prescribing the symptom." Both cases concerned "uncontrollable" children who in fact did control their environments, albeit maladaptively, and who then learned ways of more adaptive control.

M. H. Erickson's (1962) patient was an 8-year-old boy who became progressively defiant and destructive following his mother's divorce. Her disciplinary efforts served mainly to further the power struggle in which the child invariably proved himself the stronger. At the same time, he unconsciously communicated his need to know that he was not all-powerful and that there was a secure reality in which he could thrive. Erickson worked

first with the mother, using double-bind techniques to enlist her cooperation to prove absolutely to her son that she was more powerful than he. Several months later, when the symptoms recurred, Erickson worked directly with
the boy, establishing his own authority by challenging the child to live up
to his boast that he could stomp the floor or stand still for extremely long
periods. This maneuver shifted the child's focus of attention so as to permit
him to benefit from reality confrontation, with resultant positive behavior
change. Follow-up after 2 years indicated that the gains were maintained.

Lazar and Jedliczka (1979) described a single session of hypnotherapy
with a moderately mentally retarded boy with cerebral palsy whose behavior
problems included ignoring his mother, making himself late for school, using unacceptable language, and deliberately waking his parents by coughing
at night. The child and his mother agreed that he was "a cripple." As a result,
she never disciplined him, and he used disruptive behavior as a means of
gaining some sense of control and probably also as a way of asking for appropriate external control.

The therapist used several techniques, including prescribing the symptom, confusion, and double bind, in order to help the boy alter his perception of the value of his behavior. For example, she asked him to spend a
certain time each day saying bad words, and she asked him to choose which
nights he would cough. In this way, she neutralized the pleasure of the bad
language and subtly suggested that the patient would also choose nights when
he would not cough. Similarly, she devalued his misbehavior in her office,
either by ignoring it or by asking him to increase it until he stopped from
fatigue and boredom. At the same time, she gave the mother very specific
suggestions as to how to demonstrate parental control to the boy. Both mother
and therapist deemphasized the identification of the boy as handicapped and
focused instead on the fact that he could experience mastery in his own development and enjoy more positive experiences with others. The child's behavior problems virtually disappeared in one week, and follow-up 20 months
later revealed no recurrence.

Though some might argue that neither of these cases really involved the
use of hypnotherapy, we consider them both examples of the breadth of hypnotherapeutic approaches to which children can respond, especially since hypnosis can occur without any formal induction.

The following case is an example of our work with young children who
have behavior disorders. Ray, a 10-year-old adopted boy, was seen for hypnotherapy regarding frequent temper outbursts that occurred both at home and
at school. These were triggered by seemingly minor frustrations, for example, being unable to accomplish a task, being denied a privilege, being asked
to go to bed (at normal bedtime). His mother perceived him as being easily
frustrated and having a short attention span, although he did well academically in school. The patient had been adopted in infancy. When he was 4½

years old, his parents adopted two biological sisters, ages 3 and 6 years. The patient had subsequently manifested frequent jealousy of his adopted sisters. He had been examined by his pediatrician and a neurologist and had been receiving psychotherapy for several months without noticeable improvement.

At the time of the first visit for hypnotherapy, Ray appeared angry and embarrassed. The therapist first demonstrated peripheral temperature biofeedback and gave him the opportunity to raise his fingertip temperature which he did successfully on the first attempt. The therapist explained that he had accomplished this because of his own control, just as he had developed controls in many performance areas such as body control when he performed on athletic teams. He was then taught a simple breathing relaxation hypnotic induction and was asked to practice this daily. He was also asked to organize practice sessions for the entire family during which they would review relaxation exercises from *The Centering Book* (Hendricks & Wills, 1975).

Because of illness in the patient, the second visit did not occur for 3 weeks. However, telephone follow-up revealed that Ray seemed much more confident and happy, reported that the family was practicing self-hypnosis at home. He said he had had no tantrums in school and only a few at home. During the second visit, after induction of hypnosis, he was taught a jettison technique for ridding himself of things that bothered him, a method to replace the tantrums.

In the third visit, the parents reported a marked reduction in Ray's tantrums. The session was audiotaped, and Ray took the tape home for review three times weekly. Telephone follow-up 1 month later confirmed that he "has pretty much quit temper tantrums." The mother said that, other than fidgeting in church services, he was doing well and feeling much better about himself.

In the case of young children with behavior disorders, some therapists prefer to work primarily with the parents. Petty (1976) used this approach with the mothers of two children, a 4-year-old girl and a 5-year-old boy, both with severe tantrum behavior. Both mothers were initially instructed to ignore the tantrums but simply could not do so. Petty then utilized hypnotic relaxation and desensitization techniques. The mothers developed hypnotic images of past tantrums without feeling anxious or disturbed, then repeated the procedure with an imaginary future tantrum. In the first case, the tantrums abated after 3 months; improvement continued during the following year. In the second case, follow-up after 1 month also revealed marked decrease in tantrum behavior. Petty concluded that, as a result of the mothers' changed attitudes and responses, the children's tantrums lost their reinforcing value and extinguished. It is important that therapists be aware that tantrum behavior beyond the first few years may reflect brain damage with problems in self-modulation. Older children who have prolonged tantrums

that do not respond to a brief period of intervention may need further diagnostic evaluation.

Behavior Disorders in Adolescents

Kaffman (1968) described a 14-year-old boy on a kibbutz who displayed a
4-year history of poor self-control and marked antisocial behavior, including lying, stealing, property damage, and physical attacks on other children.
Both the referring therapist and the boy's teacher had recommended residential
treatment. Although the boy had refused to cooperate with earlier psychotherapy lasting 2 years, he now quickly accepted the suggestion of a 10-session
trial of hypnotherapy, with the knowledge that the decision for residential
treatment would be temporarily postponed. According to Kaffman, "hypnotic suggestions included the strengthening of his will to be and behave like
other children, emphasis on his own responsibility and capacity to achieve
this aim in the area of school, work, and social interaction, together with
increased motivation to cooperate in treatment" (p. 733). From that day forward, the boy's behavior problems ceased. He completed the 10 hypnotic
sessions, and continued in psychotherapy every 2 to 4 weeks. At the end of
2½ years, he had maintained his gains, described by the author as "remark-
able." Although the behavior change indeed may have resulted from the introduction of hypnotherapy, we wonder about the effect of the serious threat
of residential treatment. This is a case in which a 5- to 10-year follow-up
would be helpful to determine whether the boy really wanted to change his
behavior or merely wanted to avoid the "punishment" of residential treatment. In the latter instance, we might expect eventual return of antisocial
behavior. On the other hand, the hypnotherapy may have given him confidence that he could change his behavior.

The question of patient motivation arises for similar reasons in Mellor's (1960) series of 14 cases of juvenile delinquents, all of whom had been
in a juvenile hall. Their acceptance of hypnotherapy was part of the requirement for probation. The patients, ages 13 to 17 years, included 2 girls and
12 boys. The average total treatment lasted 6 hours, with successful results
in 13 of 14 cases. Follow-up ranged from 7 to 17 months, with 4-year follow-
up in 1 case. The one treatment failure was a narcotics addict who showed
no motivation for behavior change after five sessions.

Mellor's technique consisted of using ideomotor finger signaling to help
the patients get at underlying emotional tensions and to elicit confidence that
they could acquire more appropriate behavior patterns. Mellor believed that
this technique facilitated regression, recall, and reorientation of thoughts and
feelings. Since the patients were maintained in a light to medium trance, they
experienced rapid integration and soon developed insight and took respon-

sibility for overcoming their problems. They moved from the ego passivity that often accompanies impulsive behavior to ego activity and true self-control. These results are certainly impressive and the relatively short-term follow-up encouraging. But, given the adolescents' histories, one would need a 5- to 10-year follow-up in order to be able to judge more clearly the value of the treatment. As with Kaffman's (1968) patient, we have to wonder whether the motivation for treatment was based chiefly on desire for change or on a wish to avoid the punishment of incarceration. Also, the concept that a therapist can judge depth of trance or "maintain" a certain depth, is in question. Based on developmental issues raised at the beginning of this section, we are more confident of the validity of the positive reports of young children with behavior disorders than of those concerning adolescents.

ANXIETY DISORDERS

This category includes children consciously aware of and distressed by excessive anxiety, as manifested by phobic reactions, post-traumatic stress disorders, sleep disorders, or social anxiety (Kellerman, 1981).

Phobic Reactions

In general, the longer a child has had a phobia, the more difficult it is to resolve. Parents and other well-meaning adults often insist that a child will soon "outgrow" his or her fears; sometimes this is true. Often, however, the child develops a series of avoidance strategies so as not to have to confront the feared situation. Parents may reinforce and even encourage such avoidance behavior, thereby unwittingly communicating to the child that the fear is valid and depriving the child of opportunities for corrective experiences and mastery. As the avoidance strategies become more complex, with increasing involvement of parents and siblings, the problem may evolve into a "folie à famille." Given the ease of resolving recently developed phobias, early intervention makes much more sense than the approach of hoping the child will outgrow them (Gardner, 1978b).

In the hypnotherapeutic treatment of phobias, our most common approach is based on desensitization, similar to the method used in behavior modification (Schowalter, 1994). In a state of hypnotic relaxation, the children develop images in which they experience safety and mastery. Then they develop a series of images related to the feared event, maintaining the feeling of mastery as they visualize each image. The therapist then gives post-hypnotic suggestions that they can increasingly experience the same feelings of mastery in related reality situations. Sometimes the hypnotherapy sessions include in vivo desensitization such as when there is a needle phobia. Research has suggested that these active participation techniques are as good as the use of imagery alone and may, in some instances, be more effective (Hatzenbuehler & Schroeder, 1978). Symptom substitution is rare.

Ambrose (1968) described another method (a jettison technique) for helping children cope effectively with anxiety. In a hypnotic state, the child is asked to make a fist and then "is told that he has all his fears and problems clasped in his fist. On the count of three he will open his fist and all his anxieties will disappear into thin air and he will feel happy, confident, etc." (p. 3). As in the desensitization method, the emphasis here is on mastery. Ambrose further stated that, especially in the case of deep-seated phobias, dynamically oriented therapy—with or without hypnosis—is necessary for lasting results. We have a notion that analytic work may be necessary more often with Ambrose's brief, almost magical, method than with the desensitization techniques in which the child can easily see the connection between therapeutic method and problem resolution. However, there are no data comparing the relative efficacy of the two methods.

School Phobia

As in all therapeutic approaches to school phobia, the hypnotherapist must first explore and understand the underlying dynamics, a task often accomplished quite rapidly. Although the problem is usually connected to anxiety about leaving parents rather than fear of school, there may be other precipitating factors (Schowalter, 1994). Crasilneck and Hall (1985) described a 7-year-old boy whose mother had impressed on him that he should "do what he was told" in school. When older children on the school playground threatened to pull his pants down, his fantasized participation, and its attendant anxiety led to refusal to go to school. In another case, a young child's "fear of school" turned out really to be fear of the school station wagon that reminded him of an ambulance and associated fear of sickness. In both cases, assurance and clarification in both the usual state of awareness and in hypnosis produced rapid symptom relief and return to school. Crasilneck and Hall further noted the importance of parent counseling in such cases in order to avoid parental behavior that either reinforces the fear by excessive comfort or is overly critical.

Lawlor (1976) described three cases of school phobia, two of which included hypnotherapeutic intervention as well as parent counseling and environmental manipulation. In both cases—a 5-year-old boy and a 4-year-old girl—the purpose of hypnotherapy was to interview the child in a relaxed state in order to gain information about the dynamics of the problem. The first child readily verbalized feelings of hostility and destructive wishes toward parents and siblings, with concurrent fears of abandonment. After reassurance from the therapist and the mother, the boy soon made a satisfactory school adjustment. In the second case, the situation was more complicated, including the mother's suicide shortly before the onset of phobic symptoms. Hypnotic interview revealed that the child blamed herself for her mother's death, feared her own death, and hoped to reunite with mother by staying home. She was placed with an aunt and uncle. The security of her new home combined with therapeutic reassurance to facilitate a good adjustment in her new school.

In both these cases, it is not clear whether the clarification of dynamics and therapeutic reassurance might have been equally successful without hypnotherapy. There were no previous attempts at psychotherapeutic intervention. In our own practices, we find rapid success with young school-phobic children using play therapy, non-hypnotic interviews, and parent counseling. It is probably reasonable to conclude that hypnotherapy is at least as useful as more traditional methods of treating school phobia in young children.

We have few data concerning hypnotherapy with older school-phobic children, a group usually much more refractory to treatment.

Needle Phobia

Needle phobia is common among both adults and children. In children the fear of being poked or stuck with a needle produces violent reactions such as tantrums, vomiting, struggling enough to require restraint for the injection, and physical assaults on the person doing the procedure. Since the injections usually cannot be postponed, requests for help from colleagues are often urgent, and sometimes circumstances demand we must work as rapidly as possible. Approaches depend on the age of the patients, their developmental stage, past behaviors during injections, and the therapist's creativity. We believe that the development of severe needle phobia can be avoided by anticipatory training in the outpatient clinic, the dentist's office, or on the hospital ward.

We reported treatment of a 7-year-old boy who required repeated intravenous infusions of plasma in the treatment of Bruton's agammaglobulinemia (Olness & Gardner, 1978). He responded with hysterical outbursts and had to be restrained by six people. The treatment was as follows:

> It was explained to the patient that his unique imaginative ability, better than that of many adults, could help him learn a method to "turn off his pain switches." When he learned the method, he could then turn off these switches prior to his injections and it would no longer be necessary

for him to feel uncomfortable or upset. The patient was taught a standard method of relaxation, visual imagery exercises, and the switch-off technique. During the first visit he demonstrated immediate ability to tolerate pin pricks in his self-anesthetized hands and arms. Subsequently, he joined a group of boys with hemophilia who met regularly for review sessions. The next visit for gammaglobulin, which occurred three weeks after his initial visit to our hospital, was calm. He proudly hypnotically turned off his switches and held out his arm for the injection. He has been followed for one year with no further difficulties, and one nurse now starts the intravenous infusion. (pp. 230–231)

Another patient was a husky, 17-year-old adolescent boy, with a needle phobia of many years duration, who was being treated for meningitis with a 6-week course of continuous intravenous (IV) antibiotics. Each time the IV had to be restarted, he became hysterical and had to be restrained by several people. When offered hypnotherapy to overcome his phobic response, he responded enthusiastically. The treatment consisted of asking the patient to focus on pleasant mental imagery and following with in vivo desensitization, beginning with a small tuberculin needle in his forearm, then increasing the size of the needle, and later injecting him with normal saline. Instead of suggesting anesthesia, the patient was told in hypnosis to recall feelings of comfort in his arm and to fill his arm completely with comfort until there was simply no room for any other feeling. He rapidly developed a strong transference to the therapist and began to share her confidence that he could conquer his phobia. His enjoyment of adolescent bravado further contributed to his motivation for success. After three hypnotherapy sessions, he tolerated restarting of his IV without requiring restraint. A few days later, with the therapist present, he tolerated a lumbar puncture with only moderate anxiety. By the end of his hospital stay, his anxiety was minimal and his cooperation excellent. He called the therapist some months later to report that he had had no difficulty when he required a tetanus shot after a minor injury.

Other methodologies include hypnoanesthesia such as revivification of a recalled local anesthetic numbness (such as a prior dental anesthesia or anesthetic for suturing) or metaphors to facilitate dissociation. A representative case history, involving hypnoanesthesia for needle phobia, follows.

Marty was 14 years old when he was referred by his pediatric endocrinologist for hypnotherapy for needle phobia associated with the need for daily growth hormone injections. Marty had long been afraid of needles but had managed to cope with intermittent blood tests or immunizations. The idea that he could self-administer injectable growth hormone seemed impossible not only to Marty but, perhaps more significantly, to his mother. When the idea that he might someday do his own injections was presented, his doctor, nurse, and mother all agreed with him that he couldn't (but really wouldn't) be expected to do this "to himself" from the start. The missed opportunity to shift his expectation, belief, and behavior from the beginning served to perpetuate his phobic response to needles.

His mother administered the injections. With each subsequent injection, his behavioral-avoidant, phobic response was more pronounced. This usually took the form of delaying tactics, the demand that everything be "just so" before beginning, and increasing anxiety, for instance, "Wait, wait, not yet, not yet. . . . I'll tell you when . . . not yet," resulting in 60- to 90-minute ordeals at home for what should have taken less than 5 minutes. Increasingly, individual injection times were complicated by the mother's growing frustration expressed as complaints and denigrations of Marty; for example, "You're taking up too much of my time," or "You're acting like a baby." She also used threats such as "I'm not going to give them, and then you won't grow." Physicians counselled the mother to stop giving the injections in order to empower Marty to do so. For almost 6 months her fear that he would not grow if she didn't personally give the injections ("He'll never do it; I know he won't; he's too afraid") served as a major barrier to Marty's slowly developing skill and confidence that he could give himself the injections.

A timid and relatively socially isolated young adolescent, Marty lacked self-confidence in most areas of his life. His favorite activities, watching movies alone all day in the theater or at home, were also isolating. During his first visits to learn hypnotherapy skills, rapport was established slowly, and hypnosis was presented in a naturalistic, Ericksonian fashion: "This is not magic, I wish it was . . . but you might be surprised to discover when you're ready that it might *seem* like magic, because I'm sure that when you're ready you'll be really surprised how effective it will be . . . you'll probably really surprise youself the most of all, don't you think?"

Marty was taught hypnosis with favorite place imagery of being at the movies or of riding his bike. Hypnotic suggestions emphasized themes of competence and autonomy for ego-strengthening, as well as the importance of practicing self-hypnosis "just to get good at feeling relaxed and comfortable whenever you need to do so. And the more you do it, the better you'll get." After several practice sessions, therapeutic suggestions were offered in menu format, again with the focus being to facilitate personal choice and a sense of control and empowerment by letting Marty choose the (hypnotic) method by which he would indeed solve the dilemma of being able to give himself an injection. Ericksonian "double-bind" types of suggestions were given often; for example, "I don't know exactly how you're going to give the injection each time, whether it will be by letting your jaw be numb like it was at the dentist and then transferring that numb feeling with your mind and your hand down to the leg that will get the injection, *or* whether you'll just imagine that your leg isn't even there — although it is — and not notice it, or whether you'll just do it some other way." After about 6 months Marty came for an appointment. In the waiting room his mother smiled broadly and said, "You won't believe it, he'll tell you about it. . . . " She was consciously unaware of the potential negative impact and power of her own words and tone, and of the confusing nature of her obvious pride mixed with her own struggle to allow her son to grow up, figuratively and literally.

Marty reported with awkward embarrassment and pride that he had given his own injection the night before and that "it took about 20 minutes, but I finally did it . . . and I could feel it, but it wasn't as bad as I thought it would be. . . . " Beyond purposely exuberant congratulations, we reviewed and reinforced success in and out of hypnosis by focusing on "How did you do it?" Marty proceeded to administer his own daily injections for the next 4 to 5 months without much difficulty or tension. The benefit to his maturation and self-esteem seemed to be dramatic.

Then he relapsed for no apparent reason. His mother quickly became reinvolved in preparing and administering his growth hormone, and, thereafter, he never gave himself another injection. To her credit the mother was able to set specific limits. She and Marty agreed that she would give his injections only if he would not argue, fight, complain, or use delaying tactics. This accomodation was said to be mutually acceptable and continued until he discontinued the growth hormone at the end of his senior high school year.

Of note, and undoubtedly complicating this case of needle phobia, was the emergence in Marty of a full-blown panic disorder. After no contact for more than a year, Marty called the therapist because of anticipatory test anxiety that became manifest during examinations in his senior year. "Too anxious" to use his self-hypnosis, he requested and benefited from anxiolytic medication, which also allowed him to access his self-relaxation skills more easily. He had three clinic visits to develop comfort with these symptoms. Most recently, his continued struggle with autonomy was reflected in the desire to drive himself to college rather than to be "stressed" by his family taking him several hundreds of miles and then leaving him. Although this initial separation seemed to work, he soon became unhappy with his first college roommate, suffered great sadness at the long separation from his girlfriend and dramatically quit college, returning home to live with his parents. At his most recent visit, he acknowledged his continuing anxiety and noted that he still turns to self-hypnosis to help himself relax, "sometimes."

Animal Phobia

Crasilneck and Hall (1985) reported a case of animal phobia in which hypnotherapy was used both to understand the dynamics and to help the child master the problem.

A grade-school girl was brought to treatment because of a persistent fear of cats and other furry animals, for which no conscious explanation could be found in her past experiences. In hypnosis, using an age-regression technique, we found that the fear had begun at a time when she had been in the outhouse privy on the farm where she was living as a child. She had been masturbating, feeling mixed excitement and guilt, when the door began to slowly open. Frightened and fearing discovery, she had run from the outhouse, only to trip over the family cat that had apparently pushed the door open. She was bruised in the fall, skinning her knees, and had gone crying to the house, ashamed to tell what had happened. At first her aversion had been to cats, though later it had generalized to other animals. As time passed, she remembered only the fear of animals, seeming to have forgotten the incident at onset.

While in hypnosis after the original traumatic situation had been uncovered, she was asked to imagine that she was the only spectator in a darkened theater. A red light came on, a buzzer sounded, and she saw a large red curtain rise, revealing a stage. It was suggested that on the stage she would see the original situation, the outhouse, herself, the cat. She was told, "Now you will see what really went on, and you will compare and contrast it to what you remember." From the point of view of her present, older ego, she watched the childhood scene unfold with a detached, more objective eye. After hypnosis was terminated, the events were discussed with her in the waking state, emphasis being placed on the way that her guilt and fear at the forbidden masturbation had been transferred to the cat, then to other similar animals. Her "phobic" symptoms rapidly improved. (pp. 182–183)*

Post-Traumatic Stress Disorders

Children, as adults, suffer complications of trauma, and these often extend for a lifetime. When one considers the number of children in the world who experience early loss of parents, first-hand experience with the terror of war, dislocation from homes into refugee camps, earthquakes, tornadoes, mental and/or physical assaults, it is clear that the residual post-traumatic stress disorder (PTSD) varies in severity depending on many factors. These may include presence of a parent or another trusted adult, coping abilities of the family, early opportunities to express their perceptions and feelings about the event, whether the event was isolated or repetitive, and whether or not there was much associated deprivation of daily needs. Hypnotherapeutic interventions have been described increasingly as helpful for both adults and children who have suffered PTSD.

---

*From Crasilneck and Hall (1985). Copyright 1985 by Allyn & Bacon. With permission.

Friedrich (1991) described case histories of four children with PTSD. He speculated that a trance-like phenomenon occurred at the time of the trauma. A second trance, in the form of hypnotherapy, was extremely helpful in integrating the trauma so that optimal, pre-trauma functioning could be obtained. Rhue and Lynn (1991) described storytelling and hypnosis in the treatment of sexually abused children. They emphasized provision of a mental safe place as well as images of personal power and control via hypnotherapy.

Crasilneck and Hall (1985) described their work with an adolescent girl suffering psychogenic amnesia (in today's nomenclature, this would be understood as part of PTSD) after a severe trauma.

> A 17-year-old girl, angry after an argument with her mother and stepfather, had walked away from her home at night, intending to walk to the house of an aunt some miles away. While crossing a long bridge, she was offered a ride by an older man whom she did not know. The man drove to a secluded area, where he repeatedly raped her. Hours after leaving home she was found by a policeman wandering aimlessly in a deserted area. Brought to the emergency room, she denied any memory after the man had picked her up. She was vague and obviously disturbed.
>
> Following an arm-levitation induction, the patient entered a state of somnambulism. She was told the following: "Recall of feeling and emotions often helps us get well even if such events are frightening. Your recent experience was so frightening that you have forgotten many facts about yourself, but under a state of hypnosis, you can recall . . . everything that you have forgotten . . . every fact . . . every emotion . . . every detail . . . and so you are going to go back in terms of time and space . . . back in terms of space and time to that experience that caused you to lose your memory . . . you are going back to the exact time and you can recall, relive . . . revive . . . feel . . . and experience everything that happened."
>
> As the patient began to talk, cry, and abreact the traumatic scene that led to her amnesia, her memory abruptly returned and she dramatically abreacted the rape scene, struggling frantically against an imagined attacker and crying out in fear and pain. As the reenactment subsided, she regained her composure, had an intact memory for the entire event, and was reunited with her family.
>
> She was followed in the psychiatric clinic afterward and given an opportunity to understand not only her repressed feelings about the assault, but also the difficulties with her family that had led to the situation. (pp. 234–235)*

In our hypnotherapeutic work with amnesic patients, we give an additional permissive suggestion for reinstatement of the amnesia: "When you come out of hypnosis, you can remember as much as you are now ready to

*From Crasilneck and Hall (1985). Copyright 1985 by Allyn & Bacon. With permission.

cope with, now ready to face. Whatever you need to forget, you will be able to forget until a later time when you are ready to deal with it." This wording does not authoritatively impose reinstatement of amnesia, a maneuver that we think often has more to do with the narcissism or anxiety of the therapist than with the needs of the patient. Instead, it communicates respect for the patient's defenses and ego strengthening by also implying that the patient may—either now or in the future—be strong enough to face and integrate the traumatic material.

Sometimes a child has good recall of a traumatic event and wants to talk about it, but he or she is unwilling to do so for any of several reasons. Here again, the combination of hypnotic relaxation and heightened positive transference often provides a setting in which the child feels free enough to communicate.

In forensic cases it is sometimes suggested that hypnosis be used to assist children in recalling details of crimes in which they were victims and witnesses. Although hypnotic interrogation is sometimes valuable in criminal investigation, the process is fraught with pitfalls that sometimes lead to serious miscarriages of justice. Both the *International Journal of Clinical and Experimental Hypnosis* (Frankel & Perry, 1994; Orne, 1990) and the *American Journal of Clinical Hypnosis* (Mott, 1990; Mutter, 1994) have published monographs on the important subjects of the uses and misuses of forensic hypnosis and the relationship of hypnosis to memory. Hypnotherapists working with children must realize that techniques suitable for helping a child recall and master an emotional trauma differ in significant ways from appropriate techniques for working with the same child in the context of criminal investigation. The most competent child hypnotherapist should obtain additional special training before engaging in forensic hypnosis. We recommend that he or she take care to understand state laws regarding forensic hypnosis. We also recommend that he or she refuse to assist in obtaining evidence from children unless there is prior agreement that the information revealed will be used to guide investigators in their search for evidence but that neither the child nor therapist will be called to testify. It is also essential that there be a neutral observer present when he or she is doing hypnotherapy with the child.

Sleep Disorders

Fear of Going to Sleep

L. Jacobs (1962, 1964) described three children, ages 6, 8, and 9 years, who suffered anxiety with going to sleep. He emphasized the importance of understanding the dynamics that, in these cases, included equating sleep with death, associating sleep with anesthesia and post-operative pain, and psychic trauma resulting in generalized feelings of insecurity. Jacobs directed his treatment to the underlying anxiety, reminding the children in hypnosis of their parents' love for them and assuring them that they could feel increasingly safe and confident. In all three cases, normal sleep patterns returned within several weeks.

Our experience with many such cases of so-called sleep onset anxiety/insomnia confirm Jacobs's report that these usually do not represent a sleep disorder but, rather, are a manifestation of anxiety expressed at bedtime. Most often the child's fears have not previously been expressed except through the symptom of insomnia. Accordingly, attention to rapport and elucidation of unexpressed worries with or without hypnosis will allow the clinician to then utilize any of a variety of hypnotic strategies to promote an easy and comfortable transition to sleep.

Although most such sleep-onset anxiety cases are simple and straightforward, some are quite complex but potentially amenable to relatively easy symptom management. A representative case history follows.

Kohen (1995a) described an 11-year-old boy who was referred with a discrete 3-month history of what his family called "panic attacks" that both occurred before he went to sleep at night, causing him to take two hours before falling asleep, and also awakened him during the night for 1 to 2 hours. He described feelings of great fear both at the time of the episodes and when he worried that the events would happen again during the night or on the following night. He reported that the first episode occurred the night after the first day of school. They had occurred nightly since then.

History taking also revealed that the family had moved recently from their home of many years and that the patient missed his friends. Furthermore, the father was back in the home part-time while remaining in a day-treatment, sexual-offender program for the molestation of the patient's sister who had been removed from the home, and that he "missed his maternal grandmother who had died 3 years earlier." He had never spoken about these events before and did so in a detached, spontaneously hypnotic fashion. In response, the therapist spoke to him in hypnotic fashion, offering positive, ego strengthening and reframing, reassuring suggestions in the absence of any formal hypnotic induction. The patient was told that the therapist was certain he could be of help and that he was quite confident that the boy would soon find it easy to go to sleep. In what may have been a pivotal and valued hypnotic suggestion, the therapist ended the first visit by assuring the boy that his mother had a picture of the grandmother that she could give to the patient as his very own and that he would keep with him at bedtime. He agreed to do so.

To investigate the possibility of partial complex seizures, an electroencephalogram (EEG) was obtained the following day and was normal. Six days later, the patient returned and reported happily that he had not had any trouble going to sleep and, for the first time in 3 months, he had not experienced any "panic attacks." He and his mother nonetheless requested medication, and a prescription for a low dose of imipramine (a medication of choice for panic attacks) was given. He returned a week later having remained free of panic attacks or sleep difficulties. The prescription had not been filled because of insurance problems. The boy spoke openly of sadness about his grandmother's death, anger with his father, and missing his friends from his hometown. At the fourth visit, he remained free of further panic attacks.

Although no formal hypnotic induction was conducted in this case, elements of hypnotic behavior and hypnotic suggestion seem to be clearly operative in beginning therapy with this youngster. Early in the clinical relationship, his diagnoses certainly included sleep-onset anxiety/panic attacks. Separation anxiety regarding the family move, prolonged grief, and bereavement regarding the death of his grandmother, and perhaps PTSD of delayed onset, regarding the sexual abuse in the family may each have contributed to his symptoms.

Nightmares

Although all children occasionally have nightmares, some children have them so frequently that they become truly disruptive, making the child afraid to go to sleep and causing the parents to be aroused at night. In contrast to night terrors (sleep terror disorder), the child usually is able to recall some details of the nightmare. If there is a known precipitating event, the child can be encouraged to recall that event in hypnosis and then be reminded that he or she is now older or safer or in some way able to deal with the problem. Whether or not there is a known precipitant, the child can be asked to experience hypnotic safety and then to redream the nightmare in hypnosis, but this time changing the ending so as to emerge the master rather than the victim of the situation. The child is then told that it is possible to do the same thing when actually sleeping, if the nightmare should recur. Children enjoy this challenge, and their nightmares usually cease after one or two sessions of hypnotherapy (Gardner, 1978b).

King, Cranstoun, and Josephs (1989) described three children (ages 6, 8, and 11 years) with whom "emotive imagery" was utilized to allay anxiety associated with nighttime fears and nightmares. In addition to self-monitoring and behavioral assessment of "darkness toleration," each child was presented with therapeutic imagery suggestions based on favorite fantasies and interests. Although the authors do not identify this work as hypnotherapeutic, a perusal of their "scripts" clearly reflects elements of positive imagery, post-hypnotic suggestions, future-oriented suggestions, and ego-strengthening suggestions for safety and comfort; for example, "What a brave boy you are, you slept in your bed by yourself all night." Two of the three children showed fewer behavioral disturbances over the intervention period. In their multiple-baseline design study, the authors concluded that a combination of treatment procedures be utilized to help children with these problems including the emotive imagery, hypnotherapeutic-like strategies, along with systematic desensitization, relaxation, and parent counseling.

Parent counseling is a reasonable and appropriate concomitant to hypnotherapeutic strategies with children. This is important for some parents who, in their efforts to help their child, have been unwittingly reinforcing a behavior. For example, some well-intentioned parents may overdo the recommendations for a comforting nighttime ritual by developing a series of measures such as a snack, a back rub, a story and/or favorite song, getting up to watch television, and/or sleeping in bed with the parents (or vice-versa). With such rewards the only surprise would be the child whose nightmares didn't continue!

Parents can be reassured that attention to underlying anxiety and the teaching of simple self-hypnotic exercises are often and usually quickly successful in eliminating the troublesome behavior. For preschool children, it may be helpful to ask parents to facilitate the hypnotic strategy through the technique of favorite stories or other strategies outlined earlier (Chapter 5).

Night Terrors–Sleep Terror Disorder

Partial arousals from sleep include nocturnal behaviors ranging from quietly sitting up in bed to so-called "bloodcurdling" screaming associated with heightened autonomic arousal. These partial arousals typically occur in the first third of the sleep cycle, usually 60 to 90 minutes after sleep onset and during completion of the first period of slow-wave sleep. During these arousals, children are "caught" between deep (slow-wave) sleep and full arousal. This state has characteristics including (1) high arousal threshold, (2) unresponsiveness to the environment, and (3) mental confusion. Although clinical symptoms vary, they include three basic categories: quiet sleepwalking, confusional arousals, and sleep terrors, or night terrors. Although symptoms vary, all of these disorders of partial arousal are similar in pathophysiology, timing in the sleep cycle, duration, clinical features, and genetics (family history is positive in up to 60%). The feature that clearly distinguishes night terrors/sleep terrors from nightmares is that children (or adults) are amnesic for night terrors.

Since children do not recall night terrors, one cannot use the hypnotic dream alteration method employed for nightmares. As with all problems, clinicians should, however, seek to clarify the history and any information known regarding possible precipitating events. Acute life-event changes or stressors are often identified as apparent triggers as are acute, febrile illnesses. However, methods for establishing a cause and effect relationship have not been defined. In taking a careful history, one can clarify the precipitating event and then employ hypnotic imagery to increase the child's sense of confidence and safety. Taboada (1975) used this method with a 7-year-old boy who had had night terrors for 15 consecutive nights after a frightening incident at camp. The night terrors ceased after one hypnotherapeutic session, with no recurrence at a follow-up 18 months later.

Kramer (1989) described hypnotic intervention for a 10-year-old boy with a 6-year history of night terrors that had themes of changing into a werewolf or of being physically mutilated or hurt. He was amnesic for the events, but his mother reported the content he expressed during the night terrors. Induction of hypnosis was accomplished with a "finger-lowering technique" in which the middle two fingers were raised, and he was given a metaphoric suggestion to watch his fingers go to sleep. Therapeutic suggestions consisted of repetitive and methodical explanation of sleep physiology, emphasizing the regularity and continual movement of the cycles of sleep. After two hypnotherapy sessions, he became free of night terrors and remained free of recurrence for 2 years of known follow-up. He was reported as happier and able to watch scary movies, which had, in the past, seemed to trigger the night terror behavior. Kramer (1989) appropriately identified the need for further research to understand how hypnosis affected the night terrors.

Koe (1989) described a 16-year-old male adolescent with sleep terror disorder that had occurred nightly for 7 years and had been resistant to interventions including benzodiazepine medication, behavior modification, and psychotherapy. A typical episode began with repetitive screaming, leaping out of bed, running around his room, often becoming violent including breaking his mother's nose during one episode and also smashing a window and furniture. Embarrassed and motivated to change, he explained the night terror as a fear of dying in his sleep but could not explain how or why the fear had begun.

Koe utilized hypnotherapy to identify that the patient utilized exernal stimuli, that is, noises, to (unconsciously) cue himself to the night terror/partial arousal. While he was in a hypnotic state, suggestions were given that he was in a deep sleep, the stage in which he usually had night terrors. In response to the hypnotic suggestion, autonomic arousal (increased respiratory rate, agitation) occurred, and the noise of a pencil tapping on the desk evoked a full-blown night terror with screaming and running about, and associated confusion. Subsequent hypnotic sessions focused repeatedly and only upon the post-hypnotic suggestion that, while asleep, he would gradually become less and less aware of outside sounds and sensations. The night terrors decreased from several per night to a total of three during the following week. Three months later he experienced no further night terrors.

Hurwitz, Mahowald, Schenck, Schluter, and Bundlie (1991) described the successful use of hypnosis in 27 adult patients with sleep terror disorders. Seventy-four percent reported much or very much improvement with the use and practice of self-hypnosis. Training required a mean of only 1.6 office visits.

We (Kohen, Mahowald, & Rosen, 1992) described the use of self-hypnosis for four children, ages 8 to 12 years, who had frequent, prolonged, or dangerous disorders of arousal documented by a polysomnogram (in a regional sleep disorders center) that showed sudden arousals out of slow-wave sleep associated with the complex behaviors of sleep terrors. After demystification of their symptoms through methodical education about sleep physiology (unlike Kramer mentioned previously, education was provided before, not during trance), and because of the dangerous or prolonged nature of their sleep terror behaviors, these children were treated pharmacologically first. Each responded to a short course of imipramine while also being taught relaxation/mental imagery (self-hypnosis). In each case the medication was discontinued while self-hypnosis was reinforced, and in each case, the children remained free of further arousals over 2 to 3 years of follow-up. Induction and deepening were individualized with favorite place imagery, and then each child was offered the opportunity to "let me know, with a finger signal, when you are ready to learn how to use this very nice feeling and imagination to reprogram that computer we call the brain to sleep very well." Superimposed on the waking-state information they received about sleep cycles and the "accidentally getting stuck" between a state of deep sleep and wakefulness, each child was given the simple therapeutic suggestion that "as you practice this each night, and before you go to sleep, remind yourself to have a peaceful, restful, quiet night's sleep in your own bed and wake up in the morning happy and proud." Audiotapes of the office hypnotic suggestions were provided for reinforcement.

As success with these four children became evident, we then offered hypnotherapy to children without prior pharmacological treatment. Successful reduction and elimination of night terrors with the hypnotic approach only occurred in six of seven children ranging in age from 21 months to 16 years. More recent data analysis (G. R. Rosen, personal communication, 1994) has revealed that polysomnograms previously believed to be diagnostic for night terrors in these children are, in fact, not distinguishable from matched siblings. Polysomnograms, also showing partial arousals from slow-wave sleep occur in the siblings of night terror patients but with *no* clinical night terror behaviors.

We concluded, as did Kramer (1989), that hypnotherapy was successful in eliminating the troubling night terror behaviors but that we do not understand the mechanism by which hypnotherapy effected the change. Research continues in this fascinating area.

Social Anxiety

For both temperamental and psychodynamic reasons, some children and adolescents feel especially insecure in social situations outside the immediate family. Many of these youngsters learn adaptive social skills as a result of participation in preschool groups, with the support of parents, teachers, and other helping adults. Some, however, continue to be generally shy and withdrawn, and their difficulties may become pronounced when there is additional social stress such as occurs with a move to a new neighborhood or a change of schools. Although long-term psychotherapy may be indicated, sometimes brief supportive hypnotherapy can help these children use their strengths to overcome the problem. The following case example illustrates the possible value of short-term hypnotherapy.

Diana, age 15 years, came into the office with her mother to request help in overcoming shyness that had become incapacitating in school and in social situations. The patient described herself as always having been introverted, especially when compared to three older siblings, but this had become more of a problem at age 13 when she entered junior high school. Previously she had attended parochial school and had known the same classmates for 6 years. In the new junior high school, she found herself unable to stand up in class and recite or raise her hand to answer questions. She preferred accepting failing grades rather than giving oral presentations. In the therapist's office, she also expressed her reluctance to initiate friendships except with her siblings and said that she engaged in social activities only when with her older sister and two older brothers.

Diana was a strikingly beautiful, well-groomed adolescent. According to her mother, she had been a good student until entering junior high school. She got along well with parents, siblings, and other relatives and a few girlfriends. Her mother volunteered that, although she accompanied her daughter for the first visit, she would encourage her daughter to come alone on subsequent visits. This and other comments suggested that the mother truly wanted her child to achieve greater independence and social participation. There was no evidence of severe family pathology.

Diana was seen three times for hypnotherapy. In the first interview, it became apparent that she was interested in becoming a model, perhaps a counterphobic reaction but still one that could be used to her advantage. Hypnosis was induced with eye fixation and progressive relaxation. Diana was asked to imagine herself feeling comfortable as a model. She was asked to practice self-hypnosis twice daily, using ego-strengthening imagery. When

seen 2 weeks later, she said she was feeling more comfortable in social situations and had been able to recite in class. During this visit, she was asked
to regress to a past experience that had been pleasant and represented success to her. She was asked to squeeze her right fist to make the recollection
of positive, happy feelings more vivid. When she did this, the therapist asked
her to let herself be aware of something that might be bothering her, to consider whether or not she could let go of this, and then to imagine sending
it off on a plane or freight train. She was told that she could repeat this imagery in her self-hypnosis exercises at home if she wished.

On the third visit, 6 weeks later, Diana reported proudly that she had
had her first date, that she was comfortable in the classroom, and was now
practicing self-hypnosis once daily. While Diana was in a hypnotic state, the
therapist asked her to imagine herself on a stage, performing in front of people whom she liked and feeling good about herself. She was followed by telephone and continued to do well at 6-month follow-up.

PSYCHOPHYSIOLOGICAL DISORDERS

The problems discussed here have in common a presenting complaint of a
physical problem for which the basis is primarily psychogenic. We include
conversion disorders, psychogenic seizures, pain where there is no identifiable organic origin, and anorexia nervosa. In some cases, the psychological disorder is precipitated by a bona fide physical problem; in other
cases, the origins are psychogenic. In all cases, however, psychological
factors play a major role in maintaining or aggravating a somatic complaint,
as noted by M. S. Smith (1983). Stressors triggering these symptoms may
be environmental or physical stressors and psychological (emotional)
stressors.

In evaluating such symptoms, Rickert and Jay (1994) have recommended
the severity, affect, family, and environment interview strategy (SAFE). The
severity of symptoms should be assessed in the beginning of the interview.
The affects of both the patient and parent/guardian should be evaluated.
Efforts should be made to understand ongoing family concerns and conflicts
as well as the patient's environment, including peers, school, and community. We have found that a helpful approach in meeting with the family together
is to ask each parent, "What does your body do when you are nervous or
anxious?" Or, "When I am anxious, my hands feel cold. What does your
body do when you are nervous or anxious?" This question is always answered,
and family members are often surprised to learn that other family members
sometimes feel anxious. Children with somatoform disorders, however, often
do not know immediately how their bodies react to distress.

Conversion Reactions

Conversion reactions have been conceptualized as expressions of neurotic conflict that may center around issues of hostility or independence or sexual wishes. Conversion reactions may occur in children and in borderline or psychotic individuals as well as in neurotic individuals. Williams and Singh (1976) reported a case of conversion reaction, manifested by hysterical amblyopia, in an 8-year-old girl. We quote their report in full, since it is an excellent example of careful diagnostic assessment, detailed description of hypnotherapeutic treatment, and appropriate follow-up.

> Maria, an eight year old Puerto Rican girl, was admitted from the emergency room to the pediatric service after an urgent referral from school, which reported a progression of visual difficulties over a three week period. These difficulties involved markedly diminished acuity in distance and peripheral vision, culminating in total inability to function in school. Neurologic, ophthalmologic, and psychiatric evaluations upon admission all concurred in the diagnosis of a conversion reaction.
>
> Precipitating environmental stresses included: (1) a 10-year-old female cousin of Maria had an enucleation of her right eye after a traumatic injury two months prior to Maria's admission; (2) the arrival of a new infant in Maria's household (already rife with sibling rivalry) one month prior to admission; (3) a television program Maria saw three weeks prior to admission, portraying an episode of hysterical blindness; (4) Maria's class was changed without appropriate explanation two weeks prior to admission; and (5) a man approached Maria on the street one week prior to admission and pulled her hair before he ran off.
>
> Maria was found to be in the mid-range of hypnotizability (grade 2-3). A hypnotic exercise was developed and utilized, together with supportive explanation and a family session to achieve several related goals. These included helping Maria to recognize and accept the connection between accumulated anxiety and loss of vision; to develop a retrospective emotional-cognitive mastery of previous traumatic experiences; and to relinquish the regressed symptom complex in favor of a more healthy (premorbid) mode of dealing with ongoing life situations and stresses. The implementation of these goals yielded marked symptom attenuation and essentially restored full visual function in two sessions over a three day period.
>
> The exercise itself, first with Maria alone and then in joint session with Maria and her mother, involved Maria's repeating out loud the following three statements while in a trance state:
>
> 1. When people are very scared and upset, they may stop being able to see.
> 2. By relaxing (with this exercise), I can overcome my scared and upset feelings.

3. As soon as I am able to see better, I can go home and do all the things I like to do.

Maria was discharged after the second session, with only a mild subjective report of "blurriness," taken as a call for continued psychotherapeutic support. She was seen in follow-up 10 days later, by which time her visual symptoms had fully cleared. During further outpatient sessions, the therapist placed emphasis on significant issues of ongoing concern within the family as well as upon Maria's school performance. He gave positive reinforcement to Maria for having overcome her visual difficulties, and this mastery was used as a paradigm for her capacity similarly to struggle with and overcome other problems.

Although there was no recurrence of visual symptoms over a three month period following discharge, the therapist recommended continued supportive psychotherapy at monthly intervals because of the somewhat turbulent family interaction. The family declined to follow this recommendation, but we have nevertheless received no reports from them or from the school of any recurrent visual problems during the subsequent 14 months. Follow-up contact with the school guidance counselor 17 months after discharge confirmed that there had been no recurrent visual or behavioral problems and disclosed that school adjustment had actually improved. (pp. 331–332)*

Williams and Singh briefly reported other cases of childhood conversion reaction: (1) a 12-year-old boy presented with a 9-month history of abdominal pain with flexion of the trunk and inability to walk. After two sessions of hypnotherapy over 1 week, the patient began walking during the following week. (2) A 12-year-old girl with a seizure disorder presented with inability to walk and blindness of 1 day's duration. Ability to see and walk were restored after one hypnotherapy session. (3) A 13-year-old girl complained of a 6-month history of polyarthralgia of hips, knees, and ankles, with gait impairment. Her joint pains resolved completely after three weekly hypnotherapy sessions. In all these cases, continued individual and family therapy were recommended. Follow-up ranged from 7 to 16 months. There were no cases of symptom substitution, although some symptoms transiently recurred, usually associated with situational stress or premature termination of outpatient psychotherapy.

Williams (1979) reported hypnotherapeutic treatment of a 13-year-old boy with lower-back pain, eventually diagnosed as a conversion disorder. His method was essentially the same as that used by Williams and Singh (1976). The pain disappeared after one hypnotherapeutic session. At the time of Williams' report, the boy had remained symptom-free for 2 years.

Sarles (1975) briefly described a 16-year-old girl who was hospitalized

---

*From Williams and Singh (1976). Copyright 1976 by Williams & Wilkins. With permission.

after sudden onset of total paralysis from her neck down. Physical examination revealed no organic disease. Psychiatric evaluation disclosed hysterical features and a precipitating event in which the girl had been berated for kissing a boyfriend and warned that her parents would "watch every step she took." During an 8-week course of family counseling and hypnotherapy that used regressive techniques to explore the dynamics of the paralysis, the girl made a complete recovery. No follow-up data were given in this report.

In a paper on pediatric hypnotherapy, Olness and Gardner (1978) included a short case report of a conversion reaction. We here present the case in more detail, with special emphasis on the use of hypnotherapy and its role in the larger treatment context.

Kit was a bright, active 8-year-old boy, the youngest of eight children in a middle-class, intact, Catholic family. He developed documented streptococcal pharyngitis and, soon thereafter, experienced pain and weakness in his extremities, progressing over 2 weeks to the point that he could not walk or use his arms and required total care. He was admitted to the neurological service of a large hospital, where diagnostic work-up revealed no organic basis for his complaints. Psychological evaluation pointed to conflict in the area of independence–dependence of which the boy was partially aware. He said he enjoyed the role of baby in the family, including special attention from mother; at the same time, he wished he was old enough to have more of the privileges enjoyed by his older siblings. Kit's mother acknowledged that she had always loved babies and derived gratification from continuing to think of Kit as her baby. Kit was aware of his mother's feelings, and his wish to please her contributed to his conflict. It seemed that the strep throat had tipped the balance, providing Kit with even more maternal attention. He unconsciously attempted to resolve the conflict by becoming a baby, thereby gratifying both himself and his mother. At the same time, the conversion reaction allowed unconscious expression of hostility toward the mother who seemed to interfere with his developmental needs.

The therapist explained the dynamics to the boy and his mother, assuring them that Kit was not malingering. The mother was shocked that her feelings could have such a profound effect on her son, and she immediately asked for help with her problems. Both Kit and his mother were relieved that there was no permanent physical disability, and they readily accepted the recommendation of brief hypnotherapy for Kit to alleviate his symptoms, followed by individual and family therapy to work through the underlying conflicts.

That afternoon, in the first of two hypnotherapy sessions, the therapist talked further with Kit about mind–body relationships, the dynamics of his conversion reaction, and the way hypnotherapy could help him get conscious and unconscious wishes in better alignment. He was fascinated with the idea that, while consciously he could not move his arms, he probably could do so in the altered state of hypnosis. As an initial demonstration, the therapist used an arm levitation hypnotic induction and with eyes open, to which Kit readily responded.

Then the therapist employed the method of combined age regression and age progression to facilitate the recovery of a lost skill. First Kit was asked in hypnosis to recall a specific time when he walked or ran with confidence and enjoyment and to relieve that past experience. Having accomplished this, he was then asked to let go of the situational details of the memory but to hold on to the good, strong feelings in his legs, now experiencing them in the present. He said, "My legs feel very strong; I don't think they could feel any stronger." It was then suggested that he could imagine using his strong legs in the future. He did so. Then he was told that, if he was ready, he could remain in hypnosis and walk across the room. Having followed this suggestion with obvious pleasure, he was given a posthypnotic suggestion that he could, if he wished, choose to retain the use of his legs when he came out of hypnosis. He did so, generally happy, but disappointed that we had not yet "cured his arms." The therapist said he could work on that the next day, planning to use the interim to observe his response to the partial recovery.

By the following morning, Kit had maintained his gains with no evidence of new problems. The second hypnotherapy session proceeded along the lines of the first, now focusing on his arms. He achieved hypnotic arm rigidity and experienced normal strength and sensation first in hypnosis and then in the waking state. He was discharged from the hospital later that day. The symptoms briefly recurred the next day but then disappeared totally.

Kit and his family were followed in outpatient therapy over several months, and the basic conflicts were satisfactorily resolved. Annual cards from Kit's mother have indicated that he has been symptom-free for more than 3 years and once more leads an active, happy life.

Sometimes cultural factors suggest that nontraditional methods in the general domain of hypnotherapy will be most useful. Carla was a 10-year-old Mexican-American girl with nonorganic total body paralysis and a diagnosis of conversion reaction. The child was hesitant to relate to Anglo-American doctors and responded only minimally to one session of traditional hypnotherapy. Although adequate history was difficult to obtain, it eventually came out that the child had been hexed. We then contacted a *curandera* (faith healer) who saw the child for three sessions. She produced a necklace and suggested that the power of the necklace could be transferred to the child. By touching the necklace, Carla regained movement of her arms and upper torso in two sessions. She also regained her ability to walk, though at a slower rate, since she had been confined to a wheelchair for 4 months. She was given the necklace to wear as a continuing reminder of her own power and as a symbol to the community that she could no longer be hexed.

One must not conclude from these reports that it is always the treatment of choice to use hypnotherapy to achieve rapid symptom relief in conversion reactions. Conversion reaction may occur in the context of a borderline psychotic state, serving a major defensive purpose. In such cases, hypnotherapy should be employed—if it is used at all—first for ego strengthening and only later and very gradually to aid in symptom removal or amelioration.

Psychogenic Seizures

In cases of psychogenic seizures, psychological problems play a major role in precipitating seizure activity. The patient may or may not also have an organically based seizure disorder. Although not conscious during a true seizure, the patient often has heard descriptions of the details of the seizure activity. Sometimes the child has witnessed true seizure in relatives or close friends. Although it is difficult for casual observers to differentiate between true and psychogenic seizures, there are distinguishing characteristics. For example, if the patient exhibits dramatic movements that look like a grand mal seizure but does not lose consciousness, has no incontinence, and experiences no stupor or lethargy immediately afterwards, one should suspect that the seizure has a psychogenic origin (Glenn & Simonds, 1977).

Gardner (1973) described her treatment of Tracy, an 8-year-old girl with familial seizures, whose first generalized convulsion occurred at age 9 months. From age 3 years, her EEG showed a petit mal variant disturbance, with seizure activity manifested chiefly by eye-fluttering spells. Seizure frequency increased markedly when the child was in kindergarten, and the problem worsened over the next 2 years despite several medication changes and a trial ketogenic diet. At age 8 years, Tracy was diagnosed as having both true and psychogenic seizures. No longer able to function either at home or at school, she was highly motivated to improve seizure control. Treatment lasted for 18 sessions, consisting of a combination of hypnotherapy, play therapy, and parent counseling.

The therapist avoided suggesting any sensations associated with the seizures, such as eye closure, drowsiness, amnesia, or time distortion. The hypnotic induction consisted of relaxation with eyes open, followed by hand levitation as a demonstration that the child could learn new ways to control her body. In hypnosis, she was given repeated suggestions that it could be fun to keep her eyes open and see what was going on. Ego-strengthening suggestions were also utilized praising her for cooperation and improvement and reminding her of the happy consequences of positive changes. She learned self-hypnosis and enjoyed home practice sessions focused on "being able to keep her eyes open more and more."

By the fifth session, Tracy showed clear improvement. She then developed a new problem, namely difficulty getting to sleep at night. This problem quickly resolved when the therapist reminded her that there were times when it was appropriate to close her eyes. Play therapy emphasized carry-over of the hypnotic behavior to the waking state and modification of low self-esteem. The parents were counseled to reinforce behavioral improvement and to ignore periods of eye fluttering. We did not deal with other complex family issues that would have required long-term therapy. At the time of termination, the seizure frequency was markedly reduced, and the child was enjoying success both at home and at school. Ten months after initiation of hypnotherapy, she continued to make good progress in all areas.

About 8 months later, Tracy's symptoms returned. In a second course of hypnotherapy, she made marked gains initially but then deteriorated again. Therapy was terminated after about 6 months. The parents sought help for the child elsewhere, and we have no further follow-up.

Glenn and Simonds (1977) treated a 13-year-old girl who had been having psychogenic seizures for about 2 weeks. There was no underlying organic seizure disorder. The child did have a 4-year history of emotional problems, apparently precipitated by the death of her father. Early in hypnoanalytic treatment she experienced a seizure concurrent with describing a vivid rape fantasy, probably related to conflicts over emerging sexual desires. The treatment included hypnotically induced seizures and training the patient to prevent the seizures by pressing her right thumb and forefinger together. She was also taught to verbalize her fantasies. She participated in an inpatient behavior modification program with emphasis on improving self-esteem. Her mother and stepfather were seen twice monthly for counseling. There were no seizures after the first week of a 4-month hospitalization, and follow-up revealed that the patient remained seizure-free for 2 years after discharge. It is not clear in this report whether hypnotherapy continued during the 2 years after discharge or was limited to the period of inpatient treatment.

Williams and Singh (1976) briefly described two cases of psychogenic seizures. In the first case, a 15-year-old girl presented with a 4-year history of both true and psychogenic psychomotor seizures, markedly exacerbated in the last month. She was seizure-free after a 10-day hospitalization that included both hypnotherapy and family therapy. During 14 months of continued outpatient therapy, both individual and family, she had only occasional seizures, associated with situational stress. In the second case, a 12-year-old girl presented with a 4-year history of mixed-type seizures, both organic and psychogenic, unresponsive to medications. After initial improvement in a hospital program including hypnotherapy, behavior modification, and family therapy, the girl's condition worsened after discharge. She improved again after readmission and maintained her gains over the next 12 months at home where she continued in supportive psychotherapy.

Psychogenic Pain

The diagnosis of psychogenic pain must be made with great care. We have had numerous experiences of evaluating children who were referred to us with the diagnosis of psychogenic pain and who later proved to have a biological basis for the pain symptom. Many of these children presented with headaches or abdominal pain or leg pain. It is also possible for children to have pain with both biological and psychological components. Williams and Singh (1976) described an 11-year-old boy with a long history of recurring abdominal pain, complicated by many factors including serious organic illness that had been misdiagnosed as psychogenic. The child was seen for brief hypnotherapy aimed at understanding sources of tension and using relaxation to reduce and eliminate pain. He was symptom-free in 48 hours. He was followed in outpatient psychotherapy for 20 months during which there was only 1 transient recurrence of abdominal pain, possibly attributable to gastroenteritis.

Sarles (1975) treated a 14-year-old girl with a 12-week history of severe hip pain determined to be of psychogenic origin, probably related to family discord. Her pain was relieved after one session of hypnotherapy, and she walked 3 days later. She successfully used self-hypnosis whenever the pain recurred. Follow-up revealed that she had returned to school and that the family was involved in family therapy.

When psychogenic pain serves major defensive functions or provides significant secondary gain, it is much less likely to respond to hypnotherapy. Kelly was a 14-year-old girl referred because of knee pain that began when she dislocated her knee 12 months earlier. Corrective surgery had been deemed successful, but the pain continued. Nerve blocks and various medications had been of little help.

In the first hypnotherapeutic session, Kelly was constricted and markedly depressed, expressing doubt that hypnotherapy would be of any value. Despite the fact that she responded well to hypnotic induction, she derived no benefit from several hypnotherapeutic approaches designed to alleviate her pain. Diagnostic interviews and psychological testing suggested that the pain might be binding severe anxiety and might also be providing significant secondary gain including passively expressing hostility and dependency needs, neither of which she could admit into consciousness. The girl vigorously denied any sort of emotional distress and responded negatively to the suggestion of extended psychotherapy. She terminated hypnotherapy after four sessions, her condition unchanged. Although her parents were hesitant to accept the idea of a psychological basis for her pain, 1 month later they did take her to a psychotherapist nearer their home.

Anorexia Nervosa

The syndrome of anorexia nervosa may result from a number of causes, including biological ones. However, regardless of the cause, the life-threatening aspects of continued voluntary starvation mandate whatever interventions insure food retention. Crasilneck and Hall (1985) begin hypnotherapeutic treatment with direct suggestions for increased food intake. When the patient begins to gain weight and the medical situation is stablilized, they then begin psychodynamic exploration, both with and without hypnoanalytic techniques. Their technique is illustrated in the following case report:

> One rather mild case began in a high school girl after a girl friend became pregnant. She noticed people watching the girl friend's abdomen as the pregnancy became more and more apparent. The patient became concerned that she, too, would mistakenly be thought pregnant since she was slightly overweight. To counter this fear, she began to eat less and less, losing to a point that caused anemia and fatigue.
>
> In spite of advice from her family physician that she must increase her food intake, the patient continued to lose weight. When it was obvious that her weight was dangerously low, we were called to see the patient with the hope that hypnotherapy might counter the negative attitude toward food intake.
>
> After we established rapport, hypnosis was accepted by the patient and she was able to enter a deep trance. She was then told, "You will be hungry. Food will taste good, and your body weight will be necessary for your own good health and welfare." The patient began increasing her caloric intake, starting with her next meal. Her body weight, although on the slim side, came into the normal range for her height. She was encouraged continually to verbalize her many feelings of shame, sorrow, and hostility concerning her girl friend's pregnancy. She was also quite aware of strong libidinous drives within herself, which had caused much guilt. When she was able to express the affect concerning her conflicts, the obsessive thoughts concerning food intake resolved themselves. One year later, although no longer in treatment, she was a slim attractive young lady who could accept the actions of others without introjecting their feelings. She understood that libidinous drives are normal in adults and that they should not lead to feelings of guilt, shame, and masochistic acts. (p. 215)*

Gross (1984) has reported the successful use of hypnotherapy in treating 50 patients with anorexia nervosa. Torem (1987, 1991) has reported similar success in using hypnotherapy as an adjunct. Most of the anorexic patients we see in a tertiary care setting are dangerously ill, often having lost 50% of their normal body weight. The threat of death demands immediate

---

*From Crasilneck and Hall (1985). Copyright 1985 by Allyn & Bacon. With permission.

increase in food intake. We therefore begin with a strictly controlled behavior modification program in which the patient either eats and retains frequent small meals or is tube-fed an equivalent amount. Hypnotherapy and/or conventional psychotherapy is used for anxiety reduction, to facilitate coping, improve self-esteem and for dynamic exploration and conflict resolution. However, malnourished individuals often have cognitive processing problems and irritability as a result of the malnutrition. We have found that it is difficult to work with severely ill anorexic adolescents until nutritional rehabilitation has begun and there is some improvement in nutritional status.

PERVASIVE DEVELOPMENTAL DISORDER

Gardner and Tarnow (1980) published a case report describing the use of hypnotherapy with Tom, a 16-year-old boy diagnosed as mildly autistic at age 3½ years. The child had made gains in traditional psychotherapy and in special education programs, though he remained socially isolated and unable to integrate new experiences. He had a long-standing habit of biting his finger in response to frustrating situations, and he had developed a large callus, with intermittent bleeding and infection.

At age 16 years, it seemed that Tom might be able to transfer to a regular high school, but his continued finger-biting behavior—refractory to previous treatment—seemed certain to elicit peer rejection and interfere with school adjustment. He was therefore referred for hypnotherapy in an attempt to eliminate this problem.

Unresponsive to traditional hypnotic induction methods, Tom mentioned that Aria No. 47 from the Bach *Saint Matthew Passion* helped him feel calm. Thereafter, when the therapist played him a tape recording of this aria, he easily entered hypnotic trance. Skilled in music, he wrote two short musical compositions for use in hypnotherapeutic treatment. He listened to the first, entitled "Frustration in C Minor," after recalling a frustrating experience, with the suggestion that recall of the music could replace the finger-biting behavior. Then he listened to the second composition, "Happiness in C Major," with the suggestion that recall could strengthen feelings of confidence and increased self-control. The therapist also discussed the construction of the Bach aria, focusing on the way it implied different possible responses to particular events. The finger biting, which had occurred two to three times weekly prior to hypnotherapy, extinguished entirely after 4 weeks, with the exception of 1 episode when both Tom's parents and his primary therapist were out of town. He maintained his gains over a follow-up period of 18 months.

Interestingly, Tom was able to describe frustrating events with greater detail and understanding when he was in hypnosis. At first, there was a marked difference between hypnotic and waking-state verbalizations. Later, the hypnotic communication skills generalized to the waking state. Improvement also generalized to other areas of behavior at home and at school where he continued a satisfactory adjustment in regular classes and became a member of the school jazz band. Throughout the treatment, the therapists emphasized competence and mastery in several ways:

> (1) involving the patient in treatment planning from the very beginning, (2) communicating to the patient that he was acceptable, while agreeing that aspects of his *behavior* were unacceptable, (3) focusing immediately on developing a *solution* rather than getting bogged down in discussing the *problem*, (4) praising the patient for cooperation and responding quickly to his efforts, e.g., using his compositions before he had achieved a hypnotic trance, (5) utilizing the patient's obsession with music as a strength on which to base therapeutic strategy rather than perceiving it negatively as resistance or as an obstacle in the way of progress, and (6) helping the patient observe his own progress, thus further enhancing his confidence in his ability to master problems in living. (Gardner & Tarnow, 1980, p. 178)

The authors concluded that hypnotherapy may be a suitable technique for youngsters with severe ego deficits, provided induction techniques are modified to suit special needs and interests and therapeutic suggestions focus on patient skills and ego strengthening rather than on stressful uncovering of repressed material.

CONCLUSIONS

Hypnotherapy can be useful for a great variety of emotional problems, both recent and of long duration, with children of all ages. Poor results are usually associated with lack of motivation, deep-seated conflicts that the patient refuses or is unable to acknowledge, severe underlying pathology for which the symptom serves as a major defense, significant secondary gain from the symptom, missed biological causes, and premature termination of treatment. Parental attitudes also play an important role, especially in cases where parents deny that physical symptoms are chiefly the result of psychological problems. When the child's problems are the most obvious manifestation of complex family pathology, hypnotherapy is likely to fail unless family therapy is also accepted as a treatment modality.

CHAPTER EIGHT

Hypnotherapy for Habit Disorders

Childhood habit problems potentially responsive to hypnotherapy include those such as habitual coughs (or so-called cough-tics), enuresis, thumb-sucking, fecal soiling, nail biting, hair pulling, verbal dysfluencies, sleepwalking and related parasomnias, certain eating disorders, and drug abuse. Although many habits may at one time have had emotional significance for the child, often the habit has long lost its original meaning and become functionally autonomous by the time the child is referred for treatment. Sometimes habits seem to develop without any identifiable underlying emotional significance or antecedent "trigger" and are perpetuated simply by repetition in association with certain situations. In this way they behave for all intents and purposes like conditioned responses. As discussed further in this chapter, these understandings are not only important but also may well be critical to discuss as such and explain to patients and families as part of the therapeutic education and communication process before moving into applying hypnotherapeutic strategies.

As with any other clinical problem, before beginning hypnotherapy for a habit problem, it is important to determine if and whether the habit (still) serves any important psychological function, that is, whether there is any continuing secondary gain from maintenance of the problem behavior. For example, does the child unconsciously achieve a position of control in his or her family through the prominence of his or her habit in family life? By reason of the habit does the child have "power," for example, to delay leaving the house in timely fashion to go certain places? Or, is there pleasure in making the parents angry in a passive way that avoids punishment? In the event that significant secondary gain seems to be present, it may be preferable to postpone symptom-oriented hypnotherapy, at least until such time as one or another form of insight-oriented individual or family-oriented psychotherapy can help the family identify, acknowledge, and work through

underlying problems. Occasionally, children are able to resolve dynamic issues concurrently with a symptom-oriented, solution-focused approach.

Even in the absence of apparent or important secondary gain, the clini-
cian/therapist must carefully assess the child's motivation for overcoming
the habit. This is often easily accomplished in the context of a comprehensive history obtained matter-of-factly and preferably from the child, who,
of course, knows the most about the problem. Such assessments can be made
either directly through verbal questioning, indirectly through naturalistic inquiries as part of history taking, or indirectly by ideomotor signaling in hypnosis. Beyond the standard and traditional obtaining of a clinical history,
we have had consistent success with naturalistic, Ericksonian-like approaches
that tend to allow for bypassing of critical judgment and the elicitation of
spontaneous, "true" responses from the unconscious. In response to direct
verbal inquiry, children's responses may or may not reflect active defenses.
In response to an indirect, humor-based, and perhaps "abrupt shift of context" inquiry, however, defenses are more likely to be equally abruptly by-
passed, thus allowing more honest and definitive answers to questions. As
an example, consider the following conversation between a child and a therapist regarding a thumb-sucking problem:

THERAPIST: So, how come you came over to see me?

CHILD: Well, see, uhhhh, well, . . . it's 'cause they [parents] said I had to.

THERAPIST: Because . . . ?

CHILD: Well . . . 'cause I suck my thumb sometimes. . . .

THERAPIST: Oh . . . when?

CHILD: Sometimes. . . .

THERAPIST: Oh. Well, mostly where are you when it *happens*? [*Note:* This
is a purposeful shift in language to the problem "happening" rather than the
child "doing" it. As an *implication* it is designed to let the child begin to shift
and to hear that I understand that it doesn't feel like he's in charge of it,
at least some of the time.]

CHILD: You mean like at home or school or . . . ?

THERAPIST: Yeah.

CHILD: Well, usually at home.

PARENTS: You can tell him, it's when you're going to bed or when you're
watching TV and Ms. Smith told me that at kindergarten sometimes you
suck your thumb during story-hour.

CHILD: MOM!!!! [anguish!]

THERAPIST: Say, are you going to miss the thumb-sucking when it's gone?

[*Note:* This represents a double or triple kind of shift and example of naturalistic suggestions and inquiry. The child has just been embarrassed through the mother's revealing that he sucks his thumb at school sometimes. Rather than take direct acknowledgment or mention of that, the therapist instead seemingly changes the subject, thus at one level helping to defuse the embarrassment. At another level the future-oriented suggestion is offered or planted like a seed that the problem *will* be gone by inquiring re: *when* (not "if") it's gone. Finally, the critical inquiry about whether the habit will be *missed* is embedded in the middle of the sentence in the abruptly-offered query, thus easing it into the unconscious, making it a question more likely (though of course not guaranteed!) to be answered spontaneously *from* the unconscious.]

Although children, of course, answer these questions in different ways, the answers, like those from ideomotor signals, seem to be more consistently reliable. Thus, in the example, if there is ambivalence, it is clearly there. Usually this will be revealed quite clearly by the nature or content of the response, or both. So, in answer to "Say, are you going to *miss* the thumb-sucking when it's gone?" many say, "No, of course not, are you kidding?" and look at the clinician incredulously for asking such a foolish question. Others, such as those ambivalent, are more likely to hesitate, hem and haw, or perhaps even to say openly, "Yeah, I need to suck my thumb to get to sleep at night" and then want themselves to change the subject. The theoretical advantage of these over ideomotor signaling responses in hypnosis is that the latter are not usually able to be introduced, of course, until hypnosis has been formally introduced and taught. With ideomotor signaling, unconscious conflict is more likely to be easily revealed, as, for example, when the child's "yes" and "no" fingers lift simultaneously in response to questions asked "to the fingers" during hypnosis.

It is valuable to determine how the child thinks life will be different when the problem is resolved. If, for example, a child still obtains much pleasure from a given habit, has little desire to give it up, and has come for therapy chiefly as a result of parental pressure, there is likely to be little benefit from hypnotherapy. In such a case the therapist might suggest that the parents postpone treatment for the child, and spend some time instead perhaps discussing realistic parental expectations. Sometimes parents expect too much of a young child who is not developmentally ready to change certain behavior. Accordingly, treatment for the child may be postponed while perhaps the clinician helps the family with issues related to unrealistic expectations.

In hypnotherapy for habit disorders, we have not found symptom substitution to be a problem, although we sometimes hear dire warnings in this regard. Our experience suggests that children either gladly give up habits or indicate a continuing need for them, sometimes despite an earnest desire to the contrary. In general, a trial of four to six sessions of hypnotherapy suffices to determine whether the child is really ready for habit change. In the case of some habits, successful treatment depends upon removal of misconceptions about the problem. Sometimes such misconceptions can be resolved by verbal explanations; while, at other times, the therapist may choose to use diagrams to explain anatomical or physiological relationships that may in turn enable a child to develop suitable images for success while in a hypnotic state. Many parents have also benefited from such explanations. In order to detect persisting confusion, it is helpful to request that the child bring his or her own drawing or diagram to the therapist on the next visit. Alternatively, it is often useful to invite the child to create his or her own drawing as part of their next session. Children and parents (and clinicians!) alike not only enjoy this opportunity but also are often pleasantly surprised to see how very much the child has learned from but a single guided explanation (even 1–2 weeks before) about how the body works (with respect to their particular problem).

Whenever a habit may be a symptom of an underlying physical disorder, it is crucial that the child be appropriately evaluated from a medical standpoint prior to the initiation of hypnotherapy. Since this possibility is most likely in cases of enuresis (bedwetting) and encopresis (fecal soiling), we include issues of differential diagnosis in our discussion of these problems. These habits may have both psychological and medical components, and too often the former are emphasized while the latter are ignored. A psychotherapist, for example, must not yield to parental pressure for hypnotherapy without proper diagnostic evaluation of the problem as indicated.

Finally, hypnotherapeutic approaches to habit problems should focus on the patient's competence and ability for mastery, emphasizing that it is ultimately the child, not the therapist, who makes the change. Hypnotic suggestions should include images of future recognition that the problem is solved. For example, for someone working on a thumb-sucking habit, one might say something like: "Just picture yourself on that video in your mind, and notice the date is some time later this year, I don't know which month, but you'll notice it . . . good . . . then notice what a nice evening you have, first finishing your homework, then playing a game with your sister. Then . . . notice yourself getting ready for bed and listening to a story and notice your hand and thumb comfortably down by your side under the covers." For their part and their role, parents should be asked to focus on family life without the problem, thus affirming their confidence and trust in their child's ability (and commitment) to overcome it.

ENURESIS

Through the ages, nocturnal enuresis has been the most common chronic behavioral problem faced by the pediatrician (Olness, 1977b). Glicklich

(1951) reported that this problem was discussed in a 16th-century pediatrics text in a section entitled, "Of Pyssying in the Bedde." One study has estimated that enuresis has occurred in approximately 20 million Americans over the age of 5 years (Cohen, 1975). It is generally agreed that the symptom does not warrant extensive investigation or treatment under age 5 to 6 years unless information from history and physical examination suggests organic causes. The majority of bedwetting beyond age 5 years is associated with no discernible organic or psychological causes and thus may be understood as equivalent to a habituated response, or habit problem. In his *Lectures on the Diseases of Children* (1882/1994), the famous pediatrician, Dr. Edward Henoch noted that so little was known of the causation of nocturnal enuresis that "there is a certain justification for the doubt whether this is a diseased condition or an acquired *habit*" (pp. 257–258). As such, enuresis may be not only best understood but also best explained to children and families as a developmental or maturational variant, or as an "accidental habit," that has become "stuck" and inadvertently perpetuated, using this kind of language in particular in order to defuse blame.

Evaluation

The approach to evaluation of enuresis varies depending on whether or not the symptom is *primary* (i.e., the child has never had a prolonged period of consecutive dry beds) or *onset* (i.e., the child had several months of dry beds followed by a relapse) (Olness, 1977b; Schmitt, 1990). It is also important to ascertain whether the enuresis is at night only, or a combination of day and nighttime wetting. The presence of concurrent day and night enuresis indicates that more intensive investigation is needed to rule out organic causes that might include diabetes mellitus, occult spinal dysraphism, urinary tract infections, congenital anomalies of the urinary tract, or seizures (Anderson, 1975; Kolvin, 1973; Olness, 1977b). Chronic constipation is a common, yet often unrecognized, cause of both day and nighttime wetting, and should be carefully searched for in any patient with enuresis. Rarely, the presence of nocturnal enuresis is caused by hyperthyroidism, diuretic medications such as theophylline given for asthma, or a child's habit of taking large amount of caffeine drinks such as coffee or colas. There is also a likely association between documented allergies and the presence of nocturnal enuresis. The mechanism is unknown (Gerrard, Jones, Shokier, & Zaleski, 1971; Olness & Immershein, 1977).

Initial evaluation of enuresis must include questions regarding the meaning of the symptom for the family. Although there may have been no original emotional trigger, emotional problems often develop as bedwetting persists. It is important to ascertain in particular the expectations of the parents regarding the ultimate achievement of dry beds. If, for example, the parents believe that "all children should be dry by age 3," it is possible that unreasonable parent pressure has contributed to the child losing confidence even when neurophysiological maturity has developed somewhat later than 3 years. In the case of onset (or secondary) bedwetting, it is helpful to know about stresses that may have triggered the symptom (Doleys, 1977). These may be events that we all would agree are or could well be stressful, such as an emergency appendectomy for the child, emergency surgery for a parent, death of a pet, death of a grandparent, or a move to a new home resulting in increased distance from bed to bathroom. Or, the stress might be something the adults in the child's life may not have perceived as a major stressor, but may well have been very stressful for the child and contributed to or triggered the symptom. These may include having been somehow embarrassed in school in front of the class, or not getting the part in the school play, or a friend moving away, or getting an unexpected lower grade on a homework assignment or examination, or any of a myriad of similar childhood life experiences. A model questionnaire for assessment of enuresis is presented in Appendix C.

Physical examination should endeavor to rule out the rare neurological etiologies of enuresis. Therefore, it is important to undertake a careful neurological assessment with emphasis on lower extremity muscle tone and strength, sensation, gait, and deep tendon reflexes. Examination of the spine and back, abdomen, external genitalia, and perineum is important. If concomitant soiling is present, it is crucial that a rectal examination be performed. Impacted stool present in the rectal ampulla might suggest constipation that is causally associated with enuresis. Poor anal sphincter tone or an abnormal anal wink response might suggest a neurological impairment The physician should also observe the urine stream of the child.

Each child presenting with the complaint of enuresis should have a urinalysis done. If there are symptoms or physical findings suggestive of a urinary tract infection, a urine culture, of course, should also be done. X-ray studies are not indicated unless physical findings suggest physical abnormalities.

General Management

Given the high incidence of enuresis and of its spontaneous remission/resolution, it seems logical that, in general, bedwetting should not be regarded as a major problem. Unfortunately, the perceptions of physicians, parents, and children often differ in defining when it is a problem; and sociocultural norms and expectations also play a role in whether this common and usually maturational phenomenon is experienced as a problem. If the youngster is less than 5 years old and has no historical or physical findings that suggest an underlying medical problem, then the possibility of developmental delay regarding nighttime urinary continence should be explained to the parents who may then accept patience as the most desirable approach. For children, bedwetting is usually regarded as a problem when the possibility of camp-outs or sleepovers develops. At this time the symptom may engender a sense of social incompetence and a feeling of being different from (or even teased by) siblings and peers.

If the parents and child wish treatment, it is important to agree on a plan that is acceptable to all parties involved, especially the child. Studies indicate that the most successful treatment methods are those reinforcing the child's own responsibility for success (Marshall, Marshall, & Richards, 1973; Schmitt, 1990). One such method is hypnotherapy.

A Hypnotherapeutic Approach

Initially we meet with the child and parents together. Statistics about the incidence of enuresis are presented along with a brief review of ideas concerning current understanding of cause. We routinely ask for the child's perception about the cause of the problem, as well as the parents' perceptions, in that order. Asking the child before the parents usually facilitates the elicitation of a more spontaneous and genuine response. We tend to frame this specifically by asking what they *wondered* might be the *reason* for the problem, or what went through their mind, rather than asking them specifically what they think was the "cause." Occasionally a child, particularly in the case of onset (secondary) enuresis, will recall some trigger event that the parents have not considered significant or even remembered.

It is our custom to focus an initial interview on obtaining a history of the presenting problem in the context of developing at least a beginning rapport with the child and family. Beyond knowing about the presenting problem, goals to be accomplished include that the child leave the first visit with (1) a feeling that he or she can trust us; (2) a belief that we are quite certain that we can be of help; (3) curiosity about what was said and in what ways we will be able to be of help; (4) a sense of having been believed, respected, and liked; (5) a beginning idea that he or she can have fun and get help at the same time. In an eclectic, often humor-based approach, an effort is made first and foremost to do what Milton Erickson said was critical in helping children, that is, to "go with the child." In trusting that the child knows best about his or her own problem, and in this case, his or her habit, questions regarding secondary gain can be asked directly and abruptly, often catching the child slightly "off guard," as such having the quality of "going directly to the unconscious," and in turn evoking a response likely to be quite honest. An example would be to ask a child with enuresis if he or she is going to miss the problem when it's gone. Perhaps predictably, most find this either confusing or amusing or both, and say, "NO, of course not!" Those who understand it and hesitate may in fact have more secondary gain than we realized, and that factor may need attention before focusing on further work on the enuresis.

We determine the child's words for urination and defecation. Anatomy is discussed with the aid of diagrams. While some like to use printed diagrams (e.g., from texts), we tend to draw a new picture like the one shown in Figure 8.1.

We believe that this personalized approach then becomes part of the therapeutic process, hopefully anchoring the rapport, increasing the focused attention, and as such facilitating understanding, interest, and commitment to creating change. We ask the child to review the diagram and our discussion about it before going to bed; and we may ask the child to bring a similar drawing for us at the time of the next visit, or to reproduce his or her own rendition of the drawing in the office as part of the next session. We explain that success will depend upon the child's involvement and commitment to practice self-hypnosis. We ask parents not to remind the child to practice, again emphasizing the child's responsibility in the treatment process. We give the parents a printed summary concerning enuresis and their part in the self-hypnosis treatment program, and ask them to leave, or prepare them for the fact that subsequent visits with their child will be in private.

In hypnotherapeutic sessions with children with enuresis, we discuss in detail the best time for practice of suggested exercises. It is usually not a good idea to practice just before bedtime if the child is very tired. We recommend practice just after dinner or an hour before bedtime. We review the path from bed to bathroom and sometimes have the child draw us a map of this path. We encourage the child to decide on a specific reminder to themselves for practice of self-hypnosis (e.g., a string around the toothbrush handle, ribbon around the neck of a favorite stuffed toy, sign on the door or the wall). We emphasize that the bladder is a muscle and that the patient has previously learned control of many muscles, such as in the many muscles required to ride a two-wheeler bicycle (Kohen, 1990). We also use the analogy of the therapist being the coach asking the patient to practice muscle control, thereby further placing ultimate responsibility on the child.

We proceed to ask the child to explain likes and dislikes, such as hobbies, interests, favorite colors, favorite videos or computer games, or favorite dreams. We then choose an induction method that seems appropriate. Following the induction, we often ask the child to show us a "yes" finger and a "no" finger, and then ask a series of questions, most irrelevant, such as "Do you like the color purple?" or "Do you like to eat chocolate ice cream?" and without changing pace, insert the question "Would you like to have all dry beds?" or "Are you ready to work on solving the problem of wet beds

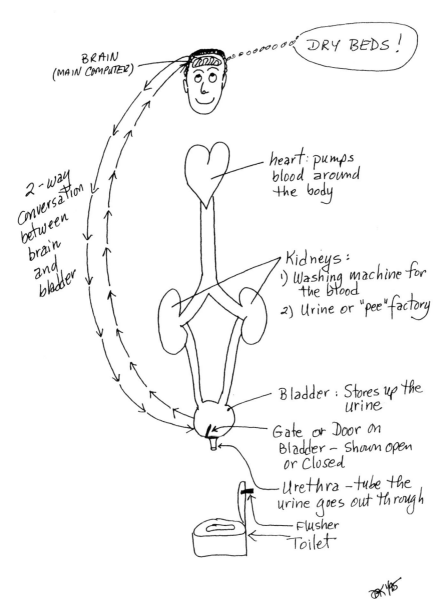

FIGURE 8.1. Simplified diagram of physiology and anatomy of urination for use with children with enuresis (see text).

today?" If the answer is "no," as it is occasionally, this suggests that the child may be receiving significant secondary gain from the problem (e.g., being allowed to get into bed with parents when own bed is wet), or simply that there is not sufficient motivation to work on the problem at this time.

Following a "yes" response, we ask the child to imagine being in a favorite place and to signal a "yes" when ready to give instructions to his or her bladder. At this point, we might say something like:

> "Tell yourself that you will sleep well tonight. Tell your bladder to send a message to your brain to awaken you when it is full of urine [or 'pee']. When you awaken, tell yourself to get out of your dry bed, walk across the room, through the door, down the hall to the bathroom, turn on the light, urinate in the toilet, turn the light off, return to your dry bed, and go back to sleep. Then think of yourself awakening in a dry bed, and go back to sleep. Then think of yourself awakening in a dry bed, knowing you will have a good day. Enjoy knowing your bed is dry because of your efforts, because you're the boss of your bladder muscle. Enjoy the good feeling of waking up in a dry bed as long as you like. Then, before you finish this nice imagination practice which you are doing so well, remind yourself that every time you practice this it gets easier and easier to do, and you get better and better at teaching yourself to wake up every day in a nice, dry bed. Then when you're ready, you can open your eyes and enjoy the rest of the day."

Both during the last portion of the hypnotic trance and after return to the usual state of alertness, the child is encouraged and engaged in a commitment to practice this self-hypnosis exercise daily. We have described similar approaches with the addition of multiple Ericksonian strategies including double-bind suggestions, metaphors for control, dissociative suggestions (e.g., for *that* bladder and *that* brain talking to each other), positive expectancy, and reframing (Kohen, 1990).

In general the initial visit takes from 45 to 60 minutes. Depending on the individual child and his or her history, a hypnosis exercise may or may not be taught at the first visit. If the complexity of the history or child/family circumstances suggest to the clinician's judgment or intuition that hypnotic rapport may take a bit longer, then formal hypnosis training as described may be deferred to the next or a subsequent visit when the child in his or her relationship with the therapist is determined to be in a readiness to learn. At a minimum, however, our first visit always includes teaching about how the body works, a commitment to keep track of numbers of dry beds at home, and a commitment to "just think about" the communication between brain and bladder prior to the next visit. Subsequent visits are tailored to the particular child. Many older children do very well after a couple of visits, and are followed by letter and phone. Younger children sometimes seem to require more professional reinforcement and may have return visits every 2 weeks for several months' time. We ask most children, and particular younger ones, to keep calendars or cumulative graphs of their successes. After termination of in-person office visits, we ask the children to mail in their calendars on a monthly basis for several months. This process of continued communication appears to be of multipurpose value in (1) providing the continuing "anchor" through connection with the clinician "coach," as such, (2) easing the termination process of a usually very positive, intimate therapeutic relationship, and (3) facilitating ongoing ego strengthening through reinforcement of the self-monitoring, practice, and self-regulation process.

Observations about Special Cases

• Occasionally, children do better with an audio cassette tape prepared during a regular office-visit hypnotherapy practice session. Ordinarily we wish to wait until the child has demonstrated understanding of and some facility with self-hypnosis practice before making a tape for home use. In theory this is to avoid or reduce the possibility of developing (complete) dependency on the clinician, and to reinforce the concept that what "happens" with hypnotherapy is both because of and inside of the child and not because of the therapist alone or the tape. Children are asked to listen to their tape each evening or to alternate practicing on their own and with the tape. We do not know any way to predict which children can benefit most from such audiotapes.

• Occasionally, children as young as 4 years old will do very well in spite of our belief and concern that many are not physiologically capable of nighttime bladder control. In one case, a therapist refused to work with a 4-year-old, saying he was "too young," but she did work with his 6-year-old brother. A week later they returned, and in the interim the 6-year-old had taught the 4-year-old, and both were dry. We have seen similar unexpected and unpredictable outcomes among other sibling pairs.

• We have worked with siblings concurrently up to a maximum of five in a single family. The siblings seem to reinforce each other in these situations, although most siblings prefer to be seen separately. From time to time even being seen separately by the same therapist can be problematic, and the clinician must be mindful of, and creative about, managing potential differential success and the risk of negative consequences of competition between and among siblings.

• A mother who is also a nurse adapted what she called the "quarter trick" (coin induction) from an article on treatment of enuresis with self-hypnosis. Her son, age 6½ years, had never had a dry bed. After 5 days of practice, he had no further wet beds. Generally, however, the process goes less well if parents teach, reinforce, or are otherwise involved in a process that we believe should be largely the child's to practice and master. Several physician–parents have reported total failures in working with their own children who then are able to do well when referred to a nonrelative for hypnotherapy.

• Occasionally, children relapse after more than 1 year of dry beds. When they review self-hypnosis, they usually recapture control quickly and easily, often after only one or two such reviews.

• Occasionally children who fail with self-hypnosis exercises will move on to use one of the several available alarm systems with rapid success. Sometimes when children will ask for our assistance in maximizing their use of alarm systems, we offer suggestions for integrating the alarm into a hypnotic approach (or the hypnotherapy into the alarm approach). One such simple suggestion is to ask the child to give him- or herself a challenging message during self-hypnosis, such as "Tonight while I'm sleeping, bladder, when you fill up with urine be sure and send the message to the brain that you're full, and brain, be sure and keep the gate on the bladder shut until you wake me up so I can get out of my dry bed, walk to the bathroom, open the bladder gate, and let the pee out in the toilet where it belongs. Brain, be sure and do that right so you can BEAT THE BUZZER, wake me up before the buzzer does." In general, we believe that self-hypnosis emphasizes more self-control than does the alarm. At present we have no way to predict which children will benefit most from hypnotherapy and which from some other form of treatment.

Results of Hypnotherapy

There are several published accounts of successful use of hypnotherapy with children with enuresis. Some are single case reports (L. Jacobs, 1962; Olness & Gardner, 1978; Tilton, 1980). Solovey and Milechnin (1959) described their hypnotherapeutic approach to the problem but presented no data concerning results.

Collison (1970) employed hypnotherapy with 9 children, ages 9 to 16 years, with onset (secondary) enuresis. Treatment lasted 6 to 20 weeks and included direct suggestion, ego-strengthening methods, and insight therapy. All nine children achieved dry beds and remained dry during follow-up lasting 1 to 5 years.

Baumann and Hinman (1974) reported improvement in 64 of 73 boys ages 7 to 13 years with enuresis who were treated with hypnotherapy in combination with imipramine and other medical management, parental instruction, and monetary rewards for dry beds. Duration of treatment and duration of follow-up were not reported.

While at George Washington University, Olness (1975) taught self-hypnosis to 40 children with enuresis, ages 4 to 16 years. Treatment focused on direct suggestions that the children were asked to review daily. Parental involvement was minimal. Of the 40 children, 31 resolved their bedwetting, most within the first month of treatment. Six others improved. Of three children who did not improve, one said he did not want dry beds and was experiencing significant secondary gain from his symptom. A second child refused to practice self-hypnosis at home. The third child had significant urological anomalies that had required surgery. The successful children required no more than two visits before improvement was apparent. Follow-up lasted 6 to 28 months. No concurrent medications were employed.

Stanton (1979) included background music along with a variety of hypnotic techniques in his treatment of 28 children with enuresis, ages 7 to 18 years. After one to three sessions, 20 children stopped wetting. Of these, 15 remained dry after 1-year follow-up. The five who relapsed were among the younger children. Characteristics of the eight who did not improve were not described.

Edwards and van der Spuy (1985) reported a study of 48 boys, ages 8 to 13 years, with enuresis who were randomly assigned to four treatment conditions: no intervention, trance plus suggestions, suggestions without trance, and trance alone without suggestions. One difficulty in interpreting this study relates to the high frequency of secondary or onset enuresis (50%) in this group. This raises the possibility, for example, that stool retention was a cause of enuresis in the secondary group. Groups were not matched for this variable. In this study, suggestions for trance with or without suggestions were given through headphones, and suggestions were tape-recorded. These were aimed at general tension reduction and enhancement of self-confidence and contained suggestions for (1) increased bladder capacity, (2) reduction of fluids before bedtime, (3) visiting the toilet before bedtime, and (4) awakening at night to go to the toilet if the bladder was full. The authors found that subjects responded equally well whether they received trance plus suggestions or suggestions alone. Those who received trance alone or no treatment showed no changes over the initial 6-week treatment period. Those who received trance induction, however, improved only to the level of the other intervention groups by the second 6-week follow-up interval. At 6 months, the nontreatment group averaged three dry nights per week, and the treatment groups averaged between four and five dry nights per week. The authors noted a greater relapse among those with secondary enuresis. The results of this study are consistent with other studies related to self-regulation of autonomic responses in children; that is, formal trance induction is not essential for suggestions to be effective. It is possible that poorer response in those with onset enuresis is related to unrecognized stool retention; or, perhaps to some other as yet unrecognized biological problem.

Kohen and associates (1984) reviewed data for 257 children with enuresis treated at the Behavioral Pediatrics Program at Minneapolis Children's Medical Center.* In all, 44% achieved complete dryness, defined as 30 consecutive dry beds and requiring a 12-month follow-up without relapse. Another 31% showed significant improvement. Most children referred had already tried two or three other treatment methods, including an alarm system, imipramine, and other drugs. Failures related primarily to lack of motivation on the part of the child and excessive involvement by parents. For example, if parents said, "We had two dry beds last week," preempting the child's own personalized report, failure was likely. If parents reminded children to practice their self-hypnosis exercises, progress was much slower. Many parents would say, "I know I shouldn't, but I can't help it." In these cases, further exploration of the parent–child relationship and/or family counseling was sometimes useful.

A recent study (Banerjee, Srivastav, & Palan, 1993) compared treatment with hypnotherapy to treatment with imipramine in two groups (25 children each) of children with enuresis, ages 5 to 16 years. Comparable results were found between groups after 3 months of treatment, with 76% of the imipramine group and 72% of the hypnosis group achieving positive responses (as defined by all dry beds or decreased frequency of wetting). After 3 months of treatment and reinforcement, imipramine was discontinued, and active follow-up visits were discontinued for both groups, while the hypnosis group were encouraged to continue self-hypnosis practice. At subsequent follow-up 6 months later, only 24% of the imipramine group had maintained a positive response, whereas in the hypnosis group, 68% had maintained a positive response, without clinical reinforcement. In an interesting finding, the authors note that in children under age 7 years hypnosis was less effective than imipramine after 3 months of treatment. Six of seven children treated with imipramine had a positive response, whereas only two of eight in this age group treated with hypnosis had a positive response. It is unclear from the author's report whether any of the children in this age group either ultimately became dry (in the hypnosis group) or were in the smaller group (24%) who sustained dryness (in the imipramine group) at the 9-month follow-up. As the authors note, methodological considerations limit the generalizability of these results and are important for future studies. In addition to random selection/group assignment, such comparative studies should consider designs that include a group or groups receiving equal time and attention to the groups receiving hypnotherapy or other treatment approaches, and/or include a group learning hypnosis (e.g., mental imagery and relaxation) without receiving specific hypnotic suggestions for enuresis control.

---

*The Behavioral Pediatrics Program is now based at the University of Minnesota. Minneapolis Children's Medical Center is now Children's Health Care–Minneapolis.

Measuring hypnotizability with the Stanford Hypnotic Clinical Scale for Children (SHCS-C), the authors found no difference in responsivity between the imipramine treatment and the hypnosis-treated groups.

Two studies (Kohen et al., 1984; Stanton, 1979) concluded that hypnotherapy is not likely to help children with enuresis if there is not marked improvement over the first three or four sessions. Prolonging treatment rarely produces gains commensurate with the investment of time and money involved, unless the focus has shifted to dealing with family dilemmas and associated parent/family counseling.

SOILING

Evaluation and Medical Management

The symptom of soiling in a child past usual toilet training age represents constipation until proved otherwise. Pure encopresis (soiling without stool retention) is rare, although parents will often insist that their child's symptoms do not represent constipation (Fleisher, 1976; M. D. Levine, 1982). The presence of primary fecal incontinence in association with urine incontinence should lead the examiner to suspect a neurological problem. Occasionally, a congenital defect (e.g., spinal dysraphism) will not manifest itself by symptoms of fecal and/or urinary incontinence until the child is 5 or 6 years of age (Anderson, 1975).

Much emphasis has been placed on the psychological concomitants of fecal incontinence (Clayden & Lawson, 1976; Halpern, 1977). There is no doubt that many secondary emotional problems develop in a child with this symptom, but the original cause is more often physical than psychological. It is important to note that psychotherapy, while often indicated for the ego damage caused by soiling, cannot unblock a stuffed colon! Practitioners may reflexly send a child with fecal incontinence to a mental health professional before undertaking a complete evaluation. Inasmuch as secondary emotional effects are common and may be profound, and inasmuch as the ongoing stress of chronicity and relapses are trying for the patient and the family, we emphasize, as do others (Buchanan & Clayden, 1992), that the initial evaluation should be carefully focused and comprehensive to prevent misconceptions about causation and treatment from contributing inadvertently to chronicity. Thus, the following information is essential before undertaking treatment:

• *How often and when does the child soil?* Children with underlying constipation are likely to soil several times a day, whereas the purely encopretic child may have a normal bowel movement once a day into a place other than the toilet.

• *Does anyone else in the family have bowel problems?* This question is important with respect to the vaguely defined entity of familial constipation, which may reflect family eating habits, or intrinsic slow motility. The question may aid in assessment of the family focus on bowel function and expectancies with respect to outcome.

• *What was the child's stool pattern in early infancy?* Constipation in early infancy may be present in the case of congenital aganglionoses (Nixon, 1964) or in the irritable colon syndrome described by Davidson and Wasserman (1966).

• *How was the child fed in early infancy?* Feeding habits established in infancy may potentiate later constipation. For example, continuation of large amounts of cow's milk into the second year of life may contribute to constipation.

• *Was there any change in diet, family constellation, caretaker, or bathroom options around the onset of constipation?* Frequently one finds that, just prior to onset of bowel problems the family moved and the bathroom changed, or the family went camping and the child didn't like outdoor toilets, or the child had a febrile illness and was dehydrated, following which he or she had a hard, painful stool, or the child suddenly began drinking an extra quart of milk a day.

• *Ask the parents to describe the child's accidents.* Information concerning size and appearance of stool aids in determining whether or not there is constipation with overflow soiling or pure encopresis. Overflow stools tend to be runny and small in amount. Occasionally, particularly after an enema or suppository, the stool of a chronically constipated child will plug the toilet.

• *Is the child taking any medicines?* Certain medications such as imipramine, codeine, and Ritalin are constipating, and their use must be considered in any management plan (Fleisher, 1976). Occasionally, parents or physicians misinterpret the problems as diarrhea and inadvertently prescribe kaopectate, which will increase the problem.

• *Has the child complained of tingling, numbness, or funny feelings in his or her legs? Is there poor coordination?* It is important to look into the possibility of lower extremity paresthesias that might suggest the presence of spinal dysraphism.

With respect to planning management, it is important to know how the child currently handles the problem, how siblings and schoolmates respond, what interventions have been tried and how they work, and what the family believes to be the cause of the soiling.

A thorough evaluation requires that a physical examination be done and that this include a careful neurological examination as well as abdominal palpation. A rectal examination is reasonable in the context of a positive rapport between the clinician and patient and after careful preparation of the child for this portion of the examination. If the examination does not confirm constipation, it may be necessary to obtain X-rays of the abdomen in order to determine whether or not stool is present, or in excess. A diagnostic anal manometry may be indicated if there is a question of rectal aganglionoses. Thyroid function tests should be done if there are any signs of hypothyroidism. If history and physical examination uncover occult spinal dysraphism or aganglionoses or hypothyroidism or other conditions requiring specific treatment, these conditions must be treated.

If a diagnosis of constipation with overflow soiling is made—as it commonly is (Buchanan & Clayden, 1992)—appropriate intervention is as follows:

1. Anatomy should be explained carefully, with the aid of drawings.
2. Mechanical problems associated with prolonged retention should be carefully explained.
3. If the patient currently has significant retention, a series of enemas for thorough evacuation should be prescribed.
4. Concurrently, the diet should be regulated. Dietary changes should be explained in detail to the child with emphasis on graduated re-entry of proscribed foods (e.g., milk, apples, bananas, rice, Jell-O, carrots) after a period of 4 to 6 weeks.
5. Unprocessed bran, or another high-fiber supplement, should be added twice daily to the child's diet.
6. The child should make a commitment to choose to sit on the toilet either after breakfast for 10 minutes or after supper for 10 minutes. This decision should be communicated to the parents.
7. In the initial period some enemas may need to be given. It is recommended that an enema be given every 48 hours if the child has not voluntarily defecated. If this rule is broken, the ultimate curative process is only delayed by the continued excessive stretching of the lower colon.

Hypnotherapy

Fleisher (1976) and Buchanan and Clayden (1992) have stressed the need for children to be given responsibility in treatment of soiling. Conventional medical and surgical management do not do this. Hypnotherapy, alone, in patients who have had the problem for many years is unlikely to affect the mechanical components. It does, however, give the child personal responsibility and the opportunity to remain in control of his or her bowels while eliminating an undesirable habit. Parents as well as children can benefit from greater understanding of the problems connected with soiling, and a workbook has been produced by the Behavioral Pediatrics Program of the Minneapolis Children's Medical Center (now Children's Health Care–Minneapolis) (Owens-Stively, McCain, & Wynne, 1986) to enable parents, physicians, and children to work together. We ask parents to refrain from reminding the child to practice self-hypnosis exercises, however, and to indicate in their praise of the child's successes that they know that their child was responsible for the happy and proud outcome.

Some children with long-standing soiling will continue to have some residual soiling, although they learn to defecate regularly. This problem may be due to long-term stretching of the anorectal sphincters.

The Behavioral Pediatrics Program at Minneapolis Children's Medical Center (now Children's Health Care–Minneapolis) offered biofeedback training of the anorectal sphincters to some of these children (Olness, 1977a). In one unpublished study from this center, 10 children from a self-hypnosis therapy group were matched with 10 children from a biofeedback group. The 20 children had each had previous medical evaluation and treatment for soiling. Children in the self-hypnosis group were taught to practice suggestions that they could keep anal muscles closed except when in the bathroom for defecation, that they could be physically and mentally comfortable and relaxed during defecation, and that they could enjoy future anticipated events without worrying about soiling. Of the children in the self-hypnosis group, there were two failures of which one was a relapse some months after doing well with self-hypnosis. This child was moved into biofeedback training and did well. In the biofeedback group there was one failure, a 4-year-old boy who seemed not to focus on the machine or his muscle control and showed no improvement after three visits. It was elected to discontinue further efforts until he was older while maintaining diet and enemas as necessary. He was matched to a 4-year-old who did extremely well using self-hypnosis. In this retrospective analysis of 20 patients, the median time from onset of biofeedback or self-hypnosis practice to dramatic improvement was 1 week in the biofeedback group and 1 month in the self-hypnosis group.

Prospective studies of hypnosis, biofeedback, and other self-regulation processes for encopresis are required. These findings may be the tip of an enormous iceberg. Common features of both self-hypnosis and biofeedback include encouragement and positive reinforcement. Some of the biofeedback subjects spontaneously reported feelings of relaxation and comfort while practicing the biofeedback exercises. These observations and results suggest several questions: Does the direct visual feedback in biofeedback sessions make it easier for children to comprehend what they must do for themselves as they sit on the toilet? Does the oscilloscope serve as a better induction of hypnosis (i.e., the equivalent of an eye-fixation technique) than verbal communication alone? Do the two together offer the potential of a cumulative benefit better than either one alone? Do both procedures stimulate and evoke imagery that becomes the reality of the bowel control that follows? Clearly, we have much to learn about the relationship between biofeedback and hypnotherapy as they relate to habit disorders.

In some clinical reports, hypnotherapy has been directed at dynamic issues with little or no attention paid to the need for medical management. While in such cases there may be improvement, the problem is rarely fully resolved.

Goldsmith (1962) described hypnotherapy with a 9-year-old girl with constipation who soiled herself several times each day. The poor bowel control was interpreted as an unconscious expression of aggression toward the mother, and hypnotherapy was directed at understanding these underlying issues, as well as including direct suggestions for symptom relief. The child was told in hypnosis that she would not be able to eliminate until she was actually sitting on the toilet. In the next week the child had no major "accidents," but experienced continuous seepage. Medical aspects of the problem were still not addressed, and the seepage was again interpreted as an expression of hostility toward the mother. Further dynamic hypnotherapy resulted in some improvement, but the child continued to have "an occasional lapse," again thought to represent hostility.

Silber (1968) did distinguish between soiling based on mechanical problems and encopresis, which he defined as psychologically motivated soiling. He employed hypnotherapy in combination with enemas with nine encopretic children, ages 5 to 9 years. Treatment, which lasted approximately three sessions, helped the child focus on anthropomorphic images related to defecation, such as the anal sphincter as an intelligent watchman. Dynamic issues were then dealt with only through these images; and all nine children were reported as cured.

Olness (1976) reported successful hypnotherapeutic treatment of four children with functional megacolon, of whom three were in the 3- to 5-year-old range. All were taught self-hypnosis and gave themselves daily suggestions regarding their ability to control their bowels in appropriate ways. Olness concluded that success was chiefly the result of the children being given responsibility for their own solution. Parents were involved only to the extent that they praised the child for improvement and reinforced emerging feelings of mastery.

SPEECH AND VOICE PROBLEMS

Stuttering

The problem of stuttering has been described from many perspectives, with treatment approaches derived from presumed neurological, educational, and psychological causes. Hypnotherapy has been found to be a helpful adjunct in the context of differing treatment approaches. A key factor in success may be the children's feelings of mastery and confidence in the hypnotherapeutic relationship. Published accounts consist of technical considerations, with isolated case reports (W. E. Moore, 1946; Falck, 1964; Silber, 1973). Silber (1973) utilized fairy tales, folklore, and symbols to help children who stutter get in touch with potential verbal fluency and self-esteem and to strengthen their ability to cope effectively with environmental stress. He used his own imaginative skills to engage the child's creative abilities in working toward a solution to the problem.

We have worked with several latency-aged children (8–12 years old) with stuttering who continued to have daily stuttering difficulties, despite years of appropriate speech therapy. As with so many people with these difficulties, their stuttering was worse during times of stress. Hypnotic approaches were geared both to creating increased internal awareness of fluency and to the modulation, control, and coping with stress. In each of the children we have seen with stuttering, their stuttering definitively and dramatically decreased or disappeared during hypnosis. Though this was a source of joy and pride and was accordingly able to be utilized as a positive affect bridge to "bring the fluent, smooth speech back with you to your usual state of mind and alertness," none made this ultimate transition with any consistency, and each gave up on the hypnotic strategy much as they had on other treatments that had helped them "a little" or "for a while."

Defects of Articulation

Silber's (1973) hypnotherapeutic approach to children with significant articulation problems again focused on imaginative use of fairy tales, folklore, and symbols. He described his successful work with a 10-year-old boy, seen for 26 sessions over a period of 18 weeks. The child continued to speak clearly 2 years later. Silber concluded that success was related to the fact that the "patient is committed by cooperation and participation in a creative endeavor of the imagination" (p. 281).

Voice Problems

Laguaite (1976) reported her hypnotherapeutic treatment of 18 children, ages 4 to 10 years, with deviant voices, usually associated with excessive shouting. In some cases, the problem was related to vocal nodules or hypertrophy of the vocal bands. Five children had normal larynges, and two could not be visualized adequately. Three children did not complete the course of treatment. For the remaining 15, hypnotherapy focused on encouraging the patients not to yell so much, ego strengthening, and insight-oriented techniques. Of these 15, all but two showed improvement in the appearance of the larynx or the complete disappearance of the nodules. Laquaite noted that another group of children, treated for nodules without hypnotherapy, also showed improvement but required an average of 14 sessions of treatment as opposed to only 10 sessions for the hypnotherapy group.

More recently Gildston and Gildston (1992) reported their hypnotherapeutic treatment of two children, an 8-year-old girl and a 12-year-old boy with voice disorders secondary to recurring juvenile laryngeal papillomatosis, caused by the human papillomavirus. In both cases the use of hypnotic strategies had multiple foci; these were to retard regress, or prevent recurrence of the papilloma(s), to facilitate vocal techniques, and to improve vocal function. In the 8-year-old girl, the papillomas diminished considerably after seven sessions and were almost gone by the 16th session; either they diminished spontaneously as these are known to do 50% of the time, or in response to hypnotic suggestion. The 12-year-old boy had had multiple surgical procedures for juvenile laryngeal papillomas between the ages of 3 and 9 years; his voice was sharply reduced in pitch and loudness and thought of as annoyingly hoarse and breathy with speech which was very difficult to understand. Hypnosis was used in an intermittent and integrated fashion with voice rehabilitation therapy. After 2 months of treatment, he was described as having achieved significant improvement in the office setting, though carryover into conversational speech was sporadic. The authors concluded that, for these two children, hypnotherapy was an excellent approach for increasing motivation and speeding up the acquisition of vocal skills.

One of our patients was an 11-year-old boy who had swallowed lye at age 21 months and subsequently underwent numerous surgical procedures. He had not spoken normally since esophageal surgery at age 9 years. When asked questions in the therapist's office, the patient whispered answers. In the preliminary conversation, he said that fishing was one of his favorite pastimes and that he looked forward to being able to sing when he recaptured his voice. He was told that there may have been a temporary organic cause of his loss of voice, such as swelling around the vocal cords associated with surgery, and perhaps he had continued to whisper as a habit. His mother said that she believed this because she had heard him speak aloud in his sleep. At the first visit, the boy learned progressive relaxation, synchronized with breathing. He then imagined himself in a favorite place. He later reported that while imagining himself in a favorite place, he went fishing and caught three walleye pike. Following the therapist's request, he then recalled a time in the past when he was enjoying singing a particular favorite song, and he carried this forward to a time in the future when he could imagine himself singing the same song aloud. He appeared very relaxed throughout the 15-minute exercise. He was asked to review it at home twice daily.

The patient returned 1 week later. After review of progressive relaxation and favorite place imagery, he visualized a calendar going backwards week by week. He used previously arranged ideomotor signals to indicate that the problem leading to his loss of voice occurred in September 1977. As the therapist described moving from week 3 to 2 in September, he coughed, had a choking expression, and tensed his left hand. Asked to return to this favorite place, he reviewed the suggestions of the first visit. In checking records of his outpatient visits to the surgeon's office, it was noted that he was seen by the surgeon on September 15, 1977, with a chart notation of "surgery to follow."

The third visit occurred 2 weeks later. The parents reported that they now heard the boy speak in a normal voice interspersed with whispering. At this visit he reviewed the progressive relaxation and favorite place imagery. He was taught the clenched fist technique (Stein, 1963) as a device for letting go of something that might be bothering him and related to the vocal loss. Following this he was asked to describe his favorite place, and he said "fishing" in a normal voice. He was encouraged to speak immediately following relaxation exercises at home and was asked to call the therapist when his voice returned.

He called 2 weeks later to say that he could speak again, but he would like to come for an additional visit. He explained that he heard himself singing loudly as he completed one of his relaxation exercises. His mother confirmed, "He's talking and doesn't need to come back, but he wants to come back once more." His mother said he was very happy after school on the day following the return of his voice. He said, "School is more fun when you can talk." However, on the second day he returned home saying, "Talking can get you into trouble." At follow-up 4 months later, he continued to speak normally.

INTRACTABLE COUGH

Many children develop cough habits that are annoying to parents, teachers, and peers and may become the focus of frustration eventuating sometimes in blame, reprimand, punishment, and ongoing conflict. Although such cough habits often represent prolongation of a response to an infectious or allergic disease, results of thorough (or even overexhaustive) evaluations typically show no evidence of underlying reactive airways disease or other physical causes. As contrasted with asthma patients who may have "nighttime cough variant asthma," children with this problem typically stop coughing during sleep. Although many children may obtain secondary gain by having to miss certain classes at school or stay home, there is no particular psychological profile that characterizes such youngsters. As with most habits, it is likely that the preceding illness or problem—like an allergy or a respiratory infection—provided the children and adolescents with an (unconscious) model for the symptom, which then became self-perpetuating. A review of the literature (Gay et al., 1987) reported follow-up information on 24 pediatrics patients with habit cough who were treated successfully with some type of suggestion therapy, 23 of whom were cough-free 1 year later. In most, successful treatment was evident even within a few days of beginning treatment.

We have noted hypnotic strategies to be very effective in helping young people with cough habits to help themselves (Kohen & Olness, 1987). The following demonstrates an approach to this problem. A 13-year-old patient was referred to us by a pediatrician for a trial of self-hypnosis in treatment of a cough that had been present for 6 months. Three months after onset of the cough, the patient was hospitalized for a bronchoscopy, the results of which were normal. He also had normal pediatric and psychological evaluations and negative allergy tests. The patient and his mother associated the onset of the cough with the time when he helped his father with a soybean harvest. He and the therapist discussed the possibility that the cough may have begun as a response to inhaled irritants from the harvest dust and had later become an annoying habit. The therapist drew diagrams of anatomy, the bronchial tree, and the cough reflex. She also explored, at length the patient's interests, hobbies, likes, and dislikes, noting that he especially enjoyed bicycle riding.

The patient was approached from the perspective of symptom relief to be achieved through daily practice of a self-hypnosis exercise. Self-induction used backward counting followed by imagining a favorite place and then increasing relaxation by imagining a long bicycle ride. When he felt relaxed, he was asked to focus on the image of his bronchial tree and cough reflex and to suggest cessation of the cough to himself. He also focused on future anticipated happy events that he could enjoy without the cough. During the exercise he did not cough. The patient practiced the exercise twice daily for 1 week and returned for a follow-up visit. He reported having no severe coughing episodes since the last visit and said he was sleeping without coughing interruptions. He continued practice for an additional month. Subsequently, the mother sent a letter which said that the patient was doing fine, and she thought his symptoms had been "like those of a virus."

GIGGLE MICTURITION

Although rare, this entity is seen occasionally by physicians and may represent a conditioned reflex as demonstrated in the following case histories.

A 14-year-old boy was referred for the problem of giggle micturition. Although he was popular among his peers and a good student, he was embarrassed by the problem of urinating whenever he laughed. His mother believed the problem had its origins in toilet training when she discovered that he would urinate if she tickled him. The patient had been evaluated by several urologists and pediatricians without improvement.

During the first visit, the boy used diagrams to understand urinary tract anatomy and bladder reflexes. After he had agreed to practice twice daily, he was taught a relaxation–imagery exercise. He relaxed by focusing on a favorite place of his choosing and also used imagery of stair descent to increase the depth of relaxation. He was asked to give himself suggestions for bladder control and to imagine himself in a laugh-provoking situation in which he could laugh freely without concurrent urination.

At the second visit 1 week later, he stated he was much improved and very pleased with his progress. He stated that he had "lost a few drops of urine" only three times while laughing. At the third visit, 2 weeks after the second, he reported only one accident.

Subsequent follow-up was by phone over the next 4 months. He was completely dry. Five months after his last call, his mother called saying he had no accidents in school but occasionally wet during group outings. He was no longer practicing the relaxation-imagery exercise. The mother was told that since he had solved the primary problem of control during school, perhaps he did not regard the residual problem as serious enough to warrant further practice. The mother was asked not to encourage him to return for therapy unless he made the request.

He returned for an additional visit 3 months later with the report that he laughed frequently and had had no accidents of any kind during the preceding 4 weeks. He spoke of his plans to become a lawyer or psychiatrist, his plans to go to summer camp, and of his recent honor grades in geometry. Follow-up over the subsequent year indicated no recurrence of giggle micturition.

A 14-year-old young woman with mild mental retardation and moderately severe speech and hearing problems was referred to Behavioral Pediatrics for help with "daytime and nighttime wetting." At the time of referral, she and her mother reported (and later recorded) a starting dryness rate of approximately 40% to 50% at night and 20% in the daytime. Thus, about 5 to 6 days a week she would have some daytime urinary accidents, and about 3 days a week she would wet the bed at night. A detailed history revealed that daytime wetting occurred most commonly when she would become involved in prolonged "laughing jags" with friends during school recess, or when "roughhousing," wrestling with her teen-age brother at home. Her mother repeatedly reassured us that the brother and sister were "very close" and the wrestling was "all in good fun." She was very embarrassed, especially by the daytime wetting. Her mother reported that pediatricians and urologists had found no physical reason for the problem; and psychologists who had followed her development suggested that the ongoing problem was related to her neuromaturational problems, and a function of inattentiveness and unawareness of "social cues."

The focus of the first visit was to develop a relationship with and assess communication abilities of this young girl. To assess understanding, motivation, and the potential role of secondary gain, she was asked directly, "Would it be okay to have dry pants every day and a dry bed every night?" and she became very excited and said, "YES!" with a broad smile. Toward the end of the first visit, a simple diagram of urinary tract anatomy and communication between the bladder and the brain was drawn. In the midst of education about the manner in which the bladder lets the brain know when it's full, she jumped up, much as a 5- or 6-year-old might, and said, "I have to go to the bathroom!" and ran out of the room, making it to the bathroom without an accident. Her mother was astonished and said that that was the first time she had ever seen her react and respond so abruptly to the need to urinate. She agreed to the simple request to "take this picture home, put it on your wall, and every night before bed just think in your inside thinking about how the bladder sends messages to the brain and the brain tells the bladder what to do, when you're awake and laughing, and when you're asleep" as well as to keep track of dry days and nights. By the second visit, 2 weeks later, nighttime dryness was improved to 70% and by the third visit 2 weeks after that, daytime dryness had improved to about 30% of days. A matter-of-fact, Ericksonian approach was utilized for reinforcement with emphasis on "being so grown up" ego strengthening and adding a more formal imagery exercise of "doing your thinking with your eyes closed sometimes." Nocturnal enuresis resolved completely over the next several months. Daytime accidents seemingly related to "not paying attention to the need to urinate" decreased steadily and after a year of monthly visits, these had decreased to no more than one to two per month. Although the giggle micturition component has been the slowest to respond, at the 18-month followup (now bimonthly), she and her mother reported only one occasion of giggle micturition during a major laughing episode at summer camp. She is proud of now being able to be tickled by her brother without urinating and enjoys "faking him out" this way.

HAIR PULLING, NAIL BITING, THUMB-SUCKING

These habits may have their origins in anxiety, emulation of a peer or an adult role model, or unsatisfied oral needs. They are nonlethal, of little physical medical significance (unless a child should ingest parasites, bacteria, or viruses in the course of biting or sucking), but they are exceedingly annoying to observers and often to the patients themselves as they develop increasing feelings of helplessness around their ability to resolve the habit. Frequent reminding from parents and resistance in the child may lead to significant family problems. The use of hypnotherapy for these problems may provide an acceptable way out.

As is true in the management of all habit problems, it is useful to structure intervention in such a way that the child's confidence, sense of personal responsibility, and mastery are reinforced. The initial interview should be structured in similar fashion to those related to problems such as enuresis and soiling. We emphasize that the original cause for the problem may no longer be important because the child is older and sees things in a different perspective. At the same time, however, we recognize that for some children the original circumstances may still be important to discuss and resolve. This must, of course, be individually assessed.

After discussion about the child's interests, likes, and dislikes, we plan an appropriate self-hypnosis exercise. Given the importance of comfort and rapport for the evolution of a successful hypnotherapeutic relationship, hypnosis would not ordinarily be taught until a second or subsequent visit, though occasionally rapport will develop rapidly, and therapist and child alike will be ready to do hypnosis at a first visit.

Following induction of hypnosis, the child is taught use of ideomotor signals and asked questions related to desire to be rid of the habit, desired rate of progress, and other details. If it is evident that the child wishes to proceed, we ask the child to devise an appropriate suggestion. These may be variations of the following:

"Whenever your hand begins to lift toward your hair or your mouth, move it instead to the other hand and give yourself a little pat for not pulling, sucking, or biting."

"Whenever your hand begins to lift, tell yourself that you can feel as comfortable as you do in your favorite place — as you do now — without any need to bite or suck or pull."

"Whenever *that* hand [dissociative suggestion] begins to lift, let that be the signal to *that other hand* to lift up and come over to help it and say, 'I'll be your friend, I'll help you' as it gently helps it down again."

"At the close of your exercise, tell yourself to sit down with a clock and suck each finger for 5 minutes in order to treat them fairly." [This often results in rapid extinguishing of the symptom.]

"You will bite all fingers but your thumb nails. When they grow out, you will let your pointer finger nails grow out" [and so forth in sequence until all are grown].

"And the final suggestion is to *see yourself without the symptom* buying nail polish and putting it on your lovely nails; hearing your friends admire your nails and color of nail polish; seeing a baby sucking his thumb and wishing you could help him the way you helped yourself; going on a trip and thinking, 'I don't suck my thumb anymore'; looking in the mirror of your mind and seeing yourself a little older, maybe a week or a month or 4 months or a year from now with your hair and eyelashes full and beautiful and just the way you wanted it; buying barrettes for your lovely hair; or going for a haircut and styling."

In general it is not a good idea to reinforce these suggestions with the image of parental praise, for that may encourage the child to resist.

Mohlman (1973) recommends that, after the patient is in trance, suggestions to eliminate thumb-sucking should be as follows: "Instead of putting your thumb in your mouth, would it be all right to put your thumb in your fist?" After receiving a yes, the therapist says, "This will be even more pleasant to you than putting it in your mouth, and also it will be easier because your fist is nearer your thumb."

M. H. Erickson (1958a) recommended prescribing the symptom of thumb-sucking to a rebellious 16-year-old girl who rapidly lost interest in the habit after 10 evenings of deliberately irritating her parents with loud thumb-sucking. Staples (1973) reported successful use of hypnotherapy in the case of a 4-year-old girl who sucked her thumb. Hypnosis was induced by having her imagine she was holding her sleeping teddy bear. Following induction of hypnosis, suggestions were made that the patient was growing bigger every day, that soon she would get so big that she would not suck her thumb anymore, that she might be big enough next week or next month. Secter (1973) has recommended a similar approach to those who suck their thumbs.

Although these approaches, stressing maturation and elimination of the symptom, are often successful, they may embarrass older children who are clearly beyond the age of thumb-sucking, bedwetting and other preschool behaviors. In the case of older children, it seems more appropriate to provide a substitute comfortable feeling for the symptom and to enhance mastery by focusing on the patient's previous successes and future anticipated events without the symptom.

Gardner (1978a) reported successful use of hypnotherapy with an 8-year-old girl who twisted and pulled out her hair, leaving obvious bald patches. As is true of many children with habit problems, she claimed to be unaware of the behavior and was highly motivated to change it. The symptom and resulting attention were interpreted as a manifestation of the child's need for power and control in her family. In hypnosis she was told that she could find a way truly to be in control of her hair. She was given suggestions for awareness of hair-pulling behavior as soon as she lifted her hand for this purpose, and she was told that she could recall the phrase "Stop, please do not hurt" from the part of her that wanted pretty hair. In the first of three hypnotic sessions, the child added her own creative details to these ideas. When she lifted her hand to begin hair pulling, it trembled as it got near her head, then returned to her lap. She reported the sensation of a "force-field," an impenetrable barrier similar to the one on the TV program "Star Trek." When not thinking of hair pulling, she could touch her head easily and enjoy new habits of good hair grooming. Although this child refused to practice self-hypnosis, she responded well to posthypnotic suggestions. After 2 weeks, the scalp lesions were healed, and there was new hair growth. After another 2 weeks, there was further hair growth, and the child was no longer wearing a bandanna. Follow-up 2 months later revealed no further hair pulling and improvement in other behavior patterns.

Kohen (1992) described a successful hypnotherapeutic approach with a 10¼-year-old boy who had several habit problems, including hair pulling and tongue-sucking. His hair pulling had begun at age 3 years, stopped briefly with home daycare in place of a large center and with giving him toys to occupy his hands, and then recurred. When his mother married, a psychologist helping with adjustment to a newly constituted family instructed the parents to use a "trigger word" to remind him when he was pulling his hair. This worked only "sometimes," and he was referred for hypnotherapy.

Like most, he professed lack of awareness of the habit — "I don't always know when I do it" — but would speculate that it happened more when he was nervous or bored. As he loved baseball, imagery of playing baseball was utilized for induction and intensification of hypnosis. A metaphor for personal control was introduced by discussing how he had learned to ride a bicycle, emphasizing *"how you did it without purposely giving out-loud instructions to each muscle about what to do to ride,"* and noting that he could now ride a bike "without really thinking about it." Playing baseball successfully was used as another metaphor for control of muscles and movement. Progressive relaxation reinforced the analogy that the brain could be the boss of the body. Dissociative suggestions for control and comfort were then introduced that "those hands can help each other, because they are friends, and because your brain is the boss of your body you can reprogram that computer we call the brain to teach those hands to help each other. Let one hand go up toward the head then use the other hand to gently push it down . . . they can be friends and help each other. . . . " At the second visit he and his mother reported improvement, and he said, "I imagine baseball, relax from my head to my toes, have one hand go up to my head and the other help it down. . . . " At the fourth visit 3 weeks later, he was proud, and his mother confirmed a dramatic disappearance of hair pulling. He proudly reported again, "I close my eyes, I relax, I think of baseball or something, *then I teach my hands."* At the fifth visit 6½ weeks later, hair pulling was

reported "90% gone," and new hair growth was evident. The hypnosis practice session was videotaped "to help other doctors and other kids learn this."
He experienced a relapse 3 months later, however, perhaps related to the
mother's continued overinvolvement. In spite of his progress she had told
him that "since you had it so long since you were 3 years old, it *might take
a real long time to get rid of* and be real *hard* to change." Although intended
to be supportive, her statement served as a strong negative suggestion, and
in hypnosis efforts were made to reframe it to "some kids are surprised by
how *easy* it turns out to be when they let their inside mind do it by practicing the way you already know you can and did." For reinforcement, he was
given an article describing how self-hypnosis had helped a famous baseball
player to improve his batting average. Four weeks later no bald spots were
evident. He was proud, his mother had stopped "bugging" him, and he had
a full head of hair by the time school began for the fall term. Three months
later, he had his first haircut in a year's time and a 2½-year follow-up showed
no recurrence.

SLEEPWALKING

The problem of sleepwalking has not been adequately studied to determine
precise etiological factors. Although the symptom may reflect anxiety, it also
seems to be associated with certain developmental periods and to be more
frequent in certain families. Although it usually is a benign symptom, those
who sleepwalk may occasionally fall down stairs and injure themselves, or
may even leave their home clad unsafely and inappropriately for the nighttime weather. This is frightening to other family members who are likely
to request investigation and treatment, while the person doing the sleepwalking is likely to at least initially remain unconcerned, largely because he
or she is usually amnesic for the event of sleepwalking. Amnesia notwith-
standing, children may become frightened simply from hearing their parents'
repeated expressions of concern and from stories about themselves about
which they have no personal memory. The following case history describes
our use of hypnotherapy in one such instance of parasomnia or disorder of
arousal:

The patient was an 11-year-old boy who had been having sleepwalking
episodes since he was approximately 4 years of age and had increased to walking around the multilevel house at least once every night. His parents were
concerned about possible injury, and having heard about his activities, he
too had become afraid to stay at homes of friends or relatives. He was taught
the coin induction method of relaxation with addition of favorite place imagery and a nice, long walk down a hill during which time he became more
and more comfortable. Prior to this, sleep levels had been discussed with

him, and since sleepwalking is thought to occur in the transition between REM and non-REM sleep, he was asked to program himself to remain in bed during this transition period. He practiced this every night prior to sleeping. There was an immediate decrease in sleepwalking incidents to two or three a week, and, within 2 months, the sleepwalking had ceased. His mother stated that she felt he was using his newly found abilities for self-control in other areas such as school and personal relationships. (See also Chapter 7.)

CHRONIC OVEREATING

C. H. Haber, Nitkin, and Shenker (1979) reported uniformly unsuccessful results of hypnotherapy with eight obese adolescents. Suggestions included maintenance of an appropriate diet, aversive response to fattening foods, increased exercise, and positive self-esteem. Four patients were not responsive to hypnotic induction. Of the other four, three experienced negative sequelae of hypnosis, including feelings of depersonalization, increased anxiety, and dissociative behavior. We have not found such a large incidence of untoward effects of hypnosis. The problems might have been due to peculiar patient characteristics.

In a previously unpublished study at George Washington University (Olness, Fallon, Coit, Fry, & Bassford, 1974), group hypnotherapy was offered to 60 obese postmenarche female adolescents. Prestudy evaluations included many laboratory studies, psychological testing, and physical examinations. Criteria for inclusion into the study included weight greater than 140 pounds, weight 20% above the weight norm for the subject's age and height, and obesity by skin-fold measurements.

Patients were divided into three groups. Group A patients were taught self-hypnosis, and Group B patients spent equal time with a control physician who gave them support and counseling, Group C patients had no treatment. All patients were seen regularly by a nutritionist and nurse clinician. After undergoing the prestudy evaluations, patients were weighed on a monthly basis for 1 year. At the end of 1 year, the subjects in Groups A and B had lost an average of 5.8 pounds, and the nonintervention Group C had gained an average of 5.0 pounds per person. However, within the group there were some significant differences that correlated with the ability of the girls to visualize themselves as thinner in the future, for example, buying clothing of a smaller size. Those girls had an average weight loss of 9.7 pounds, compared with an average loss of 0.6 pounds for the others in the group. Although this study officially ended after 1 year of follow-up, the girls in Groups A and B were weighed again after a second year. Those in Group A had maintained weight loss or continued weight loss, including those who had not lost appreciably during the first year. Those in Group B had gained weight in similar fashion to the control group.

A report (Kohen et al., 1984) of 505 children with behavior problems treated with hypnotherapy mentions five children with obesity who lost weight during periods when they practiced self-hypnosis. However, only one child maintained significant weight reduction. Treatment approaches followed those of other habit problems.

Specific suggestions included the following: enjoying eating the appropriate amount of food for health and correct weight; feeling comfortable between meals without eating snacks; and visualizing looking thinner, buying smaller sizes, being complimented for appearance, and seeing one's height and weight as compatible on a growth chart.

Our clinical impression is that it is important that obese children review the self-hypnosis exercises several times daily for several weeks and that frequent visits in the first months of treatment are essential, and much more necessary than in management of other habit disorders.

TICS AND TREMORS

We find that children with tics and tremors are frequently referred for a trial of hypnotherapy and that these referrals often come from pediatricians or neurologists, but also from psychologists and other counselors and therapists. Increasingly, referrals also come from school personnel, that is, school nurses, social workers, or psychologists. These symptoms, perhaps more than many habit problems, seem to be the symbolic expression of unresolved conflicts. For this reason, we recommend psychological evaluation with emphasis on family interaction. This may be accomplished by the primary treating clinician skilled in family assessment and treatment (pediatrician, family physician, psychologist) or by consultation and collaboration with an appropriate therapist. Although it may not be necessary or appropriate to mention the hypothesis of psychogenic determinants of the child, it is essential to have a reasonable working hypothesis before beginning hypnotherapy.

Approaches are similar to those for all habit problems with the addition of the jettison technique in which the child releases tension and problem from his or her clenched fist. Suggested imagery should emphasize mastery and the child's own control, and should include a focus on future happy events in which the patient no longer has a tic or tremor. The following case demonstrates a jettison technique.

Alison D. was a well-developed, pretty 14-year-old girl who was referred by her pediatrician for "hypnosis to control a hand tremor." She described a series of psychophysiological complaints including headaches, epigastric pain, and lower abdominal pain for each of which she had had extensive medical evaluations. She was a good student who mentioned a desire to finish school and study medicine. As she described her previous symptoms and evaluations through grade school, she said, "I always knew there wouldn't be anything really wrong, I was just nervous."

When asked why she thought she was nervous, Alison hesitated and said, "Well, I'm nervous about my mother's boyfriend who attacked me when I was around 8 or 9." She stated that she had never discussed these episodes of sexual abuse with her mother, and that her mother continued to see the boyfriend whom she said she couldn't stand to be around. She said she was angry at her mother who "knew what was going on and did nothing." She stated that she had been asked out by a boy for the first time a few weeks before, and that the hand tremor had begun at the same time. She did not wish to discuss the problem with her mother or the boyfriend. Alison was taught progressive relaxation and favorite place imagery, and she was then taught the clenched fist technique for releasing what bothered her. During the first session she opened and closed her fist several times. On return visit, 2 weeks later, she said she had no recurrence of the tremor and was coping much better.

The therapist hypothesized that the hand tremor represented aggressive and/or sexual impulses but did not share this idea with Alison, since such insight might produce unnecessary conflict about discussing the problem with her family.

Heimel (1978) reported a case that required a longer course of hypnotherapy for a tic disorder. Erik P., a 10-year-old boy, had a tic consisting of shaking movements of the head and shoulders that occurred repeatedly each day for a 9-month period prior to presentation in the pediatrician's office. He was seen on 15 occasions over 16 months.

Since Erik found it very difficult to discuss his problems with the therapist, the dynamic meaning of the tic remained unclear for quite some time. Eventually, some information became available through the use of ideomotor signaling in hypnosis. The patient had a very poor self-image and feelings of nonacceptance by his parents, grandparents, and peers. He believed that his sister was much more accepted by family members. His father seemed to be very passive and played no active role in the patient's life. As these feelings were shared with his parents, they made efforts to improve the family relationships. The dynamics of Erik's tic were never entirely clear; the head shaking might have served as unconscious expressions of hostility while at the same time assuring increased attention and concern from the family. The relatively long duration of the symptom, together with the ongoing emotional difficulties, made rapid resolution unlikely.

Initially in hypnotherapy, Erik was taught progressive relaxation and given ego-strengthening suggestions. When there seemed to be no response after a few weeks, the hypnotherapist offered Erik the jettison technique— "wrapping or packing up what was bugging him and sending it far away on a freight train or plane." During these sessions, the patient was noted to smile several times as he clenched his fist in the process of eliminating troublesome thoughts or ideas.

After addition of this technique, Erik's parents and teachers noted a 90% reduction in frequency of the tic. However, when the tics disappeared, the patient developed a chronic cough. Consultation with an otolaryngologist was obtained, and no pathology was found. Erik was again offered hypnotherapy, which he accepted. He was confronted with the possibility that he had used the cough as a substitute for the tic. The coughing disappeared within a few weeks after two hypnotherapy sessions. In follow-up 3 years later, the family stated that Erik was adjusting well as a sophomore in high school, that he had no tics, coughs, or other habit symptoms, and that he seemed happy and relaxed.

A boy was referred to us just before his 10th birthday, with a history of a lip-licking tic/habit that had begun 2 years before as a sniffing and coughing habit and disappeared until 5 months prior to referral when this began. At the time of the first visit, the tic had been gone for 3 weeks. There was no other history of tics. During further history-taking at the second visit, the patient and his mother were asked to think back to the September when the tic had begun and asked if anything important or worrisome or bad had happened or was going on around the same time. They said no. They were asked to consider the preceding month, August, and they also said no. When they were asked to think back to July they were both about to similarly say no when the mother abruptly gasped, "Oh . . . " and put her hand to her mouth as a look of recognition and remembrance came across her face. She and her son looked at one another, she said, "Remember?," and they both began to weep. Mother then told the story of how the patient and his sister were with their grandparents while the parents were visiting their close friends on their farm. They were out for a horse and buggy ride when a car traveling at high speed ran into them broadside, killing both close friends and seriously injuring and hospitalizing the parents in two different hospitals. When he visited his father in the hospital, the patient was terrified at his father's confused state of mind. Tics began 2 months later. Visits to the pediatrician and allergist eventuated in referral to Behavioral Pediatrics. Seventeen months after the accident, the father continued to be out of work, and the mother, though back to work, continued to have problems with memory. The patient had tics, became withdrawn and was tearful, and "kept everything inside." Supportive counseling was provided for the patient and his parents. An Ericksonian approach was taken in helping the child to develop mastery over his tic behaviors. He was told methodically and matter-of-factly that "back then," when he was younger, he was *appropriately* so scared and saddened by the sad and scary things that happened that he didn't know even how to talk about it, so he kept it inside *because* he was so young *back then*. *Now* that he was older and could talk about and understand how strong those feelings were to a *younger* child, the feelings didn't have to come out in *different* ways (such as tics). In hypnosis additional metaphors were provided for the manner in which the brain controls the movements of muscles of the body (e.g., "You don't have to think about walking, do you? Your brain sends messages to all of the right muscles to move in the right way at the right time, without even thinking about it. . . . "). His tics disappeared, and though there was a brief recurrence for a few weeks 9 months later, a subsequent 2-year follow-up showed no recurrence. (See also discussion on hypnotherapy for Tourette syndrome, Chapter 11.)

HABITUAL DRUG ABUSE

Baumann (1970) reviewed his experience with adolescents, from grades 6 to 12 in school, who abused a variety of drugs. With most of these patients, the hypnotherapeutic approach focused on asking the youngsters to develop a "hypnotic high" in which they used their own imaginative abilities to experience feelings even better than the similar feelings they had had following actual drug ingestion. Other forms of psychotherapy were also employed with many patients. Initially pleased with the finding that 50% of 80 marijuana users were no longer using the drug 1 year after hypnotherapy, Baumann reviewed data for 80 more marijuana users who had not been treated for this problem. Again, about half had stopped drug use after 1 year. Neither group considered the drug physically harmful, and those who stopped did so from boredom, lack of satisfaction, or fear of the law. Baumann concluded that hypnotherapy could not be considered an effective therapeutic modality for this group.

Among adolescents who used drugs that they thought to be physically dangerous, Baumann (1970) found his methods more successful. Of 30 teenagers who had only "good trips" with LSD, 26 stopped taking the drug completely and 4 reduced the frequency of usage. There was little change, however, for 12 other patients who had experienced "bad trips" with LSD; it was difficult to adapt the technique in these cases. Of 17 adolescents who were "shooting speed" (amphetamines), all stopped injecting the drug, although 4 turned to oral amphetamines. Of 28 users of oral amphetamines, 6 stopped altogether, 20 decreased usage, and 2 remained unchanged. Of 10 patients who frequently used overdoses of barbiturates, 9 showed significant improvement following hypnotherapy. Since this group had no "high" experiences, imagery was directed more toward helping the youngsters satisfy other needs more appropriately. The treatment was not considered effective for two patients who used heroin or for two others who used multiple drugs.

Baumann (1970) concluded that hypnotherapy can be a useful adjunct in the management of adolescent drug abusers, provided that they are well motivated for habit change. The greatest motivating factor seemed to be fear of physical damage to the patients themselves or to their children.

We have had little experience with adolescent drug abusers. However, we have sometimes adapted Baumann's imagery technique to help patients get rapid and maximal effect from prescribed sedatives and analgesics. Some of our patients have used hypnotic sedation and comfort to obviate the need for preoperative sedation or postoperative chemical analgesia. The technique might also be adapted in the hypnotherapeutic treatment of other habit disorders, providing the child with emotional gratifications and obviating the need to engage in the habit. Gardner's (1978a) emphasis on giving the child with hair pulling a sense of controlling her hair is one example in which the basic need, that is, control, was not changed, but rather rechanneled in more appropriate directions.

CONCLUSIONS

Hypnotherapy appears to be valuable in the treatment of a wide variety of habit disorders, provided (1) there is no underlying organic problem, (2) the child is well motivated, and (3) the child is willing to assume primary responsibility for change. As compared with many other approaches, hypnotherapy is less expensive, less time-consuming, and less dangerous. Therefore, it would be advantageous to consider a hypnotherapeutic approach early rather than as a last resort as has so often been the case. On the other hand, some of the better-controlled studies have found that patients who resolve a habit problem after hypnotherapy may not do it because of hypnotherapy, but rather for different reasons. Accordingly, we need better-controlled, prospective studies in order to determine which children with which habit problems are most likely to benefit the most from which hypnotherapeutic strategies.

CHAPTER NINE

Hypnotherapy for Problems in Learning and Performance

Many children experience problems both in learning certain material and skills and in performing or demonstrating that they have mastered the material or skills. Increasingly, children, adolescents, and their teachers, coaches, and parents turn to hypnotherapy for help, spurred on by encouraging reports in the press and in professional journals.

Many reports of hypnotherapy for learning problems contain a measure of optimism that is not really warranted by the data. Hypnotherapy can often be beneficial as either a primary or an adjunct therapy in treating emotional problems such as low self-esteem or anxiety that may impede learning. However, a clinician utilizing hypnotherapy must take care to distinguish these emotional problems from true learning disabilities. Diagnostic evaluation should include psychological and psychoeducational evaluation (of child and family), and in some cases a child will also require and benefit from evaluation by a speech pathologist, a neurologist, and an ophthalmologist.

When clinical evaluation suggests that hypnotherapy might be helpful for patients with learning difficulties, we think it is of critical importance that they understand that the process is under their own control and that they are, in large part, accordingly responsible for the outcome. Integral to this emphasis is our recommendation for the daily practice of self-hypnosis with appropriate suggestions. This approach serves to help identify children who are not (yet) really motivated for change, or who derive so much secondary gain from their problem that other counseling/psychotherapy is indicated before self-hypnosis could be expected to be of particular value.

Prior to embarking upon hypnotherapy, the clinician should discuss specific goals with the child, for example, to pass third-grade requirements, to increase reading level by 6 months, to complete arithmetic homework, to increase classroom participation, to pass a particular test, or to achieve some particular benchmark or milestone of performance. Generally the emphasis should first be on small goals, and there should be clear feedback to the child. Often the clinician conducting hypnotherapy training will need frequent consultation with the child's teachers to facilitate understanding and agreed upon, consistent reinforcement in the classroom.

When it seems clear the hypnotherapy will not be or has not been helpful, the patient and/or parents should be counseled as to more appropriate avenues of help. Parental pressure may make this referral process very difficult, particularly if the parents feel "at the end of the line," or if they were inappropriately led to believe that hypnotherapy could or would provide some sort of quick, magical, or miraculous solution to their child's ongoing learning/performance dilemmas.

The Behavioral Pediatrics Program at Minneapolis Children's Medical Center (now Children's Health Care–Minneapolis) conducted two pilot stress-reduction programs in local elementary schools. Both were successful. The most recent program consisted of 10 sessions a week apart and included review of stress-reduction strategies by teachers on a daily basis (Rusin & Wynne, 1987).

A prospective study compared two groups of sixth-grade children who participated in the stress-reduction program. One group of children was in a regular classroom; the second group was in a special classroom because of their disruptive behaviors. The Piers–Harris Children's Self-Concept Scale and the Nowicki–Strickland Internal/External Locus of Control were administered to each child prior to the initial session and following the 10th session. In beginning sessions, Dr. Rusin talked with children about definitions of stress, how to recognize stressors in daily life, and how to strengthen inner controls. All children learned self-hypnosis exercises and had opportunities to play computer games that were linked to their autonomic responses.

All children had the opportunity to learn and practice peripheral skin temperature biofeedback and galvanic skin resistance feedback. There was no difference between the Locus of Control test results in pre- and post-testing. Both groups showed similar and significant changes in reduction of anxiety (Piers–Harris Self-Concept Scale) from week 1 to week 10. The special classroom group demonstrated a peripheral temperature increase of 9.5 °F compared with an increase of 4.5 °F in the regular classroom group. This significant difference may reflect a greater degree of chronic arousal present in children in the special classroom. Training in self-regulation via self-hypnosis and providing feedback from autonomic functions by using computer games may be very helpful to children who frequently demonstrate out-of-control behaviors (Culbert et al., 1994).

APPLICATIONS OF HYPNOTHERAPY
IN THE CLASSROOM

It is clear that classroom experiences may be very stressful for children and may result in the development of undesirable autonomic responses and fear that may continue to affect them as adults. Many adults recall conscious memories of unhappy experiences related to elementary school, such as reading aloud, taking a timed math test, participating and "performing" in a spelling bee, and being teased by peers. Perhaps even more adults have repressed such memories, yet they manifest behaviors that have evolved from these or similar stressful grade school experiences.

There are many popular books, relaxation tapes, and teacher's manuals that provide methods aimed at classroom stress. Many of these use verbal instructions similar, if not identical, to those used in hypnotic inductions and hypnotherapeutic verbalizations. These may be very helpful to some children. The difficulty is that—like most teaching aids—they do not allow for flexibility and individual differences. Although most do, not all children have the ability to use visual images; some have auditory-processing disabilities that make it difficult for them to follow or recall verbal instructions.

Rusin and Wynne (1987) have developed a model system for teaching stress reduction in the classroom, which has been used successfully in entire classrooms. Its objectives are to help children recognize that their bodies respond to thoughts, that such body changes are measurable, and that the children can learn to control undesirable body changes and feelings by changing their thoughts.

Prior to experiential training, the teacher spends time in conversation with the student regarding what stress is or feels like. Subsequently, Rusin demonstrated, by means of computer game feedback, how quickly the body changed as the child's thinking changed. Each child had the opportunity to be connected to the biofeedback apparatus, which monitored peripheral temperature, and electromyographic, or galvanic skin-resistance changes. As the children experimented with the response of the computer games to their efforts to relax, they rapidly gained control of these autonomic responses.

It might be very helpful to children if, during their early elementary school years, they could have the opportunity to experience and recognize the effects of thinking on body processes. Computer game biofeedback units should soon become inexpensive and readily available, and they may be hooked into home computers. We believe that they should become standard equipment in children's museums and in hands-on science museums around the world. Prototypes of such units have been developed and are now beginning to appear in museums (see Chapter 14).

Grynkewich (1994) has developed a system of incorporating mental imagery strategies into cognitive behavioral strategies that are used in classroom education. She defines five components of mental imagery strategy instruction:

1. Student motivation, goal setting, and commitment to learn
2. Student determination of effective mental images through interview with the counselor
3. Student learning of effective relaxation techniques
4. Incorporation and practice of relaxation techniques with effective mental images
5. Self-management and regulation

Grynkewich recommends determining effective mental images by asking students to identify favorite activities, places, vacations, books, movies, and people. In addition, it is helpful to know what thoughts, images, feelings, or sensations are perceived when the student experiences personal successes and problems. She notes that it is a mistake to recommend specific imagery based on general knowledge of students of the same age. Grynkewich recommends similar individualization in choice of relaxation methods.

HYPNOTHERAPY WITH MENTALLY RETARDED CHILDREN

Parents of mentally retarded children sometimes turn in helplessness or desperation to unusual or even bizarre treatment methods that have no known efficacy and may actually do more harm than good. Probably because of its magical appeal and reports of dramatic cures in other areas, hypnotherapy similarly has been sought out with the hope it could help children with mental retardation. Clinical hypnosis researchers have also investigated this area, focusing on two issues: whether mentally retarded children are hypnotizable, and whether it is possible to increase their performance on intelligence tests and related learning tasks. All researchers do not agree on the definition of mental retardation. Consistent with prevailing beliefs, we define mental retardation as an intelligence quotient (IQ) below 70 on a standardized test, when the obtained IQ is interpreted as a valid reflection of the child's intellectual ability and not primarily the result of depression, anxiety, refusal to cooperate, or other behavioral or cultural variables.

It is important to remember that an intelligence test score measures a child's current intellectual functioning. In some instances, the response patterns on individual test items or subtests suggest that the child's potential may be higher. However, limited areas or "islands" of normal functioning in the midst of general performance at a mentally retarded level are not sufficient to conclude that a child's overall intelligence is really well above the obtained IQ score. In the past, this mistake was often made in evaluations of autistic children. Even when these children made significant gains in the emotional sphere, most of them did not achieve expected parallel gains in intellectual functioning.

One of the most commonly recognized characteristics of retarded learners is their suggestibility, but there is little empirical data to support this hypothesis. Many retarded students have long histories of failure and low expectancies of success. These factors combine to produce passive behavior; the student approaches tasks reluctantly, and this may reinforce the feeling of helplessness. A study of mildly retarded and nonretarded children (Shuck & Ludlow, 1984) between 10 and 16 years old, classified by groups according to suggestibility, were exposed to positive, neutral, or negative suggestions regarding their performance of a learning task. Highly suggestible retarded students showed greater improvement from the first task to the second; this finding permits the inference that suggestibility may enhance the learning of retarded learners. Group mean scores showed a trend toward better performance by subjects receiving positive suggestions than by those receiving neutral or negative suggestions. The fact that no difference was found between neutral and negative suggestions implies that students in general have low expectancies for success in tasks and that predicting that a task may be difficult does not affect performance any more than saying nothing at all about it. Prior reinforcement history may be the key determinant in conceptualizing success or failure.

Hypnotic Responsiveness

The normative studies of hypnotic responsiveness cited in Chapter 3 did not include retarded children and therefore contribute nothing to the question of whether such children can experience hypnosis. L. Jacobs and Jacobs (1966) concluded that children with very low intelligence were generally not hypnotizable. However, that study did not utilize any standardized measure of hypnotizability.

Sternlicht and Wanderer (1963) addressed themselves specifically to the question of whether mentally retarded children are hypnotizable. Unfortunately, however, their study also had significant methodological limitations. The subjects were 20 "certified mentally defective" children who were institutionalized at the Willowbrook State School near New York City. The children's chronological ages ranged from 7 to 15 years (mean age = 11 years). All children had been tested with the Revised Stanford–Binet Intelligence Scale, Form L, with IQs ranging from 37 to 68 (mean IQ = 52), and mental ages from 3 to 9 years.

The authors argued that use of a standardized hypnotizability scale, such as the Children's Hypnotic Susceptibility Scale (CHSS; London, 1963), would be inappropriate because the emphasis on verbal instructions would put mentally retarded children, with their typically poor verbal skills, at a disadvantage as compared to subjects of normal intelligence. In place of a standardized scale, the authors used a "progressive anesthesia" induction technique (Watkins, 1962). The children were told that parts of their bodies would become more still and rigid and would be without any feeling. When this effect was achieved in the entire body, the children would then be "in a deep state of sleep" (p. 106). These verbal suggestions were enhanced with tactile stimulation on the children's fingers and hands. The children were first asked to move a finger in which they felt altered sensation. They were then asked to report how deep a state of sleep had been achieved by giving a number on a scale in which 0 meant none at all and 10 meant deeper asleep than ever before.

Of the 20 children, 8 did not pass the initial finger-moving test and were declared "nonhypnotizable." For the remaining 12 children, the scores were negatively skewed, with 10 reporting scores in the 7 to 10 range and the other 2 reporting a score of 1. The authors concluded that 60% of their sample were hypnotizable. We cannot agree. The authors acknowledged the problem of using subjective reports of hypnotizability but defended their choice as the best available. We note the U-shaped curve of scores and come to a different conclusion. Institutionalized mentally retarded children tend to fall into two groups, those who demonstrate minimal cooperation and those who exert tremendous effort to cooperate and to please adults, apparently thriving on bits of social reinforcement so often lacking in larger institutions. All 20 children in this study counted from 1 to 12 for the examiners, as part of the process of establishing rapport and in order to demonstrate ability to use the scoring system. We wonder whether they got verbal or nonverbal reinforcement for each higher number or for completing the task. If so, they may have concluded "the higher, the better" as do young children. If they were given this sort of reinforcement, they might have simply been seeking further praise by giving a high number when later asked to estimate their depth of "sleep." We become even more suspicious of the high scores when we notice the emphasis on "sleep," in light of the repeated findings that children often respond negatively to hypnotic induction methods that suggest sleep.

In short, we think these data have more to do with social reinforcement and demand characteristics than with hypnosis, and we cannot conclude from the data that retarded children are hypnotizable. Obviously the study suffers from other concerns, including the lack of a control group of institutionalized children with normal IQ and the lack of any evidence that the children really understood the anesthesia instructions. It may be notable that none of the 12 "hypnotizable" children responded to suggested age regression.

Before leaving the question of hypnotic responsiveness in mentally retarded children, we should mention the issue of pseudoretardation. That is, a child may test and function at a retarded level but may actually have normal intelligence. For example, Gardner (1973) reported IQ data on an 8-year-old girl with psychogenic epilepsy. At the beginning of treatment, when she was virtually in petit mal status, her Stanford–Binet IQ was 72, in the borderline retarded range. Eighteen months earlier, before exacerbation of her symptoms, her IQ on the Binet had been 93 (average), and 3 months after initiation of psychotherapy, her Binet IQ was 103 (average). The fact that she was hypnotizable when her measured IQ was 72 obviously says nothing about the relationship between hypnotizability and intelligence, since the IQ score was not a true measure of her intellectual ability. In future research on hypnotic responsiveness of children with low intelligence, one must be careful not to include such cases of pseudoretardation.

Can Hypnotherapy Increase IQ?

We know of no long-term studies that utilize hypnotherapy as an adjunct in the educational programs of mentally retarded children. The results were disappointing in one study (Woody & Billy, 1970) that included a single session of "clinical suggestion." Since the study was published in a hypnosis journal, we assume that the authors believed that they employed hypnosis but avoided that term — as did many authors cited in this chapter — perhaps because they feared it might not be acceptable in the school setting where the study was conducted.

Woody and Billy (1970) located 28 mentally retarded boys, ages 9 to 13 years, in special-education classrooms. All had been given an individual intelligence test on which their IQs ranged from 50 to 75. The authors selected 32 nonretarded boys from regular classes in the same schools. Each of these groups was then divided into an experimental and a control group, equated for age and IQ. The retarded and nonretarded control groups were given the Peabody Picture Vocabulary Test (PPVT) on two occasions, 2 weeks apart. Apparently these groups received no intervening treatment or special attention. The two experimental groups received a "clinical suggestion session" immediately prior to the second PPVT administration. The suggestions focused on enhancing physical relaxation, minimizing anxiety over past test performance, and heightening motivation for and expectation of good performance. Neither of the nonretarded groups showed any change in PPVT scores. The mean IQ increase for the retarded "clinical suggestion" group was 4.79 points, whereas the mean gain for the retarded controls was 3.21 points. Although the authors indicated that the difference for retarded experimentals and controls is statistically significant, neither difference is greater than the standard error of measurement for individual IQ tests. The authors concluded that differences of such small magnitude are hardly likely to have any practical significance. Further statistical analysis led the authors to state that "it does not appear that clinical suggestions are any more effective for retarded boys than they are for non-retarded boys" (Woody & Billy, 1970, p. 270). They wondered whether several clinical suggestion sessions might have yielded different results.

Based on the data from this study, we find no evidence that hypnotic suggestions can increase IQ in children with primary mental retardation. Despite its several methodological weaknesses, it is probably the most carefully controlled study of this issue to date.

The Utility of Hypnosis in Counseling with Retarded Children

Although we do not think it has been demonstrated that mentally retarded persons are hypnotizable, neither has it been shown clearly that they are not hypnotizable. Even if they do not seem to respond to hypnotherapeutic suggestions for enhanced intellectual performance, perhaps they can utilize hypnosis as an adjunct to counseling and psychotherapy.

Woody and Herr (1967) surveyed 102 psychologists in clinical and academic settings, all trained in the use of hypnosis, concerning their opinions as the possible utility of hypnosis in counseling the mentally retarded. The 84 who responded tended to be uncertain rather than having clear positive or negative opinions; most had no experience using clinical hypnosis with this population.

Lazar (1977) reported successful hypnotherapy with a moderately retarded boy with behavior problems (see Chapter 7). Of course, in this and other single case reports, it is impossible to be certain whether the positive results should be ascribed to hypnotherapy or to some other aspect(s) of the therapeutic intervention. Lazar (1977) did not measure her patient's hypnotic responsiveness by any standardized scale, and one could conceptualize her techniques for extinguishing undesirable behavior as belonging more in the realm of behavior modification than in that of hypnotherapy.

Based on available research and our own clinical experience with mentally retarded children, we conclude that their capacity to respond to hypnotic induction is, at best, quite limited. In cases of true mental retardation, we doubt that hypnotherapy can significantly enhance intellectual functioning. In treating such children for emotional and behavioral problems, we think behavior modification and parent counseling are probably the most effective approaches; though it certainly makes sense to consider the addition of strategies of relaxation and mental imagery (hypnosis) to counseling and behavior modification in given individual situations. It should be possible to design methodologically sound research studies that would further clarify these issues.

HYPNOTHERAPY FOR CHILDREN WITH LEARNING DISABILITIES

Attentional Disorders

Among educators, psychologists, and others who work with children with learning difficulties, there are varied opinions as to the cause, frequency, diagnosis of attentional disorders, most recently, frequently, and consistently referred to as attention-deficit/hyperactivity disorder (ADHD). Though the prevalence of this group of attentional disorders is estimated at 3 to 5% of the school-aged population, they remain among the most frequently renamed and redefined problems presenting to child health care providers. Although their precise nature and best treatment approach remain a matter of ongoing debate and study, there is now general agreement on diagnostic criteria. Reiff, Banez, and Culbert (1993) note that children with attentional disorders share core symptoms of (1) inattention, (2) impulsivity, and (3) overactivity inappropriate for their developmental level and interfere with optimal functioning. Some investigators believe additional primary deficits include difficulty adhering to rules and instructions and excessive day-to-day variability in performing tasks or following directions. In this context, most clinicians agree (1) that these children have normal intelligence with specific learning deficits (if any), (2) that they experience repeated failure in school because of their academic and behavior problems, and (3) that these difficulties result in low self-esteem, anxiety, depression, and poor attitudes toward learning. These children then may decrease their own efforts to succeed in school, thus lowering academic performance even more, and creating a vicious cycle of ever-increasing problems. An awareness that ADHD and related variants are now understood to represent biological disorders allows the further understanding that the attendant learning difficulties may be primary or secondary and associated emotional problems are most often secondary.

   A wide variety of special group and individualized educational strategies have been developed to remediate the variety of learning difficulties— "general" and specific—associated with attentional disorders; and evaluation, special education, and individualized educational plans (IEPs) are now widely available and mandated by law (Public Laws 94-142 and 101-476). Sometimes, however, the children's low self-esteem, negative attitudes toward learning, and related emotional problems may combine to make it almost impossible for them to benefit from remedial training. We agree with Crasilneck and Hall (1975) that hypnotherapy is not a primary treatment for attentional disorders, then known as minimal brain dysfunction, or MBD. We also agree that hypnotherapy can often help the child with ADHD or related difficulties to (1) lower anxiety, (2) increase capacity to recognize lability, (3) develop strategies for controlling emotional outbursts, (4) manage associated problems such as sleep and/or interactional difficulties, and (5) modify attitudes toward learning in general and school in particular.

Crasilneck and Hall (1985) described their treatment of an 8-year-old girl with attentional disorder whose secondary emotional problems were manifested not only in school but also at home and with her peers. Diagnostic evaluation revealed no evidence of neurological damage or primary emotional disorder. Intelligence was average, with indications of higher potential. The child benefited from hypnotherapy designed to ameliorate the secondary problems. The chief contribution of this single case report consists of the inclusion of details of the hypnotic suggestions given and the results obtained.

> Hypnosis was instituted on a trial basis to decrease anxiety and instill a sense of confidence in the child. She was told that she would find herself wanting to study more and would find pleasure and gratification in doing the very best job possible. She was told in the trance that some of the energy that was causing her trouble would be re-directed into more useful work. She would find herself capable of making better grades in school. Such a suggestion for improved grades would not have been made had it not seemed, on balance, that the reality of her situation was such that she had been using her full capabilities. She was next told that she would be able to concentrate much better and would begin to enjoy getting along in school and with her parents.
>
> Following each hypnotic session, the child was encouraged to discuss her fears, her fantasies, her feelings about past failures, and any unusual problems or successes that she had experienced since the last visit.
>
> At the end of nine weeks her report card had come up one letter grade, on average. Her attention span seemed improved, and her ability to concentrate seemed more stable. She was enjoying school more and showed marked improvement on her examinations. Her interpersonal relations with her parents, her schoolmates, and her teachers indicated good adjustment. Six months later her grades were above average, and she had become more happy. Her anxiety was rarely sufficient to cause any of her past difficulties.
>
> Throughout her treatment great care was taken not to set goals that were unrealistically high for her apparent abilities, as this would have induced a further conflict of perhaps greater severity than her presenting complaints. This precaution makes accurate clinical assessment of great importance in using hypnosis for such cases. (p. 193)*

---

*From Crasilneck and Hall (1985). Copyright 1985 by Allyn & Bacon. With permission.

Over the past decade there has been great interest generated in the use of a variety of biofeedback strategies as adjunctive or primary treatment for attentional disorders. The potential value of biofeedback and its relationship to hypnotherapy are discussed in detail in Chapter 14. In a critical review of the literature, S. W. Lee (1991) reviewed 36 studies in which biofeedback was used as a treatment for hyperactivity. He concluded that biofeedback treatments alone have not been effectively evaluated and that methodological difficulties with existing studies limit any generalizations that may be made from individual studies or patients to so-called hyperactive populations. He also concluded, as do we, that in conjunction with other self-regulation strategies such as hypnotherapy, biofeedback is very promising in its potential for modulation of some of the behavioral concomitants of attentional disorders.

Recently Blanton and Johnson (1991) described their use of computer-assisted biofeedback to help three children with ADHD to develop self-control. Two sixth-grade boys (11 years old) and one fourth-grade boy (10 years old) were selected by teacher and principal interviews as showing the most off-task behaviors in terms of being out of their seats and touching others, failing to pay attention, and failure to complete work assignments. They each were treated with biofeedback sessions lasting 20 minutes, including a baseline of 2 minutes, verbal instruction of 2 minutes, relaxation tape of 8 to 12 minutes, and relaxation period of 2 minutes. Electromyographic (EMG) readings were monitored during the baseline. Results indicated that all students were able to relax through the use of computer assisted biofeedback, and one student in which on-task behavior was collected demonstrated an increase in on-task behavior after implementation of the biofeedback. As described in detail in Chapter 14, most if not all biofeedback clinical studies and descriptions include and involve descriptions of relaxation and some form of imagery — analogous if not identical to what we know and define as hypnotherapy. In this report by Blanton and Johnson, they refer to "psychophysiologic relaxation training and biofeedback techniques," describe the "biofeedback sessions" in which key features (of the longest duration) are an 8- to 12-minute relaxation tape with imagery suggestions, and conclude that the results are a function of "implementation of the biofeedback." Whereas this is a reflection of the methodological dilemmas S. W. Lee (1991) has noted in many studies, Blanton and Johnson's work is of interest for its demonstration of the value of creativity in the combination of self-regulation strategies (biofeedback, imagery/relaxation) to promote improvement of behavior and learning in children with ADHD.

In a more recent study, Tansey (1993) reports the stability of EEG biofeedback results for "a hyperactive boy who failed fourth grade [in a] perceptually impaired class." The 10-year-old subject presented with a "developmental reading disorder" along with hyperactivity and an educational classification as being "perceptually impaired" since the second grade. He was trained in EMG biofeedback and with an EEG 14-Hz biofeedback training regimen, became symptom-free within three sessions, and was reported to have remained free of motoric overactivity, high distractibility, low frustration tolerance, and poor self-control for over 10 years following. The author explains that the EMG session can be understood to introduce the child to a state of motoric calm, thought by the author to be a reflection of 14-Hz dominant posture from which 14-Hz brainwave training proceeded to functionally rectify the brain state activation abnormality reflected by the hyperactivity. Following the biofeedback training, this youngster is described as having shifted to a normal classroom with disappearance of learning difficulties, hyperactivity, and related (negative) behaviors. The author describes the biofeedback apparatus and procedure clearly, methodically, and in precise detail; and the results are impressive. The author also describes, however, the following concomitant "Instructions" presented verbally to the patient (Tansey, 1993):

> Instructions during the EEG biofeedback training sessions were presented to the youngsters while they were in a reclining position with their eyes closed. The instructions were: "Now, let yourself become hollow and heavy. Just let yourself be a hollow, heavy rock; quiet, hollow, and heavy — and let the music come out." Intermittent, positive reinforcement (verbal praise for "music" production and signature shifting) was provided, such as "That's very good. The better the music, the better your brain works. The better your brain works, the better your ability to be calm and learn." (p. 40)

To the trained hypnotherapist this verbalization clearly includes and reflects elements of a hypnotherapeutic intervention, that is, hypnotic induction (eye closure), positive and permissive deepening imagery with a kinesthetic focus ("*let* yourself be a hollow heavy rock"), ego-strengthening suggestions ("That's very good"), and post-hypnotic suggestions ("The better your brain works, the better your ability to be calm and learn"). However, this is not identified as hypnosis, and the author concludes, we believe mistakenly that the described biofeedback process is responsible for the outcome described. Although we don't doubt the efficacy or potential value of biofeedback, we wish to emphasize the at least potential role and value of the hypnotic-like language described. As discussed in detail in Chapter 14, the time is certainly ripe for carefully designed studies that will help elucidate the relative contributions of hypnosis and biofeedback in these and other conditions.

Illovsky and Fredman (1976) utilized hypnotherapy with 48 children, ages 6 to 8 years, selected from among 180 children referred to a clinic because of behavior and learning problems in a school. Excluding children with major psychiatric disorders or perceptual difficulties, the authors selected children manifesting short attention span, acting-out behavior, and distractibility. All of these children had a history of good school attendance, an IQ above

85, and parental consent. Concurrently with hypnotherapy, the students received remedial academic instruction, as they had before the hypnotic sessions were begun, albeit with little success. On 55 occasions—no child was present for all sessions—the children listened to tape-recorded hypnotic suggestions under the supervision of one of their reading teachers. The taped hypnotic induction included eye fixation, eye closure, general relaxation, counting from 1 to 10, and imagining a pleasant outdoor scene. The suggestions for improved learning and increased ability to cope with emotional problems were as follows:

> From now on you are going to think of what to do for yourself. If you think of something bad that happened to you before, think about whether you could have done it better. If you could have done it better, then, think that when the same thing happens again, you will do it better . . . Go into a deeper and deeper relaxation . . . deeper and deeper . . . There is nothing to disturb you and there is nothing to bother you . . . You are feeling nice and relaxed and you are sinking into a still deeper relaxation. . . .
>
> If you think that someone wants to do something bad to you, imagine that you are in his place and you want to do the same thing to him. Then think about why you would be doing it in his place. Then think that he was also not doing it to hurt you but for some other reason. Go into a deeper and deeper . . . etc.
>
> You feel like talking to people, because you want to know what they think and you want to learn something from them and also you want people to like you. For this reason, you feel like talking to people. There is nothing to disturb you . . . etc.
>
> Think also about why you should be good to people and how much you will like it, when people are nice to you . . . Go into a deeper . . . etc.
>
> If you feel sad or angry, think of something nice that you can remember that happened to you. If you cannot remember anything nice, then think of something nice or good that you wish would happen to you. While you are thinking about these nice things, the sadness or anger is leaving you and you will feel nice, calm, and good . . . Go into a deeper . . . etc.
>
> I want you to listen to me some more. From today you are going to think and dream about why you should learn in school and at home. You feel also that you want to learn and this will make you feel good. You feel that you are as good and smart as the other children and you can learn and read just as they can learn and read. When you are reading, you will feel nice, good and calm inside. Go into a deeper and deeper . . . etc.
>
> As soon as you start to learn anything, you will feel good and like reading and learning more and more. Remember, as soon as you start to learn, you will only think about the words and letters in front of you. Go into a deeper and deeper . . . etc. (p. 90)*

---

*From Illovsky and Fredman (1976). With permission.

At each session, the teacher rated every child for the presence or absence of "relaxation," manifested by eye closure and motionless behavior, with the appearance of sleep. There was no measure of hypnotic responsiveness, and the authors themselves questioned whether relaxation and hypnosis should be equated.

Teacher ratings of improved self-confidence correlated positively with the number of sessions attended by each pupil but correlated negatively with the percentage of sessions in which each pupil was judged to be relaxed. Ratings of relaxation were positively correlated with improved attention in class but were not related to five other academic and behavioral variables. The authors urged caution in interpreting the data because of teacher bias, lack of a control group, and lack of any real indication of hypnotic responsiveness.

Noting the emphasis on eye closure in the induction, the young age of the children, and the fact that the sessions were supervised by teachers with whom the children may have had a relationship marked by failure and negative attitudes, we too doubt the validity of equating relaxation with hypnosis, and are really not surprised at the paucity of positive results. In the last analysis, this study really tells us very little about the value of hypnotherapy for learning-disabled children with behavior problems in school.

Young, Montano, and Goldberg (1991) described a hypnobehavioral procedure that integrated self-monitoring, self-hypnosis and progressive relaxation, and response prevention training. The combination of these self-regulation strategies were applied to helping a 10½-year-old boy to manage and overcome an adjustment disorder manifested by anxiety secondary to learning disabilities affecting his written language output.

Evaluation in a multidisciplinary clinic revealed the boy to have an anxiety-induced tremor in one arm with no other abnormalities on examination. On the Wechsler Intelligence Scale for Children — Revised (WISC-R) he had an IQ of 111, but significant interscale scatter was noted and reading was at grade level. Reversals were noted in cursive writing. In addition to educational recommendations that included guidance in task completion and study skills, and use of recorded texts to improve comprehension, the evaluating team recommended training in self-management to hopefully reduce the negative effects of anxiety on school performance. Self-monitoring consisted of requesting that he keep track of the thoughts he had before anxiety-related experiences at home and school. This resulted in identification of three cues preceding anxiety-related thoughts and behaviors, that is, fine tremors in the left hand, thoughts of failure, and feelings of anger. Self-hypnosis training began with practice of imagery and progressive muscle relaxation and initial follow-up sessions focused on reinforcing favorite place/activity imagery and on training in rapid induction of self-hypnosis. Response prevention was integrated into his hypnosis through instructions to imagine himself getting ready to write, becoming aware of the sensations associated with tremors and anticipatory anxiety, and then imagining himself doing the rapid induction of self-hypnosis to relax his arms and eliminate the anxiety response. By the fourth treatment session, the patient's anxiety level was significantly decreased: he reported no anxiety on 6 of 14 days, and on 6 other days, he reported the easy conversion of anxiety to comfort through the techniques he had learned. His parents corroborated his improvement and reported dramatic improvement in handwriting productivity. Even though his learning disability per se remained the same at follow-up 18 months later, he had maintained the effective application of his self-management skills, found school and writing much easier, was on the honor roll at school, and was engaged in many positive social activities. We agree that the description of Young and associates (1991) supports their conclusion that such hypno-behavioral, integrative approaches offer the clinician the opportunity to target specific behavior(s), to identify the approach to altering that behavior(s), and to easily assess both overall and individual strategy effectiveness. As they suggest, such combined approaches have promise as procedures to be evaluated within larger, systematic research studies.

Margolis (1990) describes a variety of self-regulation strategies in a recent literature review from which he concludes that what he overall refers to as "relaxation training" has promising results in reducing symptoms of anxiety, impulsivity, hyperactivity, distractibility, and emotional lability of exceptional learners, while also positively influencing their self-concept, academic achievement, and classroom behavior. While hypnotherapy per se is not mentioned, he briefly describes so-called common forms of "relaxation training" to include progressive muscle relaxation, visual imagery, autogenics, and meditation.

Portes, Best, Sandhu, and Cuentas (1992) recently described the effects of relaxation training on anxiety and academic performance. Their study examined relationships among state anxiety, trait anxiety, and performance; it also estimated the value of a brief session of relaxation with music as compared to a lecture treatment across two subject areas. No improvement in performance was found for either treatment. The lecture condition was found to lower trait anxiety. They concluded that both state and trait anxiety may be reduced by autogenic (experiential) and lecture "treatments" with no improvement in test performance.

Reading Disability

Illovsky (1963) studied the effect of group hypnotherapy with five nonpsychotic adolescent boys confined to a state hospital because of delinquency and severe behavior disorders. Five similar adolescent patients served as no-treatment controls. All subjects were nonreaders, with reading skills at or below first-grade level at the beginning of the study. Every day, before class began, the experimental group listened to a hypnotic induction followed by several suggestions for increased motivation, concentration, and performance in reading. Although no standardized hypnotizability scale was administered, these boys all responded to several informal measures similar to items from the Stanford Scales. One boy in this group cooperated minimally and was not included in the data analysis. After 6 months, the four remaining boys in the hypnotherapy group had gained an average of 2 years and 3 months in reading skills; the no-treatment controls had gained an average of 9 months. The author concluded that "hypnosis through its well-known hypermnesia can maintain and even enhance the reading ability of the hypnotized subjects" (Illovsky, 1963, p. 65). Such a conclusion seems unwarranted, in view of uncontrolled factors such as attention. At follow-up 2 months later, two boys in the experimental group showed no further improvement.

Jampolsky (1975) reported his hypnotherapeutic work with a small group of third- and fourth-grade children who were having difficulty learning to read. In a unique effort to overcome the negative reinforcement to which such children are repeatedly subjected, Jampolsky also used imagery techniques with the teachers and parents, encouraging them to visualize the children as successful readers. The research included a control group of poor readers who apparently received no treatment but were tested at the beginning and end of the study.

The experimental group participated in an 8-step program over a period of three 45-minute sessions: (1) since the children had already demonstrated problems with traditional visual learning, the group hypnotic induction minimized suggestions for visualization and focused instead on kinesthetic techniques such as feeling a weight pull their arm down or feeling fur on their face; (2) the children then imagined being in a pleasant place of their own choosing and concentrated on rhythmic breathing; (3) they were encouraged to get rid of painful associations to learning by mentally washing such bad feelings, dirt, and grime out of their brains; (4) they imagined themselves writing a small book about their favorite subject; (5) they used suggested tactile, auditory, and visual imagery to picture themselves on a motion picture screen reading their books with fluency, success, confidence, and joy, thus creating an ego ideal; (6) they climbed into their images on the screen, merging with the ideal self; (7) they imagined the new self permeating all body tissues; and (8) they were asked to repeat this process daily for 5 to 10 minutes before going to school and before going to sleep. Jampolsky emphasized that this is a holistic approach to learning rather than the bit-by-bit process usually employed.

Over a 1-month period, the experimental group averaged an increase in reading skill of 1½ years, whereas the control group gained only 1 month. Self-esteem was markedly increased in the experimental group, and the parents and teachers reported decreased tension and increased energy. When the experimental group was retested 1 year later, their progress continued to be excellent, as compared to that of the control group. Jampolsky's results are encouraging, although the study contains methodological problems similar to those of the Illovsky study. Jampolsky presented no evidence that the subjects were really in hypnosis and, if so, that hypnosis and not some other variable accounted for the results.

Johnson, Johnson, Olson, and Newman (1981) studied the impact of group hypnotherapy and self-hypnosis on the academic performance and self-esteem of learning-disabled children, using the Jampolsky study (1975) as a model but extending the type of data gathered and analyzing it for more explanatory power. The authors suspect that, in practical application, group treatment may be highly feasible, but the effectiveness of the procedure may be better evaluated by individual techniques such as multiple correlation.

Krippner (1966) studied 49 children, ages 8 to 17 years and generally of average intelligence, enrolled in a 5-week remedial reading program. Hypnotherapy was utilized adjunctively with nine children whose parents specifically requested it. The median amount of reading improvement for the entire group was 5 months, as measured by a standardized reading test. In the hypnosis group, 8 children scored above the median and 1 at or below the median; in the control group, 16 children scored above the median and 24 at or below. The difference between the two groups was statisticially significant, although the difference in actual amount of improvement (6 months vs. 5 months) was too small to be of much practical value.

For the hypnosis group, Krippner tailored the induction to the expectations and needs of each child. The suggestions pertaining to reading focused on three areas: reducing tension and anxiety, enhancing the motivation to read, and increasing concentration and attention span.

> Tension: As you relax, you begin to stop worrying. You stop worrying about reading. You begin to think how much you would like to read better. You begin to think how much you would like to improve your reading ability. You know that you can read better if all the muscles of your body are relaxed. If all of your muscles are relaxed, you will be able to pay closer attention to what you read. You want very much to relax your muscles while you read and to be completely at ease. You want very much to relax all the little muscles in your eyes while you read. This will help you to read with your eyes wide open so that you will not miss any of the letters. If your eyes are wide open, you will not miss any of the words. If your eyes are wide open, you will read much, much better.
>
> Motivation: Every time you read a word or a sentence correctly, you will feel very good inside. You will feel proud of yourself because you read so well. You will enjoy the feeling that reading well gives you. You will want to read some more words and sentences. You will become interested

in reading books and magazines and newspapers. Every time that you read something correctly, and understand what you read, your interest will increase. You will want to read another book, or another magazine, or another newspaper. Sometimes you will make mistakes while reading. These mistakes will not bother you because we all make mistakes. None of us is perfect. However, when you read a word or a sentence very well, you will be pleased and happy. You will want to read more and more.

Concentration: When you open your eyes, you and your clinician will select a story in a book that interests you. After looking it over for a few minutes to make certain that it is really interesting, you will start to read the story. You will find that you are able to pay very close attention to the story. You will pay close attention for many, many minutes. It will be just as if your eyes are glued to the page. In fact, you will not want to take your eyes away from the story until you have read several pages. Perhaps you will even finish the whole story. When you have trouble with a word, your clinician will help you out. But this will not affect your attention which will be very, very strong. At the same time, your concentration will be better than it has been for a long, long time. You will think about nothing but the characters in the story and what is happening to them. You will understand what you are reading. You might even see the characters in your mind's eye. You will enjoy what you are reading. Your concentration and attention will be so good today that you will find it even easier to concentrate and to pay attention tomorrow. (pp. 263–264)*

In discussing his results, Krippner noted the need for cautious interpretation. It is possible that parents in the hypnosis group were especially cooperative and optimistic about the entire remedial program, with unknown effects on their children's progress. The effect of special attention from the hypnotherapist in the experimental group is also unknown. Finally, it is possible that the suggestions might have been equally effective in the absence of any hypnotic induction.

Although Crasilneck and Hall (1985) have not attempted a research study, their clinical results are optimistic, yielding moderate to marked improvement in approximately three-fourths of their child patients presenting with dyslexia. They do not mention the length of required treatment, although they mention one adolescent with very severe dyslexia, previously diagnosed as retarded, who appeared to them to have normal intelligence and no severe emotional problems. "After extensive hypnotherapy lasting a few years, she graduated from high school, passed both the written and practical part of her driver's license tests, and has become more functional" (Crasilneck & Hall, 1985, p. 190). Presumably most of their dyslexic patients were not this severely affected. In their hypnotherapeutic work with dyslexia patients, suggestions include the following:

---

*From Krippner (1966). With permission.

Your vision is simply going to improve. . . . You can recognize words with much more ease. . . . Once you have learned the word, it will make an impression upon your unconscious brain and mind and recall of this word in the future will be much easier. . . . Your memory for words that you learn will become implanted in your mental processes and will be recalled in a smooth, coordinated fashion. There will be an excellent coordination between your eyes, your brain, and your memory . . . and your reading capabilities will continuously improve until they return to normal. . . . You will be much less anxious and much less afraid in your reading and learning habits. . . . Your reading is going to improve consistently. (p. 190)

We have heard some therapists say the material "will burn itself into your brain." Because of the tendency for people in hypnosis to take words literally, we prefer the more neutral phrase "make an impression" as used by Crasilneck and Hall.

Prichard and Taylor (1989) reported a study of 32 remedial reading students who participated in a SALT program modified to include a creative writing exercise as a substitute for one-half of the relaxation/visualization activities normally employed by their classroom teachers. Students were pre- and post-tested with the California Achievement Test. The average gain per month of instruction was 2.375 months, indicating a considerable decrease from the 3.86 months gain/month average. The authors believed that the most likely reason for the drop in reading success was the reduction by one-half of the opportunities for students to employ their visual imagery modality. The substitution of a creative writing activity, while enjoyed by students and thought worthwhile by teachers, appeared not to have exerted as strong an accelerative learning effect as did the full complement of relaxation/visualization exercises employed in previous years. These data were felt to provide support for instructional programs that set out to create a strong positive-suggestive atmosphere and to employ relaxation/visualization activities on a daily basis. Again we note that hypnosis and hypnotherapy are not mentioned in this report; nonetheless, the operative ingredients of the study are indeed those of hypnotherapy as we understand and describe it, that is, of imagery and relaxation, and of the concomitant awareness of the importance and value of the "positive suggestive atmosphere."

Number Reversals

Jampolsky (1970) studied 10 children in grades 1 to 3, ages 6 to 9 years, who manifested number reversals. All the children had abnormal EEGs and various signs of attentional difficulties, then called minimal brain dysfunction. The five children in the experimental group had a single hypnotic induction focusing on kinesthetic and tactile imagery and including suggestions that they would learn to write numbers properly. There was no determination of whether these children were actually in hypnosis. The single hypnotic session was followed by 2 weeks of remedial training in writing numbers, using a variety of special techniques for learning-disabled children. The five control children received no hypnotic induction and no remedial training. After 2 weeks, number reversals were entirely eliminated in the experimental group; the control group showed a slight increase in reversals. The design of the study makes it impossible to determine whether the difference was due to hypnotherapy, to remedial training, or to other factors.

Test Anxiety

We sometimes see children whose IQs are at least average, whose study skills are adequate, and whose teachers insist that they have mastered classroom material as evidenced by workbook assignments, learning games, and other classroom activities. Yet, when these children are confronted with a formal test of their knowledge, they become markedly anxious and perform at a level much lower than would be expected.

When children with test anxiety come to our office, they usually are quite aware that their anxiety is unwarranted, and they are most often highly motivated for help. Sometimes the test anxiety is a clue to a more pervasive problem requiring intensive psychotherapy, and accordingly, as always, a careful diagnostic assessment is essential. Often, however, the problem can be treated quite directly, usually with gains then spreading to other areas of the children's (commonly adolescents') lives. Our approach includes the following steps:

Step 1. Having established the children's understanding of the irrationality of their anxiety, and their motivation for assistance, we teach them to go into hypnosis by whatever method seems most appropriate and the best match for them.

Step 2. In hypnosis we invite them to visualize themselves in some activity unrelated to school, in which they know they are competent and perform with minimal or no anxiety.

Step 3. Having achieved a feeling of competence, they are then taught to let go of the specific content of the imagery, retain the feeling, and visualize an idealized self with the same good feelings in a classroom. This can be accomplished in many ways: It is often easily done with a split screen idea, or letting a screen be full, then blank, then full again with the new image.

Step 4. They then experience a series of images, in a manner similar to systematic desensitization, beginning with a very brief and simple performance task, such as distributing homework sheets. They move through images of more difficult tasks, culminating in an image of taking a major test or final examination, always retaining the feeling of confidence and competence, and merging with each positive image as it becomes clear. If at any point anxiety develops, they may drop back to an easier image before progressing, and/or they utilize the imagery equivalent of thought-stopping by equally abruptly imagining, for example, a STOP sign to abruptly interrupt the feelings of anxiety.

Step 5. They are informed that this kind of rehearsal in fantasy often carries over into the actual situation.

Step 6. They are given the post-hypnotic suggestion that when actually required to perform, for example, take the examination, they can recall and reexperience the same good feelings as in the therapeutic sessions; they can do the same when preparing for the examination.

Step 7. They are taught self-hypnosis, with the specific suggestion to review the positive images at an appropriate time and place, preferably twice daily for 5 to 10 minutes. They are encouraged as a post-hypnotic suggestion and also out of hypnosis that "the more you practice the better you get." In a future projection suggestion, they are encouraged to picture themselves successful before, during, and after an examination and being proud of that accomplishment.

Step 8. Finally, they are reminded that no one performs perfectly all the time, and they are encouraged to set realistic expectations and to perceive failures as opportunities for new learning.

We find that two to five sessions are usually sufficient to master the problem, provided there is no significant psychopathology in the patients, their families, or the school environment itself.

CONCLUSIONS

Clearly, research and clinical reports are rife with methodological problems that prevent us from concluding much about the value of hypnotherapy for enhancing learning and performance. Some of the more detailed approaches contain therapeutic suggestions that are interesting and might indeed prove valuable, but both clinicians and researchers must distinguish between "interesting" and "valuable." It is unfortunate to find this distinction lacking in some of the research reports. For example, Woody and Billy (1970) begin their paper with a brief literature review, including the statement that "Krippner (1966) successfully used clinical suggestion and/or hypnosis to decrease tension and increase motivation with children enrolled in a reading clinic" (p. 268). Our own evaluation of Krippner's (1966) research found no basis for such a conclusion.

At the same time, it has not been shown that hypnotherapy is not helpful in learning and performance problems in children. We therefore suggest that clinicians continue to treat such problems with hypnotherapy, with proper modesty in the claims they make to prospective patients, and with an eye toward the creative integration of hypnotherapy with other self-regulatory strategies as reflected in the efforts of Young and his colleagues (1991). As recent investigators have begun to do, we hope that both clinicians and researchers will continue to consider methodological issues carefully and, in so doing, avoid making nonverifiable claims and "much ado about nothing" in published reports.

CHAPTER TEN

Hypnotherapy for Pain Control

Historical accounts of hypnotherapy include many reports of its use for pain control including that of James Braid, an English surgeon, who, in the mid-19th century, applied hypnotic training techniques to alleviate the pain of major surgery (Braid, 1843/1960). Given that children generally have more hypnotic talent than adults *and* the ability to control pain with hypnotic suggestion is positively correlated with hypnotizability (E. R. Hilgard & Hilgard, 1975), it should come as no surprise that children have been found to be more adept than adults in using hypnotherapy for control of pain (Wakeman & Kaplan, 1978).

Although these findings are true in terms of group comparisons, of course there are individual differences. Advantages to children who learn these methods of self-regulating pain include enhancement of self-confidence, personal participation in the therapeutic process, reduction of side effects, and increased ability to participate in normal daily activities. Articles report successful use of self-hypnosis techniques by children with a variety of chronic illnesses, including malignancies, hemophilia, diabetes, sickle-cell disease, migraines, and juvenile rheumatoid arthritis (Dahlquist, Gil, Armstrong, Ginsburg, & Jones, 1985; C. J. Erickson, 1991; Olness, 1985a; Olness & MacDonald, 1987; Russo & Varni, 1982; Varni & Gilbert, 1982; Varni, Katz, & Dash, 1982; Zeltzer, Dash, & Holland, 1979). Hypnotherapeutic interventions may be helpful as adjunct therapy in the management of childhood pain. Some children may prefer to use self-hypnosis at some times and not at others. The following case report illustrates these complexities; it also reveals the power of the spoken word in a hypnotherapeutic context.

Frank L., age 13, suffered electrical burns over much of his body after trying to retrieve a kite that had landed on a high-voltage wire. In the course of his hospitalization, he was taken to the department of physical medicine for a special test to determine the extent of nerve damage to his hand. During the test, he reported to the hypnotherapist a pain level of 8, on a 0 to 10 scale, in his right arm and back. He responded very well to suggestions for reduction of the pain in his arm, lowering it to a 0 level in a minute or so. He could not, however, do anything about the pain in his back. When questioned about this, he said that he did not want to relax and lie down on his back because his back would then stick to the sheet, and he would have to go through the severe pain of getting unstuck in order to get back to his own room and back to his bed. This pain was so severe that Frank could not use hypnosis at all to modify it. The therapist agreed with his logic and casually remarked, "That's okay. I'll go back upstairs with you and you can get rid of the back pain after you are in your room and back in your own bed."

Since the therapist knew that Frank had had little success using self-hypnosis for severe pain, of course she intended to communicate that she would help him. She accompanied Frank back to his room. A few minutes after he was in bed, she told him that he could now begin work to get rid of the pain in his back. He smiled and said that, as soon as he got into bed, the back pain disappeared. He had indeed taken the therapist's casual remark as a post-hypnotic suggestion. Interestingly, he then reported return of pain in his arm, which disappeared after a brief session of about 5 minutes. He was possibly responding to the demand characteristics of the therapist's seeming expectation that he would still have pain when he got into bed.

Hypnotherapists sometimes approach the problem of pain in children in a trial-and-error fashion, randomly trying hypnoanalgesic techniques with which they are most familiar with little thought as to why one method might be preferable to another in a particular instance. Research in school-age children (Ross & Ross, 1984) indicates that perception of pain in children is dependent on past experiences, education about pain, and the psychological and social contexts in which pain occurs. The following material deals with aspects of a child's experience of pain that might influence choice of technique.

VARIATIONS IN THE EXPERIENCE OF PAIN

Age

The neonate can perceive pain as is reflected by crying and by autonomic changes. However, because of its incomplete cortical development, there may be no conscious memory of painful experiences in the neonatal period. Fortunately, much research was done in the 1980s on pain experienced by newborns, including premature infants (Fitzgerald, Millard, & McIntosh, 1988; Anand, 1990; Schecter, Bernstein, Beck, Hart, & Sherzer, 1991). This has led to increased efforts to provide analgesia and/or anesthesia for these infants. By the end of the first year of life, the child can identify and localize pain, and by the end of the second year, there is clear evidence of memory. Young children quickly learn to avoid painful stimuli such as a hot bulb on a lamp or Christmas tree, and they may begin to cry at the mere sight of a doctor who has previously given some painful treatment. Since most children as young as 2 years have developed skills in imagery and in receptive language and can perceive adults as sources of help, these factors together with motivation to avoid pain should make young children receptive to hypnotherapeutic techniques for pain control. The main problems involve a poorly developed sense of time and of cause and effect. Thus a 2-year-old probably could not benefit from a statement such as "If you will do this or think about that, then the pain might go away." However, more naturalistic techniques, such as storytelling, which capture the child's attention and therefore focus attention away from pain, will often be successful (Kuttner, 1991). Generally, a child of 4 or 5 years should be able to utilize hypnotic suggestions for pain control unless past or present experience has taught a contrary expectation.

Individual Differences in Tolerance

Children vary greatly in their ability to tolerate pain; they vary more than do adults. Given three children who have apparently equal amounts of pain, the first may continue playing, the second may ask someone to "kiss it and make it all better" and will then continue playing, and the third may experience complete disruption of play and behave as if a catastrophe had occurred. In Petrie's (1967) terms, these children are reducers, moderators, and augmentors, and they tend to distort perceptions of pain. In a study of adolescents and adults, Petrie (1967) found that juvenile delinquents and youngsters involved in contact sports tended to be reducers. Alcohol and aspirin, both of which are associated with increased tolerance of pain, significantly lessened pain for augmentors but had little or no effect with reducers. Likewise, we would speculate that hypnotherapy for pain control might be more effective for augmentors than for reducers. However, the moderators might prove to be the most responsive to hypnotherapy, especially if the augmentors have some emotional investment in experiencing or expressing the experience of pain. It is not clear whether the differences among Petrie's groups reflect biological or psychological differences or both.

Schecter has reviewed neuroanatomical and neurochemical factors that may ultimately explain individual differences in pain perception (Schecter, Berde, & Yaster, 1993).

Emotional Significance

For some children, pain has little emotional significance and is perceived mainly as a nuisance or a bad experience to be terminated as soon as possible.

For other children, pain may have a variety of meanings and may serve a variety of psychological functions: (1) punishment for real or imagined sins; (2) getting attention and love, especially for children who tend to be ignored when "everything is okay"; (3) identification or merging with a loved one who has had similar pain, especially if there has been real or threatened abandonment by that person; (4) avoiding feared or unwanted situations that would be inevitable if the child were not in pain; (5) remaining close to a loved one whom the child feels a need to protect or in whose absence the child does not feel secure (most school-phobic pains fall into this category); (6) gaining status in certain families or cultural contexts where expressions of pain are socially acceptable and highly valued; (7) unconscious expression of hostility toward parents or siblings ("I'll make you feel bad to see me in pain"); (8) controlling others, especially for children with passive–aggressive tendencies ("I'll make you stay home with me. I'll ruin your day, and you can't get mad at me because you have to feel sorry for me because I'm in pain"); (9) assuring continuation of life, especially in sick children who have been taught that God uses death to take away pain; and/or (10) fulfilling the will of God, especially in children who have been taught that people must suffer for their sins and that continued suffering makes one somehow special in the eyes of God.

These are only a few of the ways in which pain can have emotional meaning; one must always be on the alert for other idiosyncratic kinds of significance. Hypnoanalgesic suggestions are likely to have no effect if the therapist has not dealt with the emotional significance of pain, either directly or indirectly.

Context of Pain

Many aspects of the child's reality affect the extent to which pain will be tolerated. Previous pain experiences may have shaped the child's expectations that the present experience will be dreadful. For many children, the repeated invasive procedures associated with chronic diseases such as cancer or sickle-cell disease are more distressing than any other aspect of illness or treatment (Fowler-Kerry, 1990; Savedra, Tesler, Holzemer, & Ward, 1989). Certain coexisting bodily states such as fatigue or physical discomfort will probably reduce pain tolerance. Coexisting psychological states are also important. Anxiety and depression usually reduce pain tolerance. Excitement and anticipatory joy, such as the time of a birthday, will often enhance pain tolerance.

A child's response to pain may depend partly on understanding of its purpose: (1) no understanding in a very small child; (2) no purpose, for example, an accident; (3) an unjust purpose, for example, a wound resulting from a fight to defend oneself; (4) a logical purpose, for example, a dressing change for burns. When a child understands the purpose or source of pain, reaction may also be influenced by the response of others. A parent who responds with anxiety and confusion will elicit a more negative reaction in a child than will a parent who responds with acceptance and with clarity about what needs to be done (Eland & Anderson, 1977).

Children's reactions to pain are often influenced by the context of their expectations concerning adults' response as much as by the response itself. Helen H., age 9 years, sustained a small laceration of her hand after a mischievous fight on the school playground. Frequently ridiculed and punished by her parents, the child was terrified that she would be punished for her misbehavior. She made no effort to report the accident and hoped to conceal it entirely by wiping the blood on her red dress. Although blood loss was minimal, she fainted a few minutes later. The fainting probably was an unconscious expression of her need to avoid "facing the consequences." The child was frankly disappointed when the pediatrician, after some deliberation, decided that sutures (painful punishment) would not be necessary. We would expect that this child would not have responded to hypnoanalgesic suggestions, had they been offered, despite her good imaginative skills.

In general, we would expect children to benefit less from hypnotherapy for pain that occurs in a negative context than from pain that occurs in a more neutral context. Therefore, we recommend that pediatricians and other child health specialists counsel parents regarding optimal ways of responding to pain in their children. Of course, doctors and other medical staff also play an important role in creating or modifying the reality context of pain in children. The doctor who communicates that pain is inevitable and may become even more severe will tend to have patients who experience a great deal of pain. On the other hand, if all members of the medical team approach the child with a calm and positive manner, then the child may well be able to fulfill the expectation that the situation is manageable and may even be enjoyable. Because children lack the preconceptions of adults, because they may be influenced positively or negatively, and because their future perceptions concerning pain may be permanently affected, it is incumbent on all adults to choose words related to pain very carefully when speaking to children.

The following is an example of a therapeutic approach to a child who had been negatively conditioned to needles and to people and places associated with needles.

Six-year-old David had become conditioned to manifest fear, tantrums, and physical resistance whenever he saw a nurse, a physician, or even the hospital doctors. David had leukemia and had been in remission since shortly after his diagnosis 14 months earlier. With respect to the disease, he was doing well; emotionally, however, he was not.

What factors could have led to his pathological fear of needles? We cannot be sure, of course, but several influences may have affected David. His father had a dental phobia, which required him to take tranquilizers before going to the dentist even for a routine cleaning. David's first nurse in the hospital had an unresolved memory of an unpleasant experience, dating from when she had first received ether anesthesia at age 6 years. The lab technician who drew blood from David the first time explained nothing to him about the procedure. We do not know what other children may have said to frighten David or if he had seen something on television that had also contributed to his fear. Whatever the causes, a finger stick became an unpleasant and dreaded experience, not only for David but for his family, the nursing staff, and the laboratory staff.

David was sedated for intravenous injections and was given general anesthesia for bone marrow exams and spinal taps. After he had an allergic reaction to sedation, his physician sought alternative approaches. David was referred to us to learn self-hypnosis for control of his needle phobia.

At the time of his initial visit, we chatted with David and his parents about his interests, likes and dislikes, fears, and learning styles. We learned about games he liked, stories he liked, and music he preferred. Then we tailored a simple relaxation exercise for David and asked him to practice his exercise twice a day until the next visit a week later.

David was a quick learner and demonstrated good retention at the time of the second visit. We reviewed the exercise with him, this time giving him the opportunity to play computer games that reflected his state of relaxation (by monitoring peripheral temperature and galvanic skin resistance). As he succeeded, we explained that he was showing that he was the boss of these body processes and that his brain was directing the changes he saw on the computer screen. We also made drawings of his nervous system and explained how nerves carried messages to his brain, which his brain then figured out. We asked him to make a similar drawing at home. He was reminded to practice the relaxation exercise once a day.

We saw David a third time a week later, and he brought the drawing with him. He was eager to play the computer game again. After one practice session with the computer, we gave David a small needle and began to rehearse procedures, using stuffed animals as models. David participated, and we asked him to review these procedures at home under his parents' direction. We also told him that he should continue to practice the relaxation exercise at home once a day.

During the fourth visit, David reviewed his relaxation exercise and then began to "program" himself to "turn on and off" the "switches" in the brain that controlled his nerves. We allowed David to let us know when he was ready, and he "turned off the switch" to his left hand. With his permission, we touched his hand with the needle. He was elated when this did not bother him. Again he practiced at home and, a week later, tolerated a venipuncture with no difficulty.

Subsequently, he watched a videotape of another child undergoing a lumbar puncture and bone marrow puncture while doing the relaxation exercises. And David underwent his next bone marrow and lumbar puncture procedures with comfort and competence.

Ross and Ross (1984), in a study of 994 school children, found no clearly defined age trends in the children's pain concept. However, they did find much evidence for early maladaptive behavior in coping with pain. These authors expressed concern that, if unchecked, such behavior might persist into adulthood. Ross and Ross also noted that the children were generally ignorant about how to cope with pain, and they suggested that pain be a topic in school science curricula.

We believe that health care professionals working with children who have pain should analyze themselves with respect to their own childhood experiences with pain, the persistence of their own fears of painful procedures, and their own strategies for coping with pain. Such analysis may not only help the therapist to understand the perceptions of the child patient, but may keep him from projecting his own negative expectations onto the child.

TOWARD UNDERSTANDING HYPNOANALGESIA

Most researchers and clinicians who work with hypnosis and hypnotherapy agree that the phenomenon of hypnoanalgesia is real and that patients and subjects are not faking in order to please the experimenter or therapist. Whereas it is possible to deny the limited pain involved in a laboratory experiment, the idea of faking becomes farfetched in severe clinical pain such as one sees in surgical procedures or in advanced cancer. Some skeptical researchers have deemphasized the role of hypnotic suggestion in favor of such constructs as role playing or expectation (e.g., Barber & Hahn, 1962; Stam & Spanos, 1980). We agree that role playing and expectation can enhance one's ability to modify pain, but we also believe that these factors are neither necessary nor sufficient for hypnoanalgesia. For example, Crasilneck and Hall (1973) demonstrated hypnotic pain reduction with naive children and with culturally unsophisticated subjects not acquainted with the expectations of the hypnotherapist. We have had similar clinical experiences.

It is one thing to accept the phenomenon of hypnoanalgesia as real: it is another thing to explain the mechanism by which it occurs. Two lines of research, one psychological and the other physiological, have been pursued.

A Psychological Lead: Alternative Cognitive Controls

It is often the case in science that new ideas occur almost by chance, beginning in unrelated areas and finding new direction by virtue of the creative ability of the scientist. Thus, the contribution of Hilgard and Hilgard toward explaining hypnoanalgesia began with a demonstration of hypnotic deafness that had nothing at all to do with pain. In a classroom demonstration, a subject who had been given suggestions for hypnotic deafness failed to respond to loud noises or to questions from classmates. Another student, noting that nothing was wrong with the subject's ears, asked if there might be some part of him that actually did hear. When the subject was asked to lift one finger, if some part of him other than the part in hypnosis knew what was going on, he lifted one finger and then asked the instructor to explain this involuntary movement. The part of him not in hypnosis was able to give a full account of pain following a signal (touching the arm). In the usual waking state, the subject was given a cue for release of hypnotic amnesia, at which point he remembered everything (E. R. Hilgard & Hilgard, 1975).

It occurred to the Hilgards that a similar mechanism might be operating in the case of hypnotic pain control, and a series of subsequent experiments demonstrated this to be true. Subjects who were capable of hypnotic pain control were asked if some "other part" of them knew more of what was going on than the part in hypnosis. In about half the cases, while the part in hypnosis reported low levels of pain, the "other part" reported pain at higher levels. The Hilgards described the "other part" as a "hidden observer," emphasizing that it is a metaphor for something occurring at an intellectual level but not available to the consciousness of the person in hypnosis.

In attempting to explain their findings, the Hilgards postulated alternative cognitive controls, which may or may not be in ascendance at any given time. These ideas also offer an explanation for the fact that subjects who are hypnotically analgesic demonstrate physiological signs of pain (e.g., increased heart rate) while reporting no felt pain. The theory of alternative cognitive controls, also called neodissociation theory, is further explicated in a book by E. R. Hilgard (1977) that we recommend to those interested in broader theoretical developments related to hypnosis and to human consciousness.

One of us (KO) successfully underwent orthopedic surgery on a finger for 50 minutes with hypnosis as sole anesthesia. Preparation consisted of listening to an audiotape of a meditation exercise for 1 hour. The coach or teacher was Dr. Kohen who reinforced my self-hypnosis. I felt comfortable throughout the procedure, which was videotaped. Physiological measures including cardiac rate, respiratory rate, and blood pressure remained steady throughout the procedure. Electroencephalographic monitoring recorded primarily theta activity, although there was a period of 15 minutes near the end of the procedure when there was no measurable alpha, beta, or theta activity. When the operation ended, the EEG recorded primarily alpha and beta activity. I used both dissociation and direct pain-control strategies and concluded that both were important to the successful anesthesia. Post-operative pain did occur, and I also controlled that with self-hypnosis. During the surgery, I felt no pain, nor did my autonomic measures suggest that some other part of me was perceiving pain. My view is that the mental strategies employed may have impacted on neurotransmitters known to be involved in pain perception. However, laboratory studies have conflicting results regarding the impact of hypnotic strategies on neuropeptides.

Neuropeptides and Pain

About 20 years ago, endorphins—endogenous morphine-like peptides—were discovered. Concurrently, another neuropeptide, substance P, was recognized to be a transmitter of pain impulses. With respect to pharmacological management of post-operative pain, opioid analgesics are the cornerstone. Opioids produce analgesia by binding to opioid receptors both within and outside the central nervous system. They are classified as full agonists, partial agonists, or mixed agonist–antagonists, depending on how they interact with opioid receptors. Many different receptors exist, and they accept various opioid agonists such as morphine and codeine. Unfortunately, most opioid agonists cause side effects including major problems such as respiratory depression and sedation and lesser problems such as constipation, nausea, and urinary retention. These side effects limit the dose that may be safely given (U.S. Department of Health and Human Services, 1992). This is why nonpharmacological treatments such as hypnotherapy may be valuable as adjuncts to opioid treatment. It is important to keep in mind that a child who has had opioids recently cannot learn self-regulation methods such as self-hypnosis as well as a child who is fully alert.

Studies to determine whether or not hypnotic strategies trigger release of endogenous endorphins have had conflicting results. It has been demonstrated that naloxone does not negate hypnotically achieved analgesia in adults (Goldstein & Hilgard, 1975). A study by Katz et al. (1982) measured beta-endorphin reactivity in the cerebrospinal fluid of 75 leukemic children who were undergoing lumbar punctures. This study analyzed beta-endorphin levels with respect to the children's reports of their pain, and of their fear, and measures of distress noted by observers. Beta-endorphin levels generally decline with increasing age of the children. Nurse ratings of the children's anxiety positively correlated with beta-endorphin levels; this suggests that beta-endorphin elevations reflected stress and might have represented the body's attempts to modulate unpleasant perceptions. This study also found that girls had higher levels of distress during lumbar puncture procedures than did boys.

Varni, Katz, and Dash (see Russo & Varni, 1982) have summarized research strategies used to elucidate the physiological, neurochemical, and behavioral implications of endorphin peptides for humans. These include administration of narcotic antagonists to displace opiates from opiate receptors; direct administration of synthetic endorphins while behavioral alterations are observed; direct assays of various endorphins in biological fluids, such as blood; and direct measurement of endorphins before and after the introduction of interventions believed to affect pain. Thus far, none of these strategies in adults or in children have led to conclusive evidence with respect to whether or not endorphin release is affected by hypnotherapy.

This area of inquiry remains an important one. Hypnotic responsiveness in children is associated with physiological changes that reflect neurotransmitter changes. It remains conceivable that the self-regulatory processes associated with voluntary pain control are mediated by release of endogenous endorphins or some other neurotransmitters.

The effectiveness of either hypnotherapy or pharmacological treatments for pain may be dependent on dietary factors, fatigue, medication interactions, or geomagnetic effects on neurotransmitters. We recognize that the following section may be much too general and that eventually we will have specific, practical methods to assess individual differences and guide the choice of pain treatment more precisely for both children and adults.

Pain-Rating Scales and Assessments

Patient self-report is the gold standard for assessment of pain intensity. Whatever the method used, it is important to use the same system at each visit with the child and to compare pain intensity between visits and from one visit to the next. Many studies in recent years have attempted to develop pain-rating scales that could be replicated and validated. Some have been observational: Others require some type of subjective assessment from the child (Eland & Anderson, 1977; Haslam, 1969; Jay, Ozolins, Elliott, & Caldwell, 1983; LeBaron & Zeltzer, 1984; Ross & Ross, 1984; Schecter et al., 1993). These methods have included color selections to represent pain intensity, visual analogue scales (such as rulers), scales made up of happy or sad faces, and the selection of pain descriptors from a list of words or audiotaped sounds.

A recent study (West, Oakes, & Hinds, 1994) compared the FACES Pain Scale (FPS) and Poker Chip Tool (PCT) in 30 children, ages 5 to 13 years, who were hospitalized in a pediatric oncology intensive care unit. Parents and patients completed these scales, and each patient's nurse completed the Objective Pain Scale (OPS). Patients' ratings on the FPS correlated significantly with parents' ratings but not on the PCT. Nurses' ratings on the OPS correlated moderately with patients' FPS ratings. The majority of children, parents, and nurses expressed a preference for the FPS. In the final analysis, child health professionals should accept the pain rating of the child rather than that of parents or other caretakers.

Varni and colleagues (Varni, Thompson, & Hanson, 1987) have developed the Pediatric Pain Questionnaire (PPQ), which attempts to assess empirically the complexities of chronic pain in children. The PPQ includes a combination of several types of pain assessments including a visual analogue scale as well as questions about the location of pain, pain history, and socio-environmental situations, which may influence pain perception. In a study of 25 children with juvenile rheumatoid arthritis, they found that correlations were highly significant for the PPQ results with respect to present pain and worst pain. This instrument may provide a step toward achieving reliable methodology for understanding the experience of and for measuring the level of pain experience in children with chronic pain.

We have developed a pain questionnaire for use with children who have chronic or recurrent pain such as migraine (Appendix B). It includes not only descriptors of pain but also information about the child's interests, likes, and preference for different types of imagery. The latter helps guide our choice of strategies for teaching the child a self-management method.

Young children may manifest pain by crying, fussing or irritability, withdrawal from social interaction, sleep disturbances, facial grimacing, guarding, inconsolability, poor appetite, and disinterest in play. These behavioral indicators should be assessed for any young child who may have pain and should be recorded.

Additional assessment of pain includes a careful medical and psychosocial history, physical examination, and a review of prior investigations and treatment. It is helpful, when possible, to include an assessment of autonomic responsivity. There are children who may not verbalize significant pain but who demonstrate changes in autonomic measures such as heart rate or electrodermal activity, and these may reflect pain.

It seems likely that the most reliable pain-rating scales will include both physiological and subjective measures. Hypnotic interventions to reduce pain may be applied more reliably after careful assessments; however this may be impractical in acute, emergency situations.

GENERAL PRINCIPLES AND GUIDELINES FOR TEACHING HYPNOANALGESIA

In working with more than 1,000 children who have learned hypnotic pain control for various conditions, we have found the following principles and guidelines to be useful.

Assess one's personal experience about pain. The clinician needs to analyze his or her own attitude toward discomfort. Most of us, by the time we reach adulthood, because of our childhood experiences and our training, have certain negative notions about pain that we may project onto our patients. A therapist who lacks faith in a child's ability to overcome pain is unlikely to succeed in helping the child.

Assess parental perceptions and expectations about pain. Expectations of parents regarding discomfort are important variables, and parents may also benefit from self-hypnosis exercises. In fact, in certain situations, it may be preferable for the parent to learn concurrently with the child. Children are less conditioned to the necessity for pain, suffering, and mental anguish if not overwhelmed by the negative expectations of their parents and other caretakers regarding how one manages pain.

Consider the impact of the pediatric treatment team. Whether interventions for pain relief are to be pharmacological, nonpharmacological, or a combination of the two, the attitudes and perceptions of adults on the treatment team may have significant effects on the outcome. Caregivers may have unresolved anxieties stemming from their own perceptions of pain suffered in hospitals or in dentists' offices as children. These can be reflected in subtle changes in voice, demeanor, or behavior when they are confronted with a child in pain or one about to undergo a painful procedure. Such anxiety may be perceived by the child and increase his or her own distress.

Consider the age and development of the child. One must decide whether or not the child is able to learn a formal technique. For the very young, music, massage, or rocking are natural adjuncts to pharmacological pain management. For the toddler, a distraction technique such as blowing may be most appropriate. Some bright, verbal 2-year-olds can learn self-hypnosis. All children think concretely; abstract reasoning skills do not develop until mid- to late adolescence. Failure to recognize this is a major impediment to successful adult–child communication. Adults tend to assume children have more abstract reasoning capacity than they actually have. Children often misinterpret expressions such as "she was fired" (interpreted as "she was set on fire") or "patching the eye" (interpreted as "sewing a piece of cloth on my eye") or "frog in the throat" (interpreted as a Kermit, the "Sesame Street" frog, in the throat). When fear seems out of proportion to the situation, the child may have misinterpreted an adult's statement as somehow threatening. The practice of hypnotherapy tends to make child health professionals more aware of the importance of word choice; this benefits all of their interactions with children.

Consider learning styles, strengths, and learning handicaps. Parents often can provide information about how their children learn best — by observing, by listening, or by reading. Many children enjoy learning via computers. Parents may also be aware of learning handicaps. Research has documented that children may develop learning handicaps after receiving cancer therapy. In a long-term follow-up of children with cancer (Olness & Singher, 1989), we found that some who learned quickly during the initial training period had developed learning disabilities after a few years and had difficulty in remembering their self-regulation methods. Information about learning also helps in choice of an appropriate pain-assessment tool. If a child does not grasp a sequence of numbers, then use of a ruler scale is not a good idea.

Consider a child's interests, likes, and dislikes. It is helpful to know what the child enjoys and does not enjoy in terms of play, environment, games, music, and sports. Does he or she like books? Which television programs does he or she enjoy? What are family interests and hobbies? The task of teaching self-hypnosis is much easier if the therapist asks the child to focus on something that he or she enjoys.

Emphasize the child's control and mastery. Learning cyberphysiological strategies provides an opportunity for children with chronic diseases, such as cancer, to develop a sense of coping ability and personal mastery. Many children with chronic illnesses have little or no control over most aspects of treatment, but they can be in complete control over self-hypnosis. We emphasize this to children from the first visit, explaining that we are like a coach or teacher, but that the child is in control just as he or she is when learning to play soccer or the piano. We provide choices such as what imagery a child will use and what reminders to use for practice. We also acknowledge the child's personal mastery when he or she succeeds. Children may not always want to use their pain-control skills depending on fatigue or secondary gain issues or other unknown factors. When this is the case, they must be allowed to have the choice of not using hypnosis. And the adults around them must understand and accept this as well.

Explain what you plan to do and what the child may do in appropriate language. The initial discussion of hypnotic pain control should be tailored to the child's interests and developmental level, the parents' wishes, and the therapists' strengths. For some adolescents, explanations may be lengthy and involve descriptions of the nervous system and pain pathways. For most young children, brief explanations are preferable. Some preschoolers benefit from watching a videotape of children of similar ages who are demonstrating hypnotic pain control. Children of grade school age understand the concept of similar sound signals being interpreted differently by the brain. For example, the sound *b* may be interpreted by the brain as "bee," "be," or "B"; the sound *c* may be interpreted as "see," "C," or "sea." Similarly, the signal from the entrance of a needle into the skin may be interpreted in multiple ways, and the child can decide how to control this.

School children can understand that one cannot focus on more than two or three stimuli at one time. This can be demonstrated easily by asking the child to pay attention to the feeling of his or her right foot inside the sock and, at the same time, to pay attention to the feeling of the shirt on the back of his or her neck, and, at the same time, to pay attention to the feeling of the watch on his or her wrist. The child cannot focus on all three stimuli at the same time. One explains that each of us is constantly choosing which stimuli we pay attention to and that we do this unconsciously. However, we can also learn to do this with our own controls such as when we learn to shut off pain signals to our brain. We then ask the child to consider what sort of a control system is in his or her brain, possibly some sort of computer system or a switch system, that allows him or her to turn signals on or off.

We also explain to the child and parents that practice is important but that parents should not remind the child to practice. They may help him or her to select a practice reminder system.

Avoid prescribing the child's images, or pain perceptions. Although it is incorrect to say that something will not hurt, it is also incorrect to say that something will hurt. It is helpful to give the child options in his or her descriptions. The therapist can say, "Some children say this feels like cold ice, and some say it feels like a thorn from a rose bush, and some say it feels like a hairbrush. I wonder what it will feel like for you." This gives the message that the child can decide how it feels and describe the feeling for him- or herself. The child's description may then be incorporated into a therapeutic suggestion; for example, "If you like, you can let that pecking bird fly away." The therapist should also avoid being too specific about when and how the pain will go away. One can rapidly back oneself into a corner by such statements as "The pain will be gone in 10 minutes" or "The hurting will go away when I count to five." If the prophecy is not fulfilled, the therapist loses credibility, and thereafter even appropriate suggestions may have no effect.

Positive Side Effects

Hypnotherapy for pain control may have a variety of side benefits, especially in the case of children with chronic or life-threatening illness. These include reduction of anxiety, enhancement of mastery and hope, increased cooperation, and increased comfort among family members and among other members of the health care team. For these reasons the use of nonpharmacological interventions including self-hypnosis, relaxation, or biofeedback is recommended by the American Academy of Pediatrics in its policy statement on the management of pediatric cancer pain (American Academy of Pediatrics, 1990).

TECHNIQUES OF HYPNOANALGESIA

The following techniques represent methods we have used with our patients. We often use several in combination. Every technique involves suggested dissociation, either directly or indirectly. For instance, notice how the phrase "that arm" rather than "your arm" facilitates dissociation. As with induction techniques, our list is by no means complete. Other hypnotherapists will prefer variations of our methods or will develop other methods.

Direct Suggestions for Hypnoanesthesia

Request for Numbness. "You know what a numb feeling is. How does numbness feel to you? [Child responds.] Good, just let that part of your body get numb now. Numb like a block of ice [or whatever image the child has used]."

Topical Anesthesia. "Just imagine painting numbing medicine onto that part of your body. Tell me when you're finished doing that."

Local Anesthesia. "Imagine putting an anesthetic into that part of your body. Feel it flow into your body and notice the change in feeling as the area becomes numb."

Glove Anesthesia. "First, pay attention to your hand. Notice how you can feel tingling feelings in that hand. Then let it become numb. When it is very numb, touch that hand to your jaw [or other body part] and let the numb feeling transfer from the hand to the jaw."

Switchbox. The therapist explains the idea that pain is transmitted by nerves from various parts of the body to the brain, which then sends a "pain message" back to the body. The therapist can describe nerves and their pathways or can ask the child to provide a color for nerves. The importance of accuracy varies with the age and needs of the child. Then the child is asked to choose some sort of switch that can turn off incoming nerve signals. The therapist can describe various kinds of switches, such as flip, dimmer, pull, or even a television computer push-button panel or control panel of lights. Having chosen a switch, the child is asked to begin practicing turning off the switches or the lights that connect the brain and certain areas of the body. It is useful to ask the child to turn off the incoming nerve signals for defined periods of time (e.g., 10 minutes, 15 minutes, or 90 minutes). The success of the exercise is judged by touching the child with a small-gauge needle or some other sharp object and asking for a comparison with feelings on the other side where the nerve signals are unchanged.

Distancing Suggestions

Moving Pain Away from the Self. "Imagine [or pretend] for a while that that arm [or other body part] doesn't belong to you, isn't part of you. Think of it as part of a sculpture or a toy or picture it just floating out there by itself." Some patients comfortably imagine having only one arm; others imagine three arms, one of which is dissociated.

Transferring Pain to Another Body Part. "Imagine putting all the discomfort of the spinal tap into the little finger of your right hand. Tell me how much discomfort is in that little finger. Give it a number rating and let me know if it changes. Good. Now let it float away."

Moving Self Away from the Pain. "You said you like to go to the mountains. Imagine yourself there now. Let yourself really be there. Just leave all the discomfort and be in the mountains. See the trees and flowers. Watch the chipmunks playing. Smell the fresh air and the pine trees. Listen to the gentle wind. Listen to the running stream. Imagine yourself running or walking, if you like." In one study of adults (R. J. Greene & Reyher, 1972), it was suggested that body-oriented imagery (e.g., feeling the warmth of the sun) was less effective for hypnotic pain control than imagery that was not body oriented (e.g., looking at scenery or skiing). We do not know if these results are applicable to children.

Suggestions for Feelings Antithetical to Pain

Comfort. "Recall a time when you felt very comfortable, very good. Then bring those good comfortable feelings into the present. Let your body feel comfortable here and now. You can let comfortable feelings fill your whole body and mind completely, until there is just no room for discomfort. You can be completely comfortable, and you can keep these good feelings for as long as you like."

Laughter. "Laughing helps pain go away. Think of the funniest movie you every saw or the funniest thing you ever did or your friend did. Each time you imagine laughing, your pain becomes less and less. You may find yourself really laughing and feeling very good."

Relaxation. "Concentrate on breathing out, for that is a relaxing motion. If you relax completely when you breathe out, you can reduce the pain. Follow your breathing rhythm. Relax more each time you breathe out. You may find that you can cut the pain in half. And then in half again. Use your energy where it will help you feel better and get better."

Distraction Techniques

Focus on Unrelated Material. Young children often obtain some pain relief if the therapist tells a story, either in its original form or with ridiculous variations such as changing the characters ("Once upon a time there were three little wolves and a big bad pig") or their roles ("Once there was a wolf who cried, 'Boy, boy' "). Older children may be distracted by discussion of areas of interest such as sports or music.

Focus on Procedures or Injury. This method is especially useful for children for whom cognitive mastery is a major coping mechanism. The therapist asks the child to describe the injury in detail, how it occurred, how others reacted, and so on. In the case of a painful procedure, the therapist describes various instruments and asks the child to assist by holding instruments or bandages, counting sutures, or checking the time at various points.

Focus on Lesser of Two Evils. If a child feels both pain and cold, the therapist can focus on the cold. If the child is having a spinal tap and also has an IV running, the therapist can focus on IV.

Directing Attention to Pain Itself

For various reasons, some children refuse or are unable to focus attention on anything but the experiences of pain. The therapist can utilize this behavior to the child's own advantage. By joining with the child and asking for a detailed description of the pain, the therapist can offer subtle suggestions for change and relief. Confusion techniques also help.

Lighted Globe. "Imagine you are inside a lighted globe, and you can see yourself walking around on the inside of a map of your discomfort. Notice that discomfort very carefully. See it right now in a color you don't like. I'll ask you to check it again later. Notice what size it is. It might be the size of a grapefruit or a grape or a lemon. Even a pinhead has a size. We'll check the size again later. And notice the shape. What shape is it right now? And what is it saying to you now? How loud is it right now? Later we'll see if you can still hear it. Look again. What color is it now? That's interesting. It seems to be changing. I wonder how you did that. How small is it now? Can you change the size too? Yes. You are really in charge there in that lighted globe. You are a good map maker. You can go wherever you want. Feel whatever you want. What shape is the discomfort now? Can you still hear it?"

Older children can benefit from a technique of focusing on breathing, then shifting focus to the area of discomfort, with emphasis on the fact that it is changing. Subsequently, the therapist can ask the child to focus on a piece of music, or a smell (e.g., by bringing an open bottle of perfume near the child's nose), and on the discomfort at the same time. The child will gradually learn that the perception of two stimuli fades as the attention is shifted to one.

Amnesia. Constructive use of amnesia along with explanation of how the body works is another way of distracting from a focus on discomfort. "I know you know that we discussed that pain is a signal to let you know that something was injured, and, in the case of after an operation, to let you know that the tissues are now healing, so it's good to pay attention to that signal, but once you know about it and pay attention to it for a while, then you don't have to bother paying attention to it any more. In fact that discomfort is so new that your brain hardly knows it very well. In fact, your brain has much *more experience with no pain or discomfort* in that part of your body than it does with this [shoulder, abdomen, head, etc.]. So, I wonder if it would be okay with you to let your brain just forget to remember about this discomfort in between times that you remember to notice it and check the level? And, so, since it remembers so well what no discomfort feels like, it's easy then to forget to remember the discomfort that used to be there anyway, and in that way it can go a way that it doesn't have to disturb — it's funny how you can program that computer we call the brain to remember to forget about the bother or to forget to remember about it, or even to remember to forget to remember or to forget to remember to forget." In addition to the confusional suggestion for amnesia, these represent invitations to the patient to perceive his or her discomfort in a different way.

Trip around the Body. This is another metaphoric storytelling and reframing approach often very useful, particularly in a naturalistic, Ericksonian approach to pain control. For example, "I knew this boy [or girl] once who was only [pick an age slightly younger than your patient] years old and he [she] liked to pretend [imagine] she was so tiny that she could go inside of her own body and take a trip around the body. She sometimes pretended she was riding on a bike on the bones or the nerves and at other times pretended that she was in a boat traveling through the bloodstream. She visited different parts of the body, went to the strong heart and watched how great it was pumping blood, and over to the lungs to admire the way they were breathing so easily, and then visited other places and took a repair kit along and just fixed things that weren't quite right." This could also be used in combination with the switches technique. For example, "And she made her way all the way to that main computer we call the brain, and when she got there, she saw all of those lights and buttons and switches, and she found the one that said [shoulder, tummy, etc.], and turned it down, sometimes part-way down and sometimes all the way off so the hurt didn't bother her at all."

Time Distortion and Reframing. Particularly with children with chronic or recurrent pain, and also useful with children with post-operative pain is teaching the use of time distortion. This can often be accomplished easily in a naturalistic and expectant fashion by appealing to the child's (and parents') sense of experience in daily life and our routine perceptions of time: "Did you ever notice how when you're having a good time, like at a party or a sleepover, or playing with favorite friends, that time *seems* to go fast? People even say that sometimes, don't they? They say things like, 'Whew, time flies when you're having fun!,' don't they? Right, and, of course, it doesn't *really* fly, but it sure *seems* like it, doesn't it? And it works the other way around, too, doesn't it? Like if you're worrying about something or can't wait for something to begin or end, it seems like time goes soooo . . . slow . . . ly. And people talk about that too, they say things like, 'Wow, this feels like it's taking *forever,* but I just looked at the clock and only 2 minutes went by; it seemed like an hour, didn't it?' You can do the same with your discomfort, like just pay attention to it for 5 minutes every hour . . . and then pay very close attention and notice what number it is on the bother scale, and keep track, especially noticing how it changes, getting better and better each time you measure it."

Reinforcement

We encourage—but do not demand—that our patients practice their skills in hypnotic pain control, using variations or new methods as they see fit. The more confident children are of their ability to use these skills, the more likely it is that they will use them whenever it is appropriate to do so. Other methods of reinforcement include selected use of audiotapes, videotapes, parents acting as therapeutic allies, group meetings, and communication with other patients who have successfully used hypnotherapy for pain control.

After several practice sessions, the therapist can ask the child which type of relaxation or imagery exercise is most helpful. This can be taped and placed over the child's favorite music, if he or she wishes, and made available on a Walkman-type recorder during procedures. The child can also be encouraged to tape him- or herself guiding him- or herself through a relaxation exercise; this can also be placed over favorite music. Therapists should also encourage children who are skilled in pain control to help the therapist coach other children. This gives confidence to the child who is teaching, and encourages the learner who can trust that other child.

CONCLUSIONS

Although pain control is one of the oldest uses of hypnotherapy, understanding of the process remains in its infancy. The next several years can be expected to produce exciting research findings that will clarify many difficult issues and allow therapists greater precision in selecting hypnoanalgesic techniques for individual patients.

CHAPTER ELEVEN

Hypnotherapy for Pediatric Medical Problems

A growing body of clinical and research data attests to the effectiveness of hypnotherapy in pediatric medicine. In many instances, children can utilize their self-regulatory talents adjunctively to reduce or eliminate disease symptoms such as nausea or pain. Although hypnotherapy may sometimes be a preferred primary therapeutic modality in certain conditions such as migraine or enuresis, presently it is more often a useful adjunct in modulating and moderating symptoms and effects of a wide variety of problems. As we develop more precision in making recommendations regarding self-hypnosis strategies, including timing, we may document the fact that specific disease processes may be altered or even eliminated.

When many children with medical problems successfully use hypnotherapy, their expressions of victory and triumph are obvious and justified. They have less need for medications that, at best, are a nuisance and, at worst, have harmful side effects such as stunting growth, damaging other body organs, causing hypoxia, and clouding consciousness. They spend less time in hospital wards and emergency rooms, and they suffer through fewer unpleasant medical procedures. They enjoy the physical and psychological benefits of normal activity. They move beyond the constricting role of "the sick one" in their families, developing a fuller sense of self based on a more balanced expression of needs and abilities. In every way, they are healthier.

For some children with chronic or life-threatening disease, hypnotherapeutic accomplishments, and expectations for them, may be limited. These children often develop behavior disorders or experience severe anxiety and depression, usually associated with helplessness, hopelessness, and low self-esteem. Such difficulties may limit capacity for constructive fantasy and preclude the positive aspects of a doctor–patient relationship that seem to underlie successful use of hypnotherapeutic skills. For example, Donald R., an adolescent boy with sickle-cell anemia, initially seemed enthusiastic that

210

hypnotherapy might allow better pain control and possibly reduce the length of his frequent hospitalizations. He had good imagery skills and enjoyed hypnotic tennis games during which his pain and depression vanished. However, he could not overcome 16 years of being infantilized by his parents and living with the assumptions that the safest place was a hospital and that comfort came from narcotic drugs. In spite of obvious relief from hypnotherapy, he refused to use his skill in the absence of the therapist. As soon as she left his hospital room, he called the nurse to request more narcotics. Repeated efforts to help him met with continued resistance, and the therapist eventually terminated visits.

There is much that we do not understand about the effects of chronic disease on perception and on the personality. A recent study designed to investigate the relationship between perceived stress, self-esteem, and "functional" pain in adolescents with and without chronic disease found, unexpectedly, that patients with chronic disease scored significantly higher on self-esteem measures and lower on stress measures (Adams & Weaver, 1986). It has long been known that living through a critical situation gives one experience in facing later problems, which also reduces the stress induced by such problems.

For some children, recent advances in medical management have allowed for cures to be achieved or for life and quality of life to be extended and improved. But new problems arise that challenge us to develop new hypnotherapeutic approaches. Children who would have died a decade ago now live, but have the added and new stress of having to cope with permanent disfigurement, or with "survivor guilt" generated by the death of peers with the same illness, or with continuing pressure to feel deserving of having received an organ transplant at the risk of harming another person. We know relatively little about these problems of survival except that we can expect them to occur with increasing frequency unless therapeutic approaches that focus on prevention are developed. The possible role of hypnotherapy as a preventive tool needs exploration.

Therapeutic methods that enhance a sense of mastery and competency are most likely to help children cope with medical problems and with the complications or effects of being cured. Children who successfully develop mastery skills may carry these skills into adulthood, becoming more able to cope effectively and reduce morbidity when illness occurs, and perhaps to prevent certain diseases. Hypnotherapeutic interventions seem ideally suited to these ends.

The following discussion presents the applications of hypnotherapy for a wide variety of medical problems, based on the existing literature and on our own clinical experiences. There are many other medical problems in which hypnotherapy might appropriately be expected to be useful, and we urge the reader to extrapolate from these examples to other problems accordingly.

ALLERGIES

Asthma

Asthma affects 6.9% of children 3 to 17 years of age (Gevgen, Mullally, & Evans, 1988). With a growing willingness to identify the problem of reactive airway disease as asthma in younger children, increasing numbers of preschool children carry the diagnosis of asthma and its attendant morbidity. In school children, asthma is the leading cause of time lost from school due to chronic disease. Nationally 20% to 25% of school absenteeism is due to asthma, and an estimated 12 million days are spent in bed rest and 28 million days in restricted activities (Gevgen et al., 1988). Additional well-known morbidities include economic stress (physician and hospital visits, medications, laboratory studies) (Marion, Creer, & Reynolds, 1985; Sheffer et al., 1991), time missed from school (Konig, 1978) and play (Francis, Krastins, & Levison, 1980) and negative effects on healthy, normal development such as maladaptive life styles (Leffert, 1980; Mattson, 1975). Recent reports have focused on education-based, self-management programs (Bauchner, Howland, & Adair, 1988; Blessing-Moore, Fritz, & Lewiston, 1985; Carson, Council, & Schauer, 1991; Hindi-Alexander, 1985; Kohen & Wynne, 1988; Rachelefsky, Lewis, & Dela Sota, 1985; Rachelefsky & Siegel, 1985; Rakos, Grodek, & Mack, 1985).

A generally agreed upon and working definition of asthma recognizes that asthma is a lung disease with three major characteristics: (1) airway obstruction that is reversible either spontaneously or with treatment (but not completely so in some patients); (2) airway inflammation; and (3) increased airway responsiveness—or hyperreactive airway—to a variety of stimuli.

Airways are typically thought of as obstructed by bronchospasm, excessive mucus production, or mucosal edema (swelling of the lining of the airways). Such obstruction is manifested clinically by wheezing. It is helpful to distinguish *extrinsic asthma,* that is, that triggered by external stimuli such as allergy, from *intrinsic asthma,* that not provoked by external stimuli. Extrinsic asthma is believed to occur as a result of inhalation, or occasionally ingestion, of an antigen that reacts with an antibody in the gamma globulin fraction of plasma (an IgE antibody). Intrinsic asthma, which is more common, may also reflect immunological mechanisms, but presently its pathogenesis is unclear (Sheffer, 1991). Hormonal, autonomic nervous system, and neurotransmitter imbalances have been postulated as being involved. For example, Henderson et al. (1979) reported experiments in which patients with asthma were compared with normal controls and with patients who had allergic rhinitis. The pupils of the patients with asthma required significantly less phenylephrine to dilate than did the pupils of the other two groups. This difference suggests greater autonomic sensitivity and/or responsiveness in the patients with asthma.

Psychological factors have long been known to play a role in asthma, especially of the intrinsic type. Though the nature, frequency, and evolution of this role has not been clearly defined, many children with asthma are described as anxious, shy, dependent, and may see themselves as passive victims of their disease. They may be convinced, for example, that they must rely on medications for control of wheezing, and some with moderately severe asthma conclude that a hospital is the only environment in which they can be safe. These children and adolescents will enter the emergency room dramatically and do not respond to drugs or psychological intervention until they are safely admitted and assured of remaining in the hospital.

The symptoms of asthma are powerful weapons, and children can use them consciously or unconsciously to control their families or to satisfy a variety of emotional needs (Kohen, 1986b). Many clinicians have seen children stop wheezing within hours after being hospitalized, thus escaping from pressures and pathological interactions at home. Such observations often lead to recommendations for residential treatment, sometimes at a great distance from home. The problem with this approach is that, while patients may improve as a result of the separation, they eventually return to the same environment, with the likelihood of the vicious cycle beginning anew. It seems more effective in some cases to work with the child in the context of family treatment (Lehrer, Sarguanaraj, & Hochron, 1992), perhaps including hypnotherapy for the entire family (Kohen, 1980a; C. L. Moore, 1980). At times, we encourage children to lead relaxation sessions with their parents, thus giving them the opportunity to exert a measure of control and influence with parents in a more constructive and positive way.

Other important psychological factors in asthma are expectation and suggestibility. Clinical observations of children and adults with asthma have demonstrated both increased and decreased wheezing in response to placebos coupled with appropriate suggestions. Laboratory studies have further documented this finding. Luparello, Leist, Lourie, and Sweet (1970) found that adults with asthma not only demonstrated increased airway resistance when given a placebo antigen but also reversed their bronchospasm when given a saline solution placebo. Thorne and Fisher (1978) found that adults with asthma experienced changes in physiological asthma, provided they were responsive to hypnotic induction. The same phenomena have been reported in children, both on the basis of clinical observations (Reaney, Chang, & Olness, 1978) and on the basis of laboratory research including pulmonary function studies (Khan, Staerk, & Bonk, 1974). The latter study included 20 children with asthma, ages 8 to 13 years. Positive response to hypnotically suggested asthma occurred in four children, all of whom scored high on the Barber Suggestibility Scale. Seven other high scorers, however, showed no change in pulmonary functions following the hypnotic suggestions. Moreover, some children reacted positively to sham allergens but not to hypnotic suggestion of bronchospasm, and vice versa. These data confirm our clinical impressions that psychological aspects of asthma are complex and that simplistic treatment approaches are likely to have a limited effect.

Hypnotherapeutic Approaches to Childhood Asthma

Kohen (1986a, 1993, 1995c, in press) has noted that self-hypnosis is helpful in management of childhood asthma. It involves reduction of anxiety during acute episodes, early rapid abatement of wheezing and reduction of frequency of wheezing episodes, as well as reduction of functional morbidity such as school absences, improvement in personal sense of mastery, possible improvement in pulmonary function, and prevention of long-term morbidity.

Although there are several reports of hypnotherapy with children with asthma, most with positive results, the actual methods used vary greatly from one study to another, making comparisons difficult. Treatment techniques have included hypnoanalytic and other insight-oriented methods, general ego-strengthening suggestions, relaxation training, teaching patients to increase and decrease wheezing, other suggestions aimed at enhancing the child's sense of control, training in self-hypnosis, and direct suggestions for symptom relief. Before reviewing this literature, we present three case reports representative of our current approaches to the problem. Generally we emphasize increased mastery and control, and we urge patients to extend hypnotic skills by training in self-hypnosis (Kohen, in press). And even though we attempt to understand underlying dynamics, insight-oriented techniques often play a relatively minor role. Careful assessment of individual adaptation and associated problems and needs is emphasized, however, since in selected cases, intensive psychotherapy may be necessary before change occurs.

Sam M. was hospitalized at age 6 years for treatment of status asthmaticus. He had experienced multiple hospitalizations in another state for asthma, which had begun at age 4 years. He was hospitalized four times in rapid succession before being referred for hypnotherapy. It was noted on the fourth admission that the patient "enjoys the hospital environment." There were significant family stresses: the parents had been divorced approximately 1 year previously; the mother had a new baby by her second husband; and the parents were fighting over custody of Sam.

Sam was seen as an outpatient six times in a period of 6 weeks for hypnotherapy. First, Sam and his family were given information about the disease, aided by drawings of the airway as "an upside-down tree" with comparison of relaxed (dilated) and tight (constricted) branches. Sam was asked to prepare his own drawings of the bronchial tree with and without asthma, again to reinforce his knowledge and mastery of the situation. In hypnosis, he enjoyed visualizing himself on a flying blanket, going where he chose, in control, and loosening up his airways. He also visualized himself in the future, free of his asthma and enjoying an active game of football, his favorite sport. In between sessions, he was encouraged to practice self-hypnosis at home. It was noted during the third visit that the patient came in with active wheezing, and a respiratory rate of 36 per minute over a 4-minute period. While in hypnosis, his respiratory rate reduced to 16, and wheezes were no longer heard on auscultation. A few minutes later, in the waiting room, he was heard to ask his mother if he could go home to play. She said that he would have to clean his room. Within 5 minutes, severe wheezing occurred that was again relieved by hypnosis exercises. Shortly after treatment began, Sam's father noted that, while at home, he was able to "stop a bad attack in 20 minutes" using his self-hypnosis. Subsequently he was seen approximately once a month for 6 months during which time, in spite of frequent acute episodes at home, he had no emergency room visits and no hospitalizations. Thirteen months after beginning hypnotherapy, he was hospitalized and during his hospitalization refused hypnosis. At this time, he seemed very upset over the conflict between his parents regarding his custody. His admission seemed to have been triggered by being grounded at home by his mother. He did not want to go home and repeatedly refused to practice hypnosis. Subsequent follow-up was by telephone only. His father stated that the patient clearly could use his self-hypnosis and did so frequently. However, the family conflict remained unresolved. The parents refused a recommendation for psychotherapy.

Hugh N. was first seen for hypnotherapy at age 7 years. His asthma had progressed to the point that he frequently had to stay home from school, and his pediatrician was about to begin steroid therapy. A cute redhead, Hugh's eyes sparkled at the idea of learning hypnotic skills. When he described his problem as not being able to get enough air into his lungs, the therapist explained that the problem in asthma is really not being able to get trapped air out of the lungs. Following good response to hypnotic induction involving progressive relaxation and hand levitation, the therapist asked, "What color are your lungs today?" When Hugh said he didn't know what color his lungs were, the therapist—with a twinkle—told him to stop talking like a grownup and to answer the question. Grinning, Hugh said his lungs were green. Then the therapist said, "Good. Now what color is the air for you today?" Still grinning, Hugh said the air was orange. The therapist then said, "Fine. Now take a nice deep breath. Watch that orange air go all the way down to the very bottom of your lungs until all you see is orange. Then breathe out and watch all the orange air come up so that your lungs are all green again, from top to bottom." After Hugh successfully used this imagery, the therapist remarked that she hadn't heard heard him wheeze and asked him to imagine a beginning acute episode of asthma. He produced a barely audible wheeze. The therapist said, "That's not much of a wheeze—can't you do better than that?" When Hugh wheezed more clearly, the therapist said, "Good. Now you have shown us that you really can control your wheezing. You can make it worse. Now control it the other way and make it go away." He did. This conversation led to further discussion of mastery, following which Hugh was taught self-hypnosis. The therapist suggested that he practice the color exercises daily and that he also use his hypnotic talent at the first sign of any wheezing. In the office Hugh demonstrated his skills to his mother, and they agreed that he would be responsible for practice. One week later, Hugh's mother reported marked improvement, and treatment was terminated after three more sessions. About 1 year later, Hugh requested another appointment, stating that he had forgotten his skills and that his asthma was getting worse again. One hypnotherapeutic review session was sufficient to put him back in control, and follow-up some months later revealed continuing gains. Steroids were never begun. In the initial sessions, Hugh's mother admitted that she feared he might die or get into serious trouble and that she knew she was overprotective toward him. However, she refused the therapist's suggestion that she obtain psychotherapy for herself. The family eventually moved to another state.

Gerald was first taught self-hypnosis when he was 9 years old. He had had wheezing as an infant, which was first officially called asthma when he was 2 years old. One of two children of a hard-working, single mother who smoked, Gerald was frequently ill with ear infections, colds, and other respiratory illnesses, many of which triggered acute episodes of wheezing. In the 3 years prior to learning hypnosis, he had been hospitalized on more than 10 occasions and had been to the emergency room almost monthly for acute wheezing. He was taught the anatomy and pathophysiology of asthma, with emphasis on the imagery of the lungs and airways as an upside-down tree and muscles around airways that can be looser or tighter. In hypnosis he was asked to imagine himself doing something he liked—like playing basketball—to then notice the very first and earliest sign of wheezing beginning and to "let that be your signal to stop, do your self-hypnosis, picture your breathing tubes and let the muscles around them get loose, soft, floppy, relaxed, and comfortable so that all the air you need can get in and out." As this was reviewed and reinforced, Gerald agreed to practice once or twice daily even when he was feeling fine "so that your muscles can learn what to do at the right time in the right way, maybe even automatically," as well as practicing whenever he had wheezing. The frequency of acute episodes, emergency room visits, and hospitalizations decreased dramatically with the practice of this cue-controlled, self-hypnosis.

Two years later, the therapist asked Gerald if he would make a videotape demonstration of his control of asthma with hypnosis. Considering its potential educational value, the therapist wondered about giving Gerald hypnotic suggestions to develop and then stop the wheezing. Having never done so in any prior hypnotherapy sessions with Gerald or other patients, the therapist casually asked Gerald what he thought of that possibility as they walked to the room where their session was to be videotaped. Gerald responded with a look of skepticism. The therapist reassured him matter-of-factly that he didn't know if he'd suggest anything like that, but if he did that it didn't matter "because you know how to get rid of wheezing when you need to anyway." A few minutes later, the interview and hypnotherapy session began (Kohen, 1982). In the interview Gerald noted that since learning hypnosis he had not had to come to the emergency room "that much" and that if he got his wheezing he would "just practice." Like many children, his internal understanding of the hypnotic experience was clearer than his verbal explanation. He noted, "When I practice I go to my room and just think. But before I do, I sit up there and think about what I'll be thinkin' about, and then when I practice I'll know what I'll be thinkin' about when I think about it" (Kohen, 1982). Gerald spontaneously suggested that the imagery be about "mountain climbing," supplying a wonderful metaphor for problem solving.

In the hypnotherapy session that followed, the therapist offered many suggestions—both direct and indirect—for control of asthma, including (1) making sure that the ropes for climbing were tied just right, not too loose and not too tight, "just like your climbing muscles and lung muscles," (2) noticing that "each time you take a turn on the path while climbing that you get more and more relaxed and comfortable," and (3) "noticing how proud you feel for what you are accomplishing." Suggestions were then given that he could notice that he came near a cloud of thick, gray smoke while climbing, and that that made breathing more difficult. He began to cough, breathe more rapidly, and to wheeze. Suggestions for increasing awareness of this response resulted in more wheezing and increased respiratory rate that were then followed by suggestions to "walk right away from that cloud and notice how much easier it is to breathe." His respiratory rate slowed again, and the wheezing disappeared.

Following the hypnotherapy session, Gerald alerted and was asked to describe what he had experienced. He reported that he had imagined climbing the mountain with a friend (though no such imagery had been suggested), and that they had "got a lot higher than half of it." He said that "when we got pretty high, I started wheezing, and I asked him what we should do, and he said we should rest, and while we were resting, I practiced, and in my practice I imagined that I was on this trip to Hawaii on this beach. . . . " The therapist was amazed and asked, "So, while you were mountain climbing in your imagination you had *another* imagination and just while you were doing that what happened to your wheezing?" and he replied, "It got clear . . . it was kind of hard to do it, but I did it. . . . " His sense of pride was clearly evident, as was his awareness that the imagery used to accomplish success was his own.

At the end of the interview, the therapist asked Gerald if he used his hypnosis for anything else, knowing that he had already solved his problems of enuresis and nail biting with self-hypnosis. Gerald demurred talking about those and instead casually described how he doesn't feel any discomfort when a nurse "gives me a shot, it doesn't hurt, I kind of just notice it. . . . " Gerald agreed to some day make a "sequel" to his video. More than 6 years later, at age 17 years, he called, needing a physical examination. The therapist had not seen him in over 2 years and asked if he would be willing to make another videotape. He agreed. In the video (Kohen, 1987c), he reported the continued utility of his self-hypnosis, particularly for exercise-induced asthma, noting that he needed only a few minutes to "get myself together" after he started wheezing. He described multisensory techniques—"I picture my lungs upside down, I hear it and when I hear it less, I know I'm better, and I feel it, you know you can massage that mucus out of there . . . "—and then spontaneously described what we have speculated about and heard from other children—"the imagination, now it's automatic, it is . . . it's like it's built in . . . " (Kohen, 1987c).

Results of Hypnotherapy with Children with Asthma

Review of research literature reveals that widely disparate hypnotherapeutic techniques result in similar dramatic improvement both in extrinsic and intrinsic asthma, though the emphasis is more on the latter. Clearly, we don't yet understand the mechanisms of change. Possibilities include enhancement of mastery, reduction of anxiety that may have some physiological effect, direct effects in relaxing bronchial smooth muscle, changes in parental attitudes and behavior, and resolution of unconscious conflicts. In any study, it is important to realize that the postulated mechanisms of change, derived from theoretical positions and related technical approaches, may or may not actually be responsible for an improved medical condition.

Diamond (1959) used hypnoanalytic techniques with 55 children with asthma who had no positive findings on skin testing or had not responded to vaccine therapy. Five children did not respond at all to hypnotic induction, and another 10 achieved only a modest response. Of the remaining 40 patients, all achieved complete remission of symptoms and remained symptom-free during a 2- to 4-year follow-up period. These children experienced hypnotic age regression to the time of the first episode of asthma, associated with emotional trauma such as severe guilt or fear of loss of parental love. They then responded to insight-oriented approaches in which they no longer needed to use their asthma as a way of getting positive parental attention and developing feelings of emotional security.

J. M. Smith and Burns (1960) used direct hypnotic suggestions for immediate and progressive symptom relief with 25 children and adolescents with asthma ages 8 to 15 years. All responded satisfactorily to hypnotic induction, and some claimed subjective improvement over the 4-week treatment period. However, repeated pulmonary function tests revealed no significant change in any of the children. The authors concluded that they had failed to demonstrate any value of hypnotic suggestion for improved pulmonary functions. We wonder whether the experimenters expected negative results and therefore communicated a subtle bias. We also wonder whether the "strongly suggested" relief was expressed in a very authoritarian way in this clinic, perhaps circumventing the children's egos and unwittingly supporting passivity.

Diego (1961) taught five boys with asthma, ages 11 to 13 years, to precipitate and stop acute episodes of asthma in hypnosis. He then gave them post-hypnotic suggestions that they would be able to stop future such episodes by hypnotic relaxation. All five patients reported rapid subjective improvement, and four continued improved for several months' follow-up. One boy relapsed after a month but improved again following a year of insight-oriented psychotherapy.

Aronoff, Aronoff, and Peck (1975) studied the efficacy of hypnotherapy in aborting acute episodes of asthma in 17 children and adolescents, ages 6 to 17 years. Subjects were given direct hypnotic suggestions for chest relaxation, easy breathing, and reduction of wheezing. In most cases, they experienced immediate improvement, as measured both by pulmonary function tests and subjective reports. The authors noted that anxiety may aggravate asthma by stimulating the autonomic nervous system, and they speculated that "hypnosis, by promoting general relaxation, diminishes vagal stimulation and consequently diminishes release of mediators felt to be responsible for the bronchospasm" (Aronoff et al., 1975, p. 361). Though the method in this study is similar to that of Smith and Burns (1960), we suspect that the general approach may have been more permissive and ego supportive.

Collison (1975) reported a retrospective analysis of 121 patients with asthma managed with hypnotherapy. This report included six patients under age 10 years and 39 under age 20 years. Collison developed four categories of response: "excellent" when there was complete freedom from episodes of asthma without medication in the follow-up period; "good" when there was a reduction of acute episodes with continuation of medications; "poor" when there was less than 50% improvement in frequency of episodes or need for medication; and "nil" when there was no change from the pretreatment assessment. Of the six youngest patients, four had excellent or good responses. Of 39 patients in the 11- to 20-year category, there were 32 excellent or good responses. In the older age groups, there were significantly fewer satisfactory responses. Since the youngest groups also were most responsive to hypnotic induction, there was some question as to whether age or depth of trance would be a better predictor of success in a prospective study. Severity of disease was also an important variable. Patients whose asthma was not so severe as to require steroids generally responded best to hypnotherapy. Collison's techniques included suggestions for ego strengthening and for general relaxation, together with exploration of psychological factors related to the disease. He deliberately avoided direct suggestions for symptom removal, fearing that such suggestions might serve only to mask medical problems and ultimately have a harmful effect. He noted the inherent difficulties in retrospective analysis and the need for prospective studies that control the multiple variables involved.

Barbour (1980) reported preliminary results of the use of self-hypnosis in adolescents with asthma. A study of six patients, over a 5-month period, indicated that the use of self-hypnosis was associated with a reduction in the severity and frequency of acute episodes of asthma. Before self-hypnosis training, skin tests with local inhalant antigens were done in four patients and demonstrated positive reactions to 14 antigens; skin tests were positive for only seven antigens after 5 months of self-hypnosis. The same four patients also had skin testing done in a hypnotic state, and no reactivity to antigens occurred in any of the patients. This finding encourages the possibility that immune responses may be modified via appropriate uses of hypnotherapy and that hypnotherapy may not only reduce morbidity from asthma but, in fact, be curative in certain patients.

Kohen (1986b, 1995c) reported a prospective study of 28 children with asthma who were randomized into groups who learned self-hypnosis techniques and controls. Although there were no differences between the experimental and control groups with respect to pulmonary function tests from the initial to post-intervention periods, there were dramatic improvements after 1 year and after 2 years of follow-up. There were dramatic improvements in FEF 25-75 in five patients at 2 months. These correlated with evidence prior to the study that these children had experience with significant, spontaneous self-hypnosis phenomena. Future studies that control for this variable are essential.

Although we do not recommend the use of hypnotherapy in childhood asthma as a substitute for usual medications, we do believe that it can reduce the need for visits to emergency rooms and hospitalizations, and, in some children, the requirement for certain medications.

Although we are not attempting a complete review of psychological approaches to childhood asthma, we want to mention that several studies involving biofeedback training have reported positive results (Feldman, 1976; Khan, 1977; Scherr & Crawford, 1978). The work of Kotses and colleagues (Kotses & Miller, 1987; Kotses et al., 1991) suggests that biofeedback (electromyographic facial biofeedback) as a method of producing relaxation in facial muscles improves some measures of pulmonary function in children with asthma and adults without asthma. In a clinical trial with 29 children with asthma, Kotses and colleagues (1991) compared the long-term effect of training to decrease facial muscle tension with training to hold it at the same level. Subjects showed improvement in some pulmonary function measurements, and those trained to decrease facial muscle tension also showed a greater improvement in their attitudes toward asthma and a reduction in anxiety, both of which may have also contributed to the observed changes in pulmonary function. Spevack, Vost, Maheux, and Bestercezy (1978) have reported that children with asthma responded well to training in "passive relaxation." We wonder about the extent to which these children may have been responding to unintended hypnotic suggestion, especially since some of the studies included training in progressive relaxation. As we have noted earlier, hypnosis can occur without hypnotic induction. At the same time, when studies purport to relate hypnotherapy to relief from asthma but fail to measure trance responsiveness, it is not clear that children who improve were actually in hypnosis. We have already seen (Khan et al., 1974) that some children with documented hypnotic talent do not respond to suggestions related to their disease. Clearly more research is required before we are able to untangle the possibilities in this complex area.

Recurrent Hives

We have noted clinically that children suffering from recurrent generalized hives or massive reactions to bee stings have had fewer difficulties and more rapid recoveries when using adjunct hypnotherapy. Suggestions given have included those for general relaxation, mastery, and imagery of the patient without the swellings. It is possible that the state induced by hypnosis does reduce the allergic response. It may be directly through effects on a mediator of immune reactions, such as the mast cell (a cell which stores granules containing potent inflammatory and repair materials released upon injury to the organism) or indirectly through reduction of heart rate, blood pressure, and/or respiratory rates. Preliminary studies of the effects of suggestions given under hypnosis on immune processes were conducted by Good (1981) in the late 1950s. Because of the important implications for patients with specific allergies and immunodeficiencies, these studies should be expanded and replicated (see also Chapter 16).

Specific Allergies

Perloff and Spiegelman (1973) reported the use of hypnotherapy in treating a 10-year-old girl's allergy to dogs. The child, acutely sensitive to dog dander, but wishing to have a dog, was taught a visual desensitization while in hypnosis. Thereafter, her sensitivity to dog dander disappeared. Barbour's (1980) study with adolescents lends credibility to this clinical report.

Madrid and Barnes (1991) presented a case report of a successful single-session hypnotherapeutic intervention for a 12-year-old girl with a 7-year history of "stuffy and running nose continually . . . since she moved to the country." With the hypothesis that their technique triggered state-dependent memory, learning, and behavior, they suggested to the patient that when her body remembered how to heal itself and starts doing it, her index finger would twitch and float in an ideomotor response. After several suggestions evoked no response, they noted, "Consider your nose is too small to be fighting off these pollens all by itself. You need to use the rest of your body to get involved in dealing with these irritants. Use your arms and chest and legs and stomach to handle these things. Your nose is so small and can't do it all." In response to this suggestion the patient's finger twitched and legs and torso jerked for 15 seconds. Reinforcing suggestions were offered that her body could remember how to do this. Her nose was clear after the session and remained clear at a 3-month follow-up.

An 11-year-old patient of ours, Sarah, had learned and applied self-hypnosis very effectively for management of her asthma, so much so that with the guidance of her allergist she was able to stop taking any medications and, instead, applied self-hypnosis whenever she had what became very infrequent episodes of minor wheezing. One day Sarah called from the lobby of the hospital and asked if she could come up to my office and talk. As there was a temporary lull in the schedule, I was able to meet with her. Sarah said matter-of-factly, "Can hypnosis help with hay fever?" I asked her why she wanted to know, and she explained that even though her asthma was "tons better," that she continued to have "major problems" with runny nose and itchy red eyes for several months during pollen season. She then asked, "What are allergies, anyway?" I followed with a brief explanation of mast cells and how upon exposure to various antigens (such as pollens in the air) they release substances such as histamine into the bloodstream that ultimately cause the allergic reaction. A bright young lady, she said, "Histamine? Oh, is that why I sometimes take an *anti*-histamine to help the symptoms?" to which I, of course, answered, "Yes." She then observed and inquired, "So, then all I really have to do with my hypnosis is keep the histamine *inside* the mast cells, and not let it go outside into the bloodstream?" Though surprised at her matter-of-fact observation, I agreed. She said, "Thanks a lot!" and left.

Several months later her mother informed me that despite the high pollen counts, Sarah's "hay fever" symptoms of allergic conjunctivitis and rhinitis had been so minimal as to require no medications. As we have noted with so many of our patients, we are unsure whether these results are a function of the self-hypnosis per se, the patient's positive expectations, the self-confidence, an understanding of the physiology involved, the specific imagery, or some combination of all of these. Even though it may not matter at the clinical level, there is much research to be done to clarify the answer to these questions (see also Chapter 16).

CYSTIC FIBROSIS

Cystic fibrosis (CF) is the most common life-shortening autosomal recessive disease of Caucasians in the United States and occurs in approximately 1:2,500 White live births and 1:17,000 Black live births in the United States. In 1992 the median projected life expectancy was 28 years in the United States. Over 95% of patients die of progressive respiratory failure. Now known to be caused by defects in a single gene on the long arm of chromosome 7, CF is characterized by chronic obstruction and infection of airways, maldigestion, and their consequences. Dysfunction of exocrine glands is responsible for a sometimes confusing and broad array of manifestations. It is the major cause of severe chronic lung disease of children and also causes most exocrine pancreatic insufficiency in early life. The current treatment of CF addresses delaying the consequences of organ dysfunction and failure rather than correcting the underlying defect. With the identification of the gene for CF in 1989, and the cloning of the DNA, it is hoped that gene therapy will provide a breakthrough in treatment.

In the meantime, those with CF require extensive therapy including (1) dozens of pancreatic enzyme pills, (2) antibiotics, (3) nutritional supplements, (4) chest percusssion by a respiratory therapist or a motorized, vibratory vest, and (5) aerosolized nebulizer medications. Clinic visits, hospitalizations, repeated pulmonary function tests, blood tests and/or IV therapies round out the framework of management for the average youngster with CF, whose life is often functionally quite different from that of his or her peers. Physical activity may be limited both by the severity of lung disease and the rigorous schedule of daily treatments.

A recently published pilot study explored the effects of self-hypnosis as a coping strategy for 12 children and teen-agers with CF (Belsky & Khanna, 1994). The authors focused the hypnotic imagery on a theme of overall mastery of the effects of chronic illness and improvements in functioning, with specific suggestions for thinner mucus, clearer lungs, deeper breathing, and improved absorption of medication. Six children with CF in the experimental group (learning hypnosis) were studied along with six comparable youngsters with CF in the control group. Results supported the authors' hypothesis that self-hypnosis would be associated with well-being as measured by five standard psychological measures. On four of five measures, the change scores from the first to the second interview showed statistically significant differences between the group learning self-hypnosis and the control group. Significant differences were noted in (1) locus of control (Nowicki–Strickland Locus of Control for Children) with children who learned self-hypnosis reflecting more internality or sense of independence; (2) children's health locus of control (Parcel Children Health Locus of Control) with the experimental group showing a positive change in attitude about control; (3) Piers–Harris Self-Concept Scale; and (4) trait anxiety with an increase in anxiety for the control group and a decrease in the experimental group. In addition, the experimental group could be distinguished from the control group by differences (improvements) in peak expiratory flow rate, a measurement of lung function. Although the authors note the limitations of generalizability of this small sample-size study, they have provided preliminary information that supports the value of self-hypnosis in enhancing psychological well-being and improving physiological functioning. Future studies can and should build upon this important research.

We have had the opportunity to work with an increasing number of children, adolescents, and young adults with CF. Each was referred for hypnotherapy to help with one or more problems associated with CF or its treatment (Kohen, 1994). Each has benefited definitively and sometimes dramatically from hypnotherapy. Applications have included (1) pain control, including distraction, dissociation, switches to turn down or turn off pain, and amnesia for previous (painful) experiences; (2) anxiety control, via distraction or dissociation, relaxation, focused breathing, the jettison technique, and various forms of imagery; (3) taste control, through the switches technique and negative and positive hallucinations; (4) nausea control through use of imagery, distraction, dissociation; and (5) general control of disease, with suggestions for the use of imagery, future projection, and self-control.

Although our patients have varied from 5 to 17 years of age, and CF has played a unique role in each of their lives, some generalizations can be made from their collective experience: The application of hypnotic strategies to help modulate the uncertainty and anxiety that are hallmarks of chronic illness is perhaps its greatest value. Our clinical observations of this are strongly supported by Belsky and Khanna's work as described above (1994). The ability to use hypnosis to reduce, manage, or eliminate the fear of loss of control has been markedly evident in the young people with whom we have worked. While a cure for CF seems to be on the not too distant horizon, the knowledge that anxiety can be managed with the aid of hypnosis is a great comfort to those already in the end-stages of this disease and suffering the anxiety with dyspnea, hypoxia, and associated sleep deprivation.

The abilities to take a measure of control of appetite, to modulate discomfort, and to exercise control of weight provide not only comfort but also potentially add life to this as yet life-threatening disease.

DERMATOLOGICAL PROBLEMS

Itching, Scratching, and Picking

Hypnotherapy provides a useful adjunct in management of many skin conditions including atopic eczema, psoriasis, and acne. In these conditions hypnotherapy may serve to reduce scratching or picking and therefore interrupt the vicious cycle of scratching–picking, discomfort, scratching–picking, exacerbation, and more discomfort. Suggestions that encourage general relaxation, a sense of mastery in controlling the disease progress, and images of coolness and wetness seem most helpful in these situations.

Mirvish (1978) reported a case history in which hypnotherapy led to relief of symptoms and improved behavior in a 10-year-old boy with chronic eczema.

Olness (1977c) reported a case of intractable itching in a 9-year-old boy hospitalized for evaluation of possible rheumatoid arthritis. The pediatric resident caring for the boy considered teaching the boy hypnosis but had not yet begun when a social worker came to request urgent help. The boy was, at that moment, clawing at himself frantically. Olness established that the social worker had good rapport with the boy and asked her to sit down with him and talk about something cool like a swimming pool or a lake. The social worker said, "He's afraid of water. In fact, he won't get in the bathtub here." Olness then suggested the concept of snow and ice and winter sports. An hour later, the social worker returned, elated. She had discovered that snow sliding was a great joy for this boy. They sat together, imagining a particular hill, its particular bumps, and they felt the snow spray as they slid down the hill. The incessant scratching stopped. Two days later, when a resident asked the patient's private physician about starting steroids, the physician, watching the boy racing down the hall, said, "He doesn't need them now. Since he started that hypnosis, he's doing fine." One might question whether or not formal hypnotherapy was used. Certainly rapport with an interested, caring therapist, imagery, and suggestion of a feeling to counter pruritus were parts of the successful outcome for this patient.

As is true in conditions associated with uncomfortable symptoms, it is often helpful to teach self-hypnosis to children who itch and to recommend that they practice when they are comfortable in order to have more facility in self-control when symptoms recur. Often a simple playful suggestion like "Just picture the itch switch in your mind's imagination . . . and when you see it clearly . . . then . . . just . . . turn . . . it . . . down until it's turned off. That's right . . . " will suffice to empower the child to practice and develop control over the troubling symptom.

Hyperhidrosis

Ambrose (1952) reported a case of a 13-year-old boy with excessive sweating who responded to hypnotherapy. The condition had begun at age 8, when the boy was evacuated during the Second World War. While hypnotically regressed to age 8, he remembered being beaten up by a gang of boys while on his way to his new school. The boy became quite tense while describing these events, which he also recalled out of trance. Following six visits, he had no further problems in control of sweating. Ambrose postulated that hypnotherapy cut off the increased release of acetylcholine at the postganglionic nerves that had previously caused excessive sweating. At this time, this hypothesis has been neither confirmed nor denied, but studies of chemical mediations coincidental with hypnotherapy are essential for comprehension of mechanisms involved in such dramatic resolution of autonomic response problems.

We saw an 8-year-old girl who was referred specifically for hypnotherapy for profuse sweating. As neither the referring pediatrician nor the consulting dermatologist was able to determine a successful therapy, they concluded that "hypnosis might be worth a try." While the mother was concerned that in the future her daughter's profuse sweating would produce an offensive odor, the girl was already distraught at being teased for having wet hands and at reprimands from teachers for smearing or smudging her school papers. Indeed, during the first visit her hands literally dripped sweat when held out palms downward. During the initial interview and development of rapport, an imagery idea presented itself. As the history of the problem was being discussed, the patient became increasingly sad and soon began to cry, first slowly and then profusely. With comforting from her mother and the therapist, the tearfulness slowed and ceased, and the sadness lightened. She was reassured at the first visit that the therapist had some good ideas that would probably help her a lot. At the second visit she was taught self-hypnosis and in the first trance asked to recall how in her mind the "faucets" for her tears had seemed to turn on all by themselves in response to her feelings and then equally quickly turned off "because somewhere in your mind they got the signal to turn off." She was asked to find the "faucet" for her sweat glands in her hands and to practice turning them down. After four biweekly visits for hypnotherapy review, practice, and reinforcement, she and her mother reported "better than 50% improvement" and a sense of growing confidence; they decided no further follow-up was required.

Warts

Warts are reported to respond to many interventions (Chandrasena, 1982). Left to its own devices, the half-life of a wart is about 1 year.

Surman, Gottlieb, and Hackett (1972) reported the successful hypnotic treatment of a 9-year-old girl who had 31 warts on her hands and face that had failed to respond to four attempts at conventional treatment. She was told that first one side would be treated for five sessions and, if the warts went away, the other side would be treated. She chose her left hand and left side of her face for initial wart removal. Hypnotic induction included eye closure, simulated stair descent, and hand levitation. The patient was then told she would feel a tingling sensation in all the warts on the left side. The left-sided warts began to disappear after the first session. By the fifth visit, she had lost 26 warts. After 3 months of follow-up, only two small warts remained.

Tasini and Hackett (1977) reported the use of hypnotherapy in three immunosuppressed children all of whom had developed numerous warts. Each of the patients had been repeatedly treated with standard wart regimens for several years prior to the successful use of hypnotherapy. Hand levitation was used for induction. The patients were asked to think of doing something they enjoyed and to relax more each time they breathed out. While in trance, the patients were told that the warts would feel dry, then turn brown and fall off. Patients were seen for three to five sessions. Dramatic regression of warts began within a few weeks in each child, eventuating in complete disappearance. There was no evidence of recurrence in follow-ups that ranged from 4 to 8 months.

Following an appropriate induction, one can ask children to give themselves the message that they are cutting off the food supply to the wart or warts. This suggestion may be included in the course of a routine physical examination, and the child is asked to reinforce the suggestion twice daily at home. We recall cases in which warts were treated topically in routine office practice only to have patients return with wart recurrences. Since we have adopted hypnotherapy as the primary mode of wart therapy, our patients have not required further topical chemicals.

In a report of 41 consecutive cases of warts treated with hypnotherapy, Ewin (1992) described 11 prepubertal children (under 12 years of age) and five adolescents. Ten of the 11 children and four of the five adolescents were described as healing in response to direct hypnotic suggestion in hypnosis, with no focus on ongoing self-hypnosis. Children ranged from 6 to 12 years of age, and most required three visits or less. One required six visits, and one required 12 visits. Clinical presentations and time-to-healing varied considerably; for example, one 7-year-old had one wart that was gone in 2 weeks, a 12-year-old had seven warts that took 25 weeks to disappear, and a 6-year-old with 32 warts had only one visit, and the warts were gone within 10 weeks. Ewin believes that daily attention via self-hypnosis detracts from natural healing processes and instead suggests hypnotically that the subconscious mind will heal the warts and that the patient should ignore the warts and get interested in other things. Compared to conventional treatment of warts, none of his child patients had any scars and none experienced recurrence of the warts.

In commenting on studies reporting disappearance of warts following hypnotherapy, Thomas (1979) emphasized the potential value of understanding what goes on when a wart disappears in association with hypnosis. He recommended further investigation in this area. Clawson and Swade (1975) speculated that the mechanism involved in wart removal via hypnotherapy is the constriction of capillary sites to the warts. Whether the mechanism is vascular or immunological, it would seem that its understanding might relate eventually to treatment of other tumors and skin diseases. We address this further in Chapter 16.

DIABETES

Ratner and colleagues (1990) reported a hypnotherapeutic intervention with seven adolescents, ages 11 to 19 years. Six of them were followed for more than 6 months. Compliance improved according to the average hemoglobin A_1C and blood glucose levels. Each adolescent had three hypnotherapy sessions with additional visits as needed.

The psychological components of diabetes are well known (Ehrlich, 1974). Parents feel guilt about genetics and resent their lack of control. Family members are anxious about possible insulin reactions or episodes of ketoacidosis. Patients resent the intrusion of blood tests, diets, and drugs by injections. Some children develop fears over injections. The daily injection of insulin may become a cause célèbre in the family unit. Hypnotherapy, presented in the context of patient mastery, can provide a solution for some of the difficulties. We have taught self-hypnosis to many children and adolescents with diabetes in individual and group sessions.

Paul B. was referred for hypnotherapy to overcome his fear of needles when he was 6 years old. A year earlier, he had been diagnosed as having diabetes mellitus. Insulin injections were given for a few weeks and stopped as he entered the "honeymoon phase" of the disease. When insulin was required again nearly 1 year later, this naturally aggressive, active, and rather dominating child was crushed. He struggled to avoid injections, screamed throughout them, and was generally depressed. His mother, father, and younger brothers were upset, torn by their sympathy for Paul's predicament and their need to cooperate with the treatment regimen. When Paul was seen initially in the office, he sat sullenly next to his young, intelligent, and obviously concerned mother. He responded with interest when handed a 50-cent piece to hold but made no comment as his mother briefly described the onset of diabetes and Paul's fear of needles. The therapist said, "I once knew a 5-year-old boy who had diabetes and was so mad that he had to have those shots every day. He was mad at his doctor and at his parents and at his brother, who didn't need to get the shots. But then he learned something that they didn't know about how to handle needles himself. He knew, but his brother didn't." Paul asked, "What was it?" The therapist answered, "It was a way to turn off switches between his skin and where the needle went in and his brain—except in the beginning I couldn't tell him that because he was too young to know what a brain was." "I know what a brain is," said Paul. "Do you know what a nerve is too?" "Yep," he said proudly. "Well, you're already way ahead of this younger kid." Paul then learned the coin technique of induction, followed by favorite place imagery, suggestions about his switch system, and how he could use it. Throughout, the therapist stressed his ability, his control, his choice to use his skill when he wished, and to share with his family as he wished. At the conclusion of the first session, Paul was comfortable when touched with an insulin needle. He agreed to practice at home daily and to return in 1 week. His mother reported that injections no longer posed problems. He "turned off" his switch before each one, and the rest of the family didn't know how he did it. Subsequently, Paul attended group sessions where he was a good teaching assistant and very helpful to children with similar problems.

It is possible that the use of hypnotherapy to enhance mastery in children with diabetes, particularly as they approach adolescence, will indirectly affect morbidity from the disease. Children who are actively participating in their therapy may also be more likely to follow recommendations regarding urine testing, eating, and insulin with fewer complications and hospitalizations.

A recent study of adult diabetes evaluated the effects of acute psychological stress on metabolic control. Those with diabetes and controls were subjected to the acute stresses of mental arithmetic and public speaking. Blood pressure rose, and plasma epinephrine and cortisol increased in all subjects; but there were no changes in blood glucose, free fatty acids, glucagon, or growth hormone. The authors acknowledge that laboratory-induced stress may not be representative of stressful life events, but they conclude that metabolic control in insulin-treated diabetic patients is not jeopardized by sudden, short-lived emotional arousal. The primary benefit of hypnotherapy may be to enhance comfort for children who must suffer injections and to enhance compliance (Kemmer et al., 1986).

DYSPHAGIA

Dysphagia, or difficulty in swallowing, is more common in adults than in children, and its variety of organic causes can usually be easily discerned through careful history, physical examination, or radiological studies. In children, dysphagia is not uncommonly the result of psychological influences, including apparent conditioned responses in which dysphagia is associated with an acute illness or episode of physical or psychological trauma and then prolonged well after cessation or resolution of the original problem. These may include circumstances as common as difficulty in swallowing in association with a tonsillitis (e.g., strep throat, infectious mononucleosis), with an injury, or with psychological trauma such as forced oral sex in sexual abuse cases (see also Chapter 7 for discussion on hypnosis and child abuse).

Elinoff (1993) described the case of a 9-year-old girl who developed an inability to swallow rough-textured foods following an episode of feeling as though a nut in some ice cream had stuck in her throat. When she refused to eat anything except liquids and soft foods, her mother became worried about her nutritional status and increased the pressure on her daughter to eat, resulting in the emergence of a power struggle and further refusals to eat. Integrated into the routine of a busy family practice visit, the author offered the hypnotic suggestion "Did you ever watch water go over a waterfall?" and added ego-strengthening suggestions to the effect that food would become easier to swallow. Four days later the patient's symptoms had worsened, the mother had become increasingly insistent that the child needed better nutrition, and the patient had lost 5½ pounds. Reinforcement of the same hypnotic imagery was accomplished through suggestions to remember that even as a baby she had known how to swallow, and that all she needed to do was to let her body do what it already knew how to do, helping it by thinking about the waterfall each time she swallowed. Two days later she began to eat solid foods, and in follow-up 1 week later and 2 years later, she remained symptom-free with no recurrence.

LaGrone (1993) described a case of a 10-year-old boy who refused to take liquid medications for his reactive airway disease, because liquid medicines were for "little kids," but who had been unable to swallow pills for many years because they made him gag and / or vomit if he was able to swallow them. The pediatrician referred the patient for assistance in being able to take pills and / or capsules. After ascertaining the absence of any major intrapsychic problems, the therapist involved the child in a commitment to a plan including imagery and relaxation, self-monitoring, and self-regulation in the form of desensitization with direct suggestion and self-reinforcement. A 10-session desensitization and hypnosis treatment plan resulted in the child's ability to comfortably swallow pills and to maintain that comfort at 1 year follow-up.

We have seen many similar patients, and our experience concurs with these reports that the problems are common, usually easily amenable to resolution with hypnotherapy, and rarely recur (refer to case history, pp. 265–266).

ERYTHROMELALGIA

Chakravarty, Pharoah, Scott, and Barker (1992) described the case of an 18-year-old woman with a 4-week history of severe, constant burning pain in her hands and feet, which was unresponsive to usual analgesics and relieved only when immersed in ice-water. Examination also revealed persistent hypertension (165–185/110–125), and within 3 days, her feet and hands had become hot, red, and swollen, typical of this unusual condition. Her pain was unresponsive to aspirin, paracetamol, nonsteroidal anti-inflammatory agents, beta-blockers, vasodilators, and tricyclic antidepressants. Psychiatric evaluation revealed no evidence to suggest conversion disorder. Hypnotic suggestions included allowing the pain to flow out of the affected extremities, leaving normal sensation behind and teaching of self-hypnosis. The patient became pain-free and remained pain-free at 6-month follow-up. Elevated blood pressure was controlled initially with medication that was discontinued after 2 weeks.

EPISTAXIS

Edel (1959) reported the case of a 10-year-old boy who had been referred for reading difficulties. After eight sessions using hypnotherapy, his reading problem disappeared, and he no longer required tutoring. Two months later, he was brought into the physician's office because of a severe nosebleed. The use of bilateral anterior nasal packs with vasoconstrictors was to no avail. The physician gave instructions for posterior nasal packing and decided to add hypnotherapy as an adjunct. He told the patient that he could stop the bleeding himself, that he should hold his head way back and relax. Within minutes, the bleeding stopped and the boy breathed easily. When his head was placed forward, no blood spilled out. The next morning the parents reported there had been no further bleeding.

Although this was a patient previously familiar with hypnosis, it would be reasonable to give similar suggestions to any child with life-threatening bleeding from any source. (See also discussions on bleeding in Chapter 12.)

HEMOPHILIA

In Czarist Russia, the monk Rasputin used hypnosis to aid the hemophiliac czarevitch in the control of bleeding. In the 1950s, hypnosis was reported to be effective in control of bleeding and pain during dental surgery in those with hemophilia. In 1975, LaBaw taught a group with hemophilia self-hypnosis and encouraged them to use this technique when faced with anxiety-provoking situations, particularly bleeding episodes. His 4-year study documented a significant reduction in the number of units of blood products required by 10 adult and child patients who practiced self-hypnosis on a regular basis.

Gustke's pilot work (1973) suggested that some patients with hemophilia were able to increase Factor VIII levels in association with hypnosis. However, there are no controlled studies to support the idea that hypnotherapy consistently reduces bleeding in people with hemophilia. As routine adjunct therapy, hypnotherapy may be as valuable for its enhancement of mastery as for what it can do to reduce pain, relieve anxiety, or reduce the frequency of bleeding episodes.

Olness and Agle (1981) have reported group practice sessions for hemophiliac patients and their families over 6 years. Although individual practice sessions are available to the patients with hemophilia, most become comfortable and prefer the group format. Sessions last 1 hour. During the initial 10 minutes, patients share experiences, ask questions, and explain to newcomers. Thirty minutes of hypnosis exercises include suggestions for general relaxation, pain control, and reduction of bleeding. Following this, adults are invited to participate in self-hypnosis exercises. Children join parents if they wish to, or go to another room for play or movement exercises with another therapist. In recent years, children have been offered the option of practice in thermal biofeedback. Graphic evidence of control of skin temperature seems to have encouraged many children to pursue their self-hypnosis exercises more regularly. A typical account of such a group session is as follows:

J. K. had taught his family to do relaxation exercises during the summer. His mother was able, for the first time with his help, to have major dental work done without general anesthesia. T. is doing very well with his intravenous injections. One morning, while he was at the Art Institute, he experienced pain associated with the eruption of a molar. His mother was concerned that they would have to leave because T. was so miserable. She asked him to sit down and "turn off his switches," which he did promptly. He and his family were happy and comfortable during the rest of their visit. D. D., age 4 years, has been doing well in "turning off his switches" for IVs and has amazed the nursing staff.

When we asked the children about the sort of imagery they were using, J. K. reported that he imagined antique cars running about his bloodstream to stop bleeds, especially in his ankle. He said this was effective. K. K. imagines planes full of bombs of Factor VIII that he dispatches to parts of his body that need them, as well as a special glue named "Super-Clot" that he squeezes out in bleeding areas. The group went through a review of the switch-off technique, a coin induction also using favorite place imagery, and an exercise in which each child visualized a package containing a special gift for that child. Dr. D. guided the parents through a general relaxation using the image of a walk along a beach. The children also participated with their parents and expressed pleasure in the experience.

It is our perception that younger children learn best from older children in the group setting. If not threatened by much individualized cajoling and attention, they seem to learn by osmosis. Some younger children (age 2 to 3 years) merely sit quietly observing for one or two sessions without giving overt evidence of participation. Parents often report evidence of their learning at home before they show cooperation in the group sessions.

The children have provided many subjective reports of decreased bleeding. For example, Lanny L. said he awakened at midnight with a stiff arm, turned off the bleeding, and that his arm was fine by morning. His parents confirmed the report. Tom H., age 3 years, said he had a stiff arm (confirmed by his parents) but "I unstiffed my arm today."

Parents involved in the hemophilia group have reported perceived benefits for themselves associated with the relaxation exercises. Not only have they learned specific pain control techniques, which they have invoked during dental procedures or surgical experiences, but they also state they have found themselves calmer in stress situations related to the hemophilia. One father attributes reduction of blood pressure (20 millimeters diastolic) over a period of several months to his regular practice of self-hypnosis.

Over this 6-year period, the boys with hemophilia had decreased their average use of Factor VIII replacement therapy. They had also become more mobile with less use of splints, crutches, and fewer days lost from school because of bleeding episodes. However, they have also become older and perhaps more careful about activities that might result in bleeding. Several have moved from hospital to home administration of replacement therapy, and two had major surgery which required large amounts of replacement therapy over a short period.

A pilot study (Ritterman, 1982) examined the use of adjunctive hypnotic techniques with families in which at least one member had hemophilia. Little systematic work has been done previously to introduce families to such techniques. This study used an open-systems approach model of hemophilia coupled with interviews to facilitate that introduction.

PERSISTENT SOMATIC COMPLAINTS

A guideline for therapists in evaluating persistent somatic complaints in children is in Appendix F. A questionnaire on this subject appears in Appendix B.

GASTROINTESTINAL DISORDERS

Recurrent abdominal pain is a common symptom among pediatric patients and one for which organic causes are often not found (Apley, 1977; Berger, Honig, & Liebman, 1977; Dodge, 1976). As a last resort, these patients are sometimes referred for hypnotherapy to relieve symptoms. Although hypnotherapy may be helpful in these situations, its use simply or only to relieve pain is less likely to be successful than in children with known organic reasons for pain. A typical case history follows:

Linda, age 15, was referred by a pediatrician for symptomatic relief from abdominal pain that had been present for 6 months. The pain was recurrent, intermittent, and not associated with any specific time of day or situation. The parents had divorced 2 years earlier, and both had remarried. The patient's mother had custody, and the patient visited her father and his new family on weekends. Evaluation had included numerous laboratory and radiological studies, the results of which were normal. The patient was losing weight, which increased uneasiness in the referring pediatrician who was concerned about an undetected malignancy. At the time of the first visit for hypnotherapy, the patient and her mother were uneasy. They spoke very little to one another and demonstrated little affect. The patient was told that she would learn a self-hypnosis exercise that she could review at home, if she wished. The patient indicated her wish to learn hypnosis but responded mechanically to the initial induction. When she returned, she claimed to have practiced but said there was no improvement. During this session, she used hypnotic age regression to recall an event that she had enjoyed and in which she had felt in control; and she enhanced the feeling of joy and mastery by squeezing her right fist. She was then asked to become aware of things that were irritating her or worrying her and to decide if she could let go of any of them. Following this session, she spontaneously said that she felt better but did not reveal any of her possible concerns. She then refused a recommendation for psychotherapy. She said she would practice self-hypnosis at home and that she was feeling better. A week later, she left her mother's home and moved into her father's home. All symptoms abated, she gained weight, and continued to come for follow-up appointments for review of hypnotherapy during the next 2 years. Though she continued to refuse psychotherapy, she had no recurrence of abdominal pain and no indication of substitute symptoms.

Williams and Singh (1976) reported the case of an 11-year-old boy hospitalized for the third time in 16 months because of recurrent abdominal pain. The results of laboratory and X-ray studies were normal. Eighteen months earlier, he had undergone surgery to correct a right hydronephrosis. Subsequent recurrences of pain triggered gastrointestinal, neurological, and metabolic evaluations with normal results. There was a strong family history of abdominal disorders. After psychiatric evaluation, hypnotherapy was recommended. The boy was an excellent subject and, while in trance, repeated the following statements after the therapist: (1) "cooped-up feelings can cause tension," (2) "tension can cause physical pain," and (3) "by relaxing I can reduce tension and eliminate the pain." The patient reported disappearance of pain during the exercise and was taught self-hypnosis to maintain his clinical improvement. In 20 months of follow-up, he had only 1 transient recurrence of abdominal pain, which was possibly due to gastroenteritis. The authors noted that this child, as is true of most with abdominal pain, no longer had any need to continue self-hypnosis exercises once the presenting symptom had resolved. We have also found this to be the case.

Marie was almost 11 years old when she was referred to us for chronic recurrent abdominal pain. She had had onset of vague complaints of intermittent abdominal discomfort 10 months earlier. Like many with similar symptoms, she had been to her doctor and to several specialist consultants and had had many laboratory and radiological studies before a large, benign ovarian cyst had been identified and removed. She had a benign intraoperative and post-operative course and was "back to normal" for about 3 months when she began to have abdominal pain again. Although examination and tests were normal, both she and her mother were reluctant to accept this in view of what they considered had been a "misdiagnosis" or at least a "delayed" diagnosis of the ovarian cyst months before. When the pain continued and she began to miss a lot of school, she was referred to us for "possible hypnotherapy." As with many youngsters with this problem, Marie had developed a well-organized belief system, the underpinnings of which included uncertainty and mistrust about physicians and an easy-to-understand fear that a not-yet-identified tumor could explain her symptoms.

In the context of Marie's fears and understandable mistrust, we focused on developing rapport—slowly!—and I made the decision to avoid any formal statement about hypnosis or hypnotherapy. Following M. H. Erickson's dictum (1958b) to "go with the patient," she was asked simply to monitor her discomfort (we never used the word "pain" even if she did) on a scale from 0 to 12, with 12 being the worst imaginable pain and 0 being none at all. She was asked to give herself a rating after school and at bedtime and to record these on a calendar. Though she continued to complain, she began to attend school and appeared to feel better, though she continued to record, present, and discuss self-ratings of "11" or "11.5" for several weeks.

After the fourth or fifth visits, I gently inquired about the apparent discrepancy between how she appeared, how she reported she felt, and what she was able to do; and I asked her to "please help me understand." She said she still had the pain, but she was dealing with it better. Using her own language, it was suggested that perhaps she should also have a "deal with it" scale from 0 to 12 and could record that alongside the recordings of discomfort. She liked this idea, and the first week's recordings of "deal with it" were all "8" or "9," while the pain ratings remained "11." Continued contact with her treating physicians revealed no positive tests or explanation for her pain. Then the "deal with it" ratings began to drop weekly, and with this, the pain ratings also began to move down. As the "deal with it" reached "4 or 5," the pain ratings dropped to "9" and sometimes "8." It was then, over 6 weeks into the therapeutic relationship, that the naturalistic hypnotic suggestion was offered: "It's interesting, isn't it, how the more you deal with it better, the less there is to deal with, and the less it bothers you . . . great." Within 3 months, the "deal with it" had become "0," and the discomfort level decreased to "1 or 2" with no functional impairment. At our last session, she was given the post-hypnotic "waking suggestion" that it was "good to know that your body will let you know when there's a problem, and in the meantime you don't have to pay much attention to it at all." She agreed and remained pain-free at 1-year follow-up.

Sokel, Devane, and Bentovim (1991) reported the successful use of hypnotherapy with 6 children, age range 7 to 14 years, who had recalcitrant recurrent abdominal pain. Each child had an extensive medical evaluation. The interval between onset of abdominal pain and referral for hypnotherapy ranged from 2 months to 6 years. Children were taught relaxation, guided mental imagery, and suggestions for pain relief that were tailored to the age and interests of each child. Examples included a switch to "turn down" the pain, "magic potions," and a pet animal that soothed away the pain. Each child was provided a cassette recording of the session and instructed to practice daily with the tape and to use the self-hypnosis when he or she felt an episode of pain beginning. Each child was seen weekly for 3 weeks, and subsequently at 2-, 3-, and 6-month intervals. Children were able to resume normal activities within a mean period of 17.6 days (range 5 days to 8 weeks). Our experiences are consistent with their description.

Whorwell, Prior, and Colgan (1987) reported on their experience with hypnotherapy for 50 patients with severe, intractable irritable bowel syndrome. Their report does not indicate whether any children or adolescents were part of the cohort. They note, however, that the response rate to hypnotherapy was best, and 100% (= no relapse for 18 months after treatment with hypnotherapy) among those under 50 years of age compared to poor responses (25%) for those over 50 years of age. Hypnotherapeutic suggestions were directed toward control of intestinal smooth muscle. We are not aware of any studies of hypnotherapy for children or adolescents with irritable bowel syndrome or inflammatory bowel disease.

We have used hypnotherapy as an adjunct in management of children with ulcers, chronic hepatitis and varices, and inflammatory bowel disease (Crohn disease, ulcerative colitis), with a focus on control of discomfort, ego strengthening, and imagery both of healthy mucosa (e.g., "Picture the lining of your intestines and see it a smooth, healthy, pink color, just like the color and texture and healthy lining of your mouth and inside of your cheeks . . . ") and of health in general. While controlled studies are recommended and needed to assess effects of hypnotherapy on morbidity and mortality in these diseases, it is our impression that the enhancement of mastery and reduction of pain contribute to more rapid improvement in these patients.

JUVENILE RHEUMATOID ARTHRITIS

Juvenile rheumatoid arthritis (JRA) is well known as a disease of exacerbations and remissions. Conventional treatment deprives the patient of many controls and may in itself trigger emotional problems. The loss of free movement associated with the disease process invariably leads to some degree of depression in both children and families.

We often recommend hypnotherapy as an adjunct with these patients not only for relief of symptoms but to enhance self-mastery and enable the patient to control a portion of therapy. The complexities of psychogenic components of this disease are demonstrated in the following case history.

Mary F., a 10-year-old girl, came with her 12-year-old sister and mother to "learn hypnosis for pain control." Both girls had been diagnosed as having rheumatoid arthritis and eczema and were under the care of rheumatologists. They suffered intermittent pain, particularly in the knee and ankle joints, and they often missed school. In addition to the problems of arthritis and eczema, the 10-year-old girl was obese. She had attended one session of a group meeting for weight control but had refused to return.

Mary said she had been taught some hypnosis by a 14-year-old friend. Her sister and mother also said they had used self-hypnosis exercises for general relaxation. When asked about her interests, the patient said she liked singing, painting, and handicrafts. Her favorite colors were blue and red. Her mother described her as very creative and added that she often wrote stories and poems for fun.

Following progressive relaxation exercises, Mary rapidly appeared comfortable. When she confirmed via ideomotor signals that she was ready to go on, she imagined herself in a favorite place, doing what she liked, enjoying the feeling of being comfortable. After 2 minutes, she appeared to be asleep. Then she became upset and began crying. The therapist told her she was safe, that she need not continue to feel upset, that she could leave her favorite place if she found it upsetting and come out of trance when she was ready. Almost immediately she stopped crying, opened her eyes and said that her favorite place was in bed, that she had fallen asleep, and that she had had this once or twice a week while sleeping—that is, a night terror. Her mother confirmed that she frequently had night terrors. The patient was asked to think about a scene in which she could be very comfortable without falling asleep and then to describe what it was when she returned for her next visit. Her 12-year-old sister went through the identical progressive relaxation and imagery exercise with no evidence of discomfort and subsequently demonstrated good evidence of pain control.

A follow-up appointment was made but not kept because of a death in the family. The sister required hospitalization, and she was able to use self-hypnosis and pain control suggestions very well. When Mary returned 1 month later, she explained that she wished to use imagining herself floating in water for an induction, to focus on pain control and weight reduction. She seemed enthusiastic, did well in the hypnotherapy session, and agreed to practice twice daily. Subsequently she lost weight, demonstrated pain control, and returned for monthly group practice sessions for children with chronic pain problems.

This patient demonstrates some of the problems that can develop in hypnotherapy. Although it is often appropriate to allow a child his or her "own favorite place" without the necessity to reveal its whereabouts, it clearly would have been better to have known in this instance. Mary's choice of her bed as a favorite place suggests depression, which would also be consistent with her obesity and other chronic problems. An additional problem was the previous uncontrolled practice of self-hypnosis at home. This practice, while possibly leading to rapid trance induction, may also have made her less responsive to heterohypnosis. She did, however, seem to be highly motivated to have some personal part in her treatment and was very pleased with her subsequent excellent response.

Whether psychogenic components of JRA are causal or reflect the disease process and its treatment is not clearly understood. Much is known about immune factors and chemistries that reflect changes in those factors. One study (Domangue, Margolis, Lieberman, & Kaji, 1985) measured self-reported levels of pain, anxiety, and depression, and plasma levels of beta-endorphin, epinephrine, norepinephrine, dopamine, and serotonin in 19 arthritis pain patients before and after hypnosis designed to produce pain reduction. Following hypnotherapy, there were clinically and statistically significant decreases in pain, anxiety, and depression and increases in beta-endorphin-like immunoreactive material. The trigger for these changes, however, remains elusive (Russo & Varni, 1982).

Cioppa and Thal (1975) reported a fascinating account of a 10-year-old girl in whom JRA had been diagnosed by a rheumatologist. She responded minimally to large doses of salicylates and physical therapy. Prior to a trial of steroids, hypnotherapy was recommended. At the time of the first hypnotherapy session, the patient was using a wheelchair and appeared severely depressed. The hypnotherapist taught her ideomotor responses and asked, "Does some part of your mind know why you have arthritis?" The ideo-

motor response was in the affirmative and the patient appeared visibly upset. The hypnotherapist then gave her a general suggestion that her legs would
feel better. The patient and her mother were upset by this approach and dis-
concerted that the session was held in the Department of Psychiatry, since
they did not believe that the arthritis had a psychological component. They
did not want to return. That evening the girl spontaneously remarked that
her legs felt different.

One month later, the patient could walk with difficulty, but deep depression persisted, and the pediatrician asked that the child undergo a second
hypnotherapy session. The patient was told that she did not have to tell the
therapist the problem as long as she knew what it was and as long as she
was certain that it would quickly resolve itself if she really wanted it to resolve.
She was given hypnotic suggestions that her joints would feel much better,
that she would feel happier, and that she would be able to play with her
friends soon. Four hours later, the patient rode her bicycle for the first time
in 3 months. Ankle swelling and pain subsided rapidly over the next few
days, and, for the first time in several months, the patient could wear shoes.
At that point, her depression began to lift. She was seen for three additional
sessions. Improvements in her condition included being able to jump up and
down with no pain, return of her sense of humor, and loss of fear both of
injections and of the hospital. Four months later, aspirin was stopped, and
a 31-month follow-up revealed no recurrence of symptoms.

It was of interest that the hospital staff, at a follow-up conference, implied that the patient had not had JRA in the first place but merely a conversion reaction with concomitant laboratory findings suggestive of JRA. Prior
to her remission, a conversion reaction had not been mentioned in the differential diagnosis. We have seen this phenomenon repeatedly among medical personnel who feel uncomfortable about "coincidental" cures that occur in
conjunction with hypnotherapy in "organic" disease.

Cioppa and Thal (1975) noted that a number of diseases could be considered to represent the conversion of a chronic tension state into an organically manifest disease state. Factors of spontaneous remission are poorly
understood, although the writings of Norman Cousins (1976) have triggered
much interest in the effects of attitude changes on remissions. Cioppa and
Thal noted that to be therapeutically effective, a reversal of attitude apparently must occur at a subconscious level. This may be brought about through
hypnotherapy.

More recently Walco, Varni, and Ilowite (1992) have demonstrated the
value of self-regulation strategies in 13 children between the ages of 4.5 and
16.9 years who had pauciarticular or systemic onset JRA. Baseline pain intensity and level of functional disability data were gathered for weeks prior
to the patients being taught self-regulatory techniques that the authors
described as "progressive muscle relaxation, guided imagery, and medita-

tive breathing." Though the words "hypnosis" or "hypnotherapy" do not appear in this report, the authors clearly describe hypnotic induction with muscle relaxation; "meditative" breathing in saying the word "relax" to themselves upon exhalation; and therapeutic hypnotic suggestion in the form of guided imagery with clearly defined aims to provide distraction and suggestion to imagine a favorite place in which they had previously been pain-free, and to reinforce images that were metaphors for the children's sensory pain experience with the intent to then alter the metaphor and thereby alter the perception of the discomfort. Practice of techniques at home was taught and encouraged with the use of audiotapes, and patients were seen weekly for eight visits.

Results showed substantial reduction of perceived pain intensity both in short-term and in long-term follow-up at 6 and 12 months later and improved adaptive functioning. The authors correctly commented that conclusions from the data, although impressive, are limited by the the absence of a placebo control group. Though there was no improvement in disease activity and no reduction of medication needs, the clear improvement in pain perception and in the concomitant functional status of the patients argues strongly for incorporation of these self-regulation strategies as adjuncts to pharmacotherapy and other aspects of comprehensive care for children with JRA.

MALIGNANCIES

Since cancer remains one of the leading causes of death in children, we have deferred discussion of studies of hypnotherapy with terminal cancer patients to a separate chapter (Chapter 13) on terminal illness. We want to emphasize here that since 1960 there has been a dramatic increase in survivors of childhood cancers. Yet although these children become free of disease, they often pay dearly in terms of psychological trauma resulting from diagnostic and treatment procedures and from the expectation of death. In addition, many have developed later learning and behavior problems associated with the very chemotherapeutic and radiation therapies designed, and successfully applied, to save their lives. Hypnotherapists must begin to attend more to these problems of survival.

It is also important that hypnotherapists consider themselves, their feelings, responses, and reexamine their perspectives from time to time. Transference and countertransference problems can be particularly intense in a therapeutic relationship with a child with a life-threatening illness. Moreover, it is possible that therapists' attitudes may affect morbidity and eventual therapeutic outcomes. Although this area is fraught with problems for the researcher, we hope to see answers take shape. Specifically, we wonder whether or not patients can use certain hypnotherapeutic techniques to facilitate biochemical, immunological, nutritional, and/or psychological interactions that lead to cure (see also Chapter 16).

MEDICAL PROCEDURES

Hypnotherapeutic approaches are very effective in helping children and adolescents prepare for, cope with, and tolerate the anxiety and discomfort associated with various medical procedures. Examples of effective hypnotic approaches to the common problem of needle phobia are described in Chapter 7. Here we note some examples of effective application of hypnotic techniques for procedures as described in recently published literature.

Broome and her nursing colleagues (Broome, Lillis, McGahee, & Bates, 1992) described the effectiveness of imagery, relaxation, and distraction for 14 children receiving lumbar punctures (spinal taps) as part of their cancer treatment. Regular practice nightly and especially 3 nights prior to the next expected procedure were integral to the training in self-management. Although fear scores in children did not change, self-reports of pain ratings decreased significantly over time.

Green (1994) described the adjunctive value of guided visual imagery, relaxation, and therapeutic touch to the intensive care management of a 17-year-old boy with muscular dystrophy and deteriorating respiratory status. The patient's ultimate acceptance of and coping with a tracheostomy seemed to be directly temporally related to the comfort he was able to achieve with the assistance of imagery and relaxation.

Marino (1994) recently described the effective use of hypnotherapeutic strategies of imagery, relaxation, and "joining" with the patient in facilitating intensive-care-unit extubation of a 12-year-old girl with severe asthma who had required 5 days of ventilator-assisted respiration. With shared imagery of their respective love of the beach, Marino's hypnotherapeutic approach included elements of information-giving (detailed description of the process of extubation and what could be expected), distraction and dissociation with post-hypnotic suggestion (i.e., she could go to her favorite beach *during* the extubation, a sure sign that she was getting better) and reframing (post-extubation cough described as a good sign of her improvement).

Pederson (1993) has produced a videotape including four vignettes of children (actors) utilizing a variety of hypnotherapeutic techniques (relaxation, favorite place imagery, dissociation, and pain switches) as an educational and research tool for children in a pediatric oncology clinic. Specific reference is made to the usefulness of these strategies for procedures, such as starting IVs, spinal taps, and bone marrow procedures.

NEUROLOGICAL PROBLEMS

Hypnotherapy has been associated with disappearance of migraine headaches, post-encephalitic headaches, tics, hiccoughs, cyclic vomiting, and urine retention. It has also been used as adjunct therapy to help children with seizures, chronic muscle disorders, Tourette syndrome, cerebral palsy, and to facilitate rehabilitation after reflex sympathetic dystrophy and severe neurological injuries. Its use in children with attentional disorders was discussed in Chapter 9.

Headaches

The frequency of headaches in children is reported as ranging from 21% to 55%; the reported prevalence of juvenile migraines ranges from 5% to 10%. Headaches may be characterized as *migraine headaches; muscle-contraction headaches* (tension); and *organic headaches* (brain tumors, malformations, or encephalopathies). It is possible that some headaches characterized as migraines or muscle-contraction headaches belong in the organic category. Careful diagnostic evaluation is essential prior to recommendation for any treatment intervention, including hypnotherapy (Olness & MacDonald, 1987). In particular, the child should be examined with respect to blood pressure measurements, neurological status, presence or absence of purulent rhinorrhea, bruits of the head, dental abscesses, temporomandibular joint status, growth velocity, and skin lesions. Environmental toxins such as lead or carbon monoxide may cause headaches. Food allergies may trigger the migraine syndrome.

In the event that the diagnosis of tension or migraine headache is reasonably well established, the child may benefit substantially from training in self-hypnosis. A number of uncontrolled clinical studies (Houts, 1982; Andrasik, Blanchard, Edlund, & Rosenblum, 1982; Labbe & Williamson, 1983; Werder & Sargent, 1984), and one prospective controlled study (Olness et al., 1987) have reported success in teaching child migraineurs self-regulation techniques for control of pain.

In our prospective study, we compared propranolol, placebo, and self-hypnosis in the treatment of juvenile classic migraine. Children, ages 6 to 12 years, with classic migraine, who had had no previous specific treatment, were randomized into propranolol or placebo groups for a 3-month period and then crossed over to the other treatment for 3 months. After this 6-month medication trial, each child was taught self-hypnosis, and this was reinforced in five visits over 3 months. The entire study was completed by 28 children. The mean number of headaches per child for 3 months during the placebo period was 13.3 as compared with 14.9 during the propranolol and 5.8 during the self-hypnosis periods. Statistical analysis showed a significant association between decrease in frequency of headaches and self-hypnosis training. There was no significant change in subjective or objective measures of headache severity with either therapy.

Engel, Rapoff, and Pressman (1992) did a long-term follow-up on 17 of 20 original participants from a prospective control-group experimental design study with random assignment to autogenic relaxation, progressive relaxation, autogenic plus progressive relaxation, or waiting-list control groups. Long-term follow-up data were obtained at an average of 51 months post-treatment. The participants from the three treatment groups had significantly more headache-free days and less severe headaches compared to the control group. Twelve of the 13 treated participants used relaxation training to relieve headaches and seven reported practicing within the past month.

Osterhaus and Passchier (1993) evaluated the outcome of a combined behavioral therapy program in a school with adolescents, ages 12 to 19 years. The program included relaxation training, temperature biofeedback, and cognitive training. Each subject received four group sessions and four individual sessions. In the group session, information was given about pain, migraine, and pain-coping strategies. The subjects also practiced progressive relaxation, autogenic relaxation, self-hypnosis, and rational emotive therapy. The four individual sessions consisted of 40 minutes of peripheral temperature biofeedback. Subjects were asked to practice the relaxation and self-hypnosis twice daily and were followed for 7 months. There was a 41% decrease in migraine frequency in the experimental group, which increased to 54% at the 7-month follow-up. The acquired capacity to raise finger temperature during biofeedback training and decreased state anxiety during the sessions was related to headache reduction after the training. Older children showed more reduction in headache duration than the younger children. The authors note that they cannot comment on the effect of the separate therapeutic strategies, although we would judge that each of the strategies, with the exception of rational emotive therapy, involves self-hypnosis.

We recommend that children who have migraine learn self-hypnosis, if they are willing, as soon as possible after the diagnosis is made. Practically, training requires three or four visits and twice-daily practice by the child for at least 1 month. Following the initial intense practice period, practice can gradually be reduced to once daily and then to twice weekly. As is true with respect to other chronic problems that benefit from some training in self-regulation of autonomic processes, it is essential that the child, not the parent, control practice. As computer game feedback programs appropriate to training in chronic pain syndromes become available, these should make regular home practice more appealing to most children.

Follow-up, by telephone or letter, is important. Children who have biological bases for pain syndromes usually do far better in achieving the desired pain control than do children who have pain that is triggered primarily by emotional experiences. Therapists must be alert to the possibility that the biological basis for the syndrome has been missed or that a biological basis has developed for continuing headaches.

Seizures

Hypnotherapy has been reported to be successful not only for psychogenic seizures (see Chapter 7) but also for seizures whose etiology is primarily organic (Puskarich et al., 1992). Crasilneck and Hall (1975) reviewed the literature concerning adults and concluded that "although the mechanism for such effect is not always clear, it may often be usefully conceptualized as a change in the balance of facilitating or inhibiting neural impulses" (pp. 205–206). They noted further that reported improvement of epilepsy after hypnotherapy "may involve some change in the excitability of the cortex around the epileptogenic focus, although experimental validation of this hypothesis is lacking" (p. 206).

Five case histories were reported in which children and adolescents with chronic seizure disorders responded well to a combination of psychotherapy and hypnotherapy. They emphasized that uncontrolled seizures produce psychological trauma for any patient and that treatment that enables the patient and family to deal with this trauma more effectively might contribute to the breaking of a cycle of seizure-inducing psychophysiological activation.

We employed hypnotherapy with a patient who had nocturnal epilepsy that was unresponsive to conventional anticonvulsants. Although the patient had significant psychological problems and was being seen concurrently for psychotherapy, the fact that seizures occurred primarily during sleep suggests an organic basis for her epilepsy. We present the case in some detail in order to underscore the difficulty of understanding both etiology and treatment mechanisms.

Katie Q. was first referred for hypnotherapy as adjunct management of nocturnal seizures at age 15½ years. The patient had first developed seizure-like activity at age 12. She was hospitalized and found to have EEGs with abnormal foci in left anterior and frontal regions of the brain. She was placed on phenobarbital and Dilantin. During a subsequent hospitalization for seizure control, her EEG was found to be normal (a finding that does not rule out organic etiology) and medications were discontinued. Her "spells" continued, usually at night and rarely during the day. She would awaken with severe muscle spasms, lasting about 2 minutes, followed by the feeling of paralysis of all of her body except her left arm and head. She frequently urinated and felt a loss of control. After many months' trial of anticonvulsants and psychiatric treatment, with little change in seizure control, the patient was referred for hypnotherapy.

Katie was seen six times for hypnotherapy. During the first session, efforts were initially made to determine her hobbies, interests, and dislikes. She indicated a preference for rock and jazz music and enthusiasm about horseback riding, bicycle riding, and walks. The therapist went on to discuss sleep stages and how they are reflected in EEG patterns. Rapid-eye-movement (REM) and non-rapid-eye-movement (non-REM) sleep were discussed. Katie was told that it would be useful if her subconscious mind could give information to her about the stage during which the seizures were triggered (i.e., from medium to deep sleep or from light to medium sleep).

Hypnosis was achieved via eye fixation on one of many rings she had on her fingers. She then focused on breathing out and coordinating that with progressive relaxation. She was given the option of closing her eyes and visualizing numbers in sequence until she found a favorite place in her mind. She used a lifted finger to signal when she felt as though she were actually in a favorite place. She rapidly indicated she was there and was given the option of relaxing even more deeply by horseback riding or bicycle riding in an area of her choosing. She chose horseback riding. She was asked to ride until she was so relaxed that her body recognized she could identify the sleep phase in which her seizures occurred. Although she appeared very relaxed, she did not, over a 10-minute period, give any further finger signals. Recognizing possible resistance, we suggested to her that perhaps she would need more practice before she was ready to obtain this information and that she should, nonetheless, program herself to "turn off the trigger" to the seizure as she was passing from one stage of sleep to another. She accepted this and, when out of trance, agreed that she would practice the exercise twice a day.

Two weeks later, Katie seemed eager to go into hypnosis. Induction was similar, and once again she was asked to continue relaxing until she was ready to identify the sleep phase in which her seizures occurred. Repeatedly, her right and left thumbs raised slightly, and after 12 minutes, the right pointer finger lifted. When asked if that was her "yes" finger, she again raised the right finger and signaled that the left pointer finger was "no." Further inquiry about sleep stages revealed no new information. The therapist reinforced the suggestion that, at an unconscious level, she had all the information she needed to control the seizures and that she could turn off the trigger as she passed from one sleep stage to another.

On the third visit, Katie seemed more relaxed than in any previous session and went through the initial induction without verbal cues. After 5 minutes, she raised her right index finger signaling that she was relaxed enough to program her autonomic nervous system to control body functions in a way that was good for her. The therapist said, "It's all right. If you wish to have pleasant dreams instead of seizures—to enjoy those dreams, let those dreams be satisfying and pleasant. When you control the seizures, you will be a stronger and happier person. Sunshine always follows rain." Following this session, Katie was relaxed, good humored, and said she thought the time passed was 5 minutes instead of the actual 25 minutes.

During the month before beginning hypnotherapy, Katie had had 15 seizures. During the next month, there were only four seizures. Between the third and fourth sessions, Katie had two nocturnal seizures, possibly associated with anxiety concerning a planned 20-mile charity walk. At the fourth visit, the therapist added positive future imagery, asking Katie to imagine feelings of physical and emotional well-being at a future time when she was seizure-free. She was then asked if she would be willing to determine her seizure aura. She agreed and went rapidly into a trance with very few verbal cues. She indicated with an ideomotor signal when she was prepared to determine the aura. After 5 minutes she opened her eyes, said it was "weird," and she didn't enjoy the part when she was getting information about her aura. She said she felt as though both legs were moving rapidly up and down. She said in the fifth session that she did not want to pursue the aura. She was taught a jettison technique after focusing on a happy memory amplified with a clenched fist. On coming out of trance, she said she had enjoyed this. Ability to jettison problems was reinforced in the sixth session. Subsequently she improved remarkably in school and home relationships. There were no further seizures over a 2-year follow-up.

Urine Retention

Positive response was reported after a single session of hypnotherapy in the case of a 10½-year-old girl with psychogenic urinary retention. This followed a herpes zoster infection in her inguinal area and placement of a suprapubic cystostomy. Urinary infections followed and life-threatening sepsis was a possibility in this patient with compromised immunological defenses. The psychiatrist noted that this patient had been traumatized and terrified by numerous bodily invasions that deprived her of autonomous control of body functions. While she was in a trance state, he had her repeat the following statements out loud: (1) "When people are very scared and upset they stop making pee-pee"; (2) "By relaxing, I can overcome my scared and upset feelings"; and (3) "The sooner I can make pee-pee, the sooner they will take the tube out." The three points were written down on a card for the patient to review during self-hypnosis. Within a few hours, after this single session, she began voiding.

We have often written reminder affirmation statements for children to use during self-hypnosis. This may be important especially in children who have stronger visual than auditory images. The following case history concerns an adolescent patient with acute neurological handicaps, including urinary retention, who developed his own creative imagery to overcome the problems.

Neal C., age 17 years, was admitted to the hospital for the sixth time in relapse with Hodgkin disease, stage IV-B. He was referred for hypnotherapy to control severe back pain, headaches, and nausea. At the time of the initial hypnotherapy session, he was pleasant, interested but frequently complained of pain and anorexia. After some discussion about his interests, likes, dislikes, and habits, the therapist chose an induction method related to his interest in electronic circuitry. He imagined himself constructing a radio until he was ready to accept suggestions for relief of symptoms. At the first visit, he was given suggestions to recall a happy meal time and enjoy feelings of pleasant hunger. At the conclusion of the first hypnotherapy session, he volunteered that his headache was "almost gone," and he added, "Strange, now I feel hungry." Chemotherapy was begun on the following day. Although the patient had expressed prior fears about vomiting, no nausea or vomiting occurred. When seen 2 weeks later in outpatient follow-up, he reported having had no nausea or vomiting throughout the recent course of treatment. He also volunteered that he used self-hypnosis to enable him to sleep easily each night. At that visit, hypnotherapeutic techniques reviewed included progressive relaxation, and imagery of computer construction. It was recommended that the patient read Norman Cousins's article in *The New England Journal of Medicine* (1976) concerning personal mastery in the face of chronic illness.

Neal did well for 9 months until he was admitted to the hospital with severe neurological symptoms including diplopia, loss of balance, absent gag reflex, and urinary retention. Consultants in neurology and oncology were unable to explain the symptoms. Results of EEG studies, computerized tomography (CT) scans, analysis of spinal fluid, and other laboratory studies were normal. Because of the patient's inability to care for himself after a week of hospitalization, plans were under way for nursing home placement. Happily, the patient dramatically improved. His dictated account, requested from him on the day following his recovery, follows:

> Early afternoon the doctors came into my room and said that unless I improved in the next 48 hours they would begin an experimental drug called ARA-C in order to remove or help restore my double vision, dizziness, bladder control, balance, and gag reflexes. ARA-C was an experimental drug and both of them agreed that it didn't provide much hope, so that night I was going to try to program my own and restore all or release some of these reflexes.
>
> The reflex that I missed most was stereo vision, and if I was going to have one eye covered in order that I would not get these headaches and nausea and see double, that was the first one I concentrated on. At 7 P.M. that night, I virtually closed off my room to the public, had a dose of Tylenol and laid back, uncovered my left eye, and looked at the ceiling

at a cat poster, which had been put there a day earlier. This cat was going to be my object and the focus for the next 12 hours while I concentrated on obtaining my vision without the headaches, nausea, and dizziness and tried to regain control of my bladder.

The way I went about relaxing or restoring these functions was very simple. I simply lowered the head on the bed back to a comfortable position, opened both eyes, and immediately I would see two cats spread apart approximately 2 feet and they were throbbing and coming in and out at me. This was confusing, but with the Tylenol the headache was tolerable. I continued staring at the cat for a period of 10 to 15 minutes when I would have to shut both eyes in order to relax for a while because I could feel the headache coming on and felt that if I pushed it too far to begin with the headache might become unbearable, and I would give up. After resting my eyes for a period of 3 to 5 minutes, I would begin opening my eyes and again concentrate on the cat, trying to maintain a single image in my mind where there was two. I would think of a single cat, and sometimes the cats would be closer together and sometimes a little farther apart. To this method, I would go through over and over and whenever I needed a rest, I'd shut both eyes in order that they both would get the same effect.

After 3 or 4 hours I began to notice that the cat was a bit closer and maybe not throbbing as much, which was encouraging, and I would rest, and I would get my Tylenol in order to help relax and relieve the headache. After about 6 to 8 hours, at about 3:30 in the morning, I could maintain a single cat without really trying very hard, but the pulsating was still there, and I fell asleep for about 2 hours. At 6:30 that morning, I again was staring at the cat; this time it was much easier to maintain a single image, and the throbbing had virtually disappeared. The pain had subsided enough that the next day I did not take Tylenol at all, and the doctors, because of this, postponed the ARA-C another 24 hours.

Also during the night that I was concentrating on my cat, I was concentrating on bladder control. I had not been able to control my bladder for about 7 days. I thought that was another function that I would be able to return to myself. The way I went about doing that was as I concentrated on the cat, I concentrated on having my bladder turned off, as an on-and-off faucet, and the faucet was turned all the way off. I felt that if I could keep the faucet "off" for 12 hours and then turn it "on" and concentrate just on going on after 12 hours, the bladder would have to be full of enough liquids that no matter what, it would go. This method proved effective except that when I turned the "on" back, it took about 10 minutes for the first stream to flow. Once again, the doctors thought this was encouraging, therefore, they would let the drugs slip by for 1 more day.

I myself felt much happier and was in brighter spirits that day because I feel like I accomplished much more than I could have with the drug. All Saturday, with my stereo vision restored and not having to wear a patch and my partial bladder control restored, the main worry was having headaches, and there was still the reflex or the gag reflex and more control of the bladder. I turned the bladder off in my mind and just concentrated that it was in the "off" position for a full 12 hours before I'd even try to go. This proved to be effective, as this time when I let my mind turn the bladder "on," I went to the bathroom almost immediately. [For] the gag reflex. I had no idea about how to go about getting this small reflex back. I had something I would try and that was just to imagine that every time I swallowed that swallowing is like a wave coming on an ocean, and this would go down my throat and when the wave would break it would hit my stomach. This I repeated over and over and over, and it seemed that that night that I was even able to swallow water. I just imagined a wave and that it would break on my stomach.

Sunday morning, I continued to show improvement in all areas, and I believe the doctors were much happier. One doctor was finally smiling, and the other didn't come in. I had gotten control of most of my functions, more control, felt weak, unbalanced, unsteady with standing up, but this may be due to being in bed for a week straight. I was in much greater spirits, and I feel that I can have a quicker recovery rate, and Sunday afternoon my NG tube was removed, and I was able to swallow clear liquids on my own.

Unfortunately, I will begin chemotherapy in another hour. I am very nervous. I will try to use relaxation. I feel that I can give better answers if I were posed questions as I am a terrible dictator. I've been very brief, and I have been unable to put into words exactly how, what, when, why, whatever happened.

Subsequently the patient underwent 5 days of chemotherapy without difficulty, and was discharged. Discharge diagnosis was (1) Hodgkin disease, stage IV-B, in partial remission, and (2) acute brain syndrome, cause unknown. The patient remained in good health for 4 months. He then developed influenza complicated by pneumonia and died after 48 hours.

Vomiting

Children are often referred to hypnotherapists for management of nausea and vomiting associated with chemotherapy or with some situation such as going to school. It is essential to evaluate the problem in terms of what triggers nausea and vomiting in the child, how the family reacts, and how medical staff react.

Vomiting is one of the most easily conditioned of reflexes. Presumed biological bases for nausea and vomiting include viral illnesses, allergies, chemotherapeutic agents, antibiotics, radiation therapy, and many metabolic disorders. The feeling of nausea or act of vomiting may be linked with environmental factors including persons, rooms, cars, buildings, colors, scents, songs, food, television programs, and so forth. The sight of a needle or of a medicine tray may induce vomiting.

An apparent example of such a conditioned response was recently reported by Sokel and colleagues (Sokel, Devane, Bentovim, & Milla, 1990) in a 9-year-old boy with vomiting. Previously well, this boy had been given a prescription for bisacodyl for treatment of constipation and developed nausea in association with this medication. Though the medication was discontinued, the vomiting persisted, leading to school avoidance in the context of having already been experiencing "bullying" at school and of increased parental attention. Intractable vomiting persisted, occurring effortlessly 5 to 10 minutes after meals, resulting in a 15% weight loss, hospital admission, and extensive radiological and laboratory studies, all of which were normal. Weight loss was reversed and vomiting reduced with nasojejunal feeding. He and his family had the vomiting explained to them as a "reflex habit" that could be treated with hypnotherapy. He was taught self-hypnosis including relaxation, guided imagery which incorporated his love of cooking and of animals, and a story of a special garden in which he found the ingredients with antiemetic powers to bake into a cake. Direct suggestions were given: "You feel your tummy becoming relaxed and comfortable so that when you eat . . . you do not vomit." The suggestions were recorded on audiotape for him to listen to before meals. Privileges in the hospital were contingent upon success, and individual counseling was also provided. Symptom relief began immediately and progressed so that the patient was able to retain food for 20 minutes by the 3rd day, until the next meal by the 11th day, and to cessation of all vomiting by the 17th day. A week later he had a relapse when he also developed chicken pox, and vomiting was eliminated by 4 weeks, with no recurrence at 12-month follow-up.

Chemotherapy-related nausea and vomiting is a distressing experience for children. Drug noncompliance due to severe nausea and vomiting is reported to be as high as 33% in children and 59% in adolescents (S. D. Smith, Trueworthy, Klopovich, Vats, & Snodgrass, 1984). Recent studies (Cotanch, Hockenberry, & Herman, 1985; Hockenberry & Cotanch, 1985) investigate the use of hypnosis as a behavioral intervention to ameliorate these side effects. Cotanch et al. (1985) suggest that chemotherapy-related nausea and vomiting in children might be reduced, and oral intake improved, with the use of a behavioral intervention.

Recently, Jacknow, Tschann, Link, and Boyce (1994) reported the results of their investigation of the effectiveness of hypnosis in decreasing antiemetic usage in children with cancer experiencing chemotherapy-related nausea and vomiting. Twenty newly diagnosed cancer patients between 6 and 18 years old with no prior chemotherapy experience were randomized to receive either a standardized antiemetic medication, or to receive hypnosis as a primary treatment for nausea and vomiting with the option of supplemental antiemetic medication on an as-needed basis. The study monitored nausea, vomiting, and antiemetic medication use during the first two courses of chemotherapy, and anticipatory nausea and vomiting at 1 to 2 months and 4 to 6 months following diagnosis. Hypnosis training was conducted in two to three sessions during the initial chemotherapy courses. Hypnotic procedures were personalized to the developmental level of the child with an emphasis on active involvement of imagination. In the initial session, children were taught imagery incompatible with the sensation and experience of nausea and vomiting. If nausea and vomiting developed, they were later also given direct hypnotic suggestions and instruction such as to "find the vomiting control center and turn it down." During both the first and second courses of chemotherapy, children learning hypnosis used less antiemetic medication than those in the control group who had not learned hypnosis. In addition, at 1 to 2 months after diagnosis, patients in the hypnosis group experienced significantly less anticipatory nausea than those in the control group who had not learned hypnosis. This effect was not sustained, however, as at 4 to 6 months no further significant differences were identified for anticipatory nausea.

Prior to recommending an intervention, the therapist must assess the child's tolerance for procedures such as intravenous injections. He or she must learn exactly when the vomiting usually occurs. If it is associated with chemotherapy, can the environment be modified somehow? Do family members or members of the treatment team reinforce the expectancy of vomiting by asking, "Are you nauseated yet?" Do family members become anxious themselves just before the treatment? How long a wait does the child usually have in the clinic?

If vomiting is associated with a procedure, and needle phobia is present, the therapist should first address the issue of needle phobia. After several sessions of heterohypnosis, the therapist may make a tape that can be listened to over headphones during procedures. Kuttner (1986, 1988, 1989) has recommended that the young child be encouraged to focus on blowing out the breath slowly in order to relax and gain control during procedures. She also encourages young children actually to blow bubbles when preparing for procedures.

Zeltzer, LeBaron, and Zeltzer (1984a, 1984b) have studied nausea and vomiting in children who have cancer and have recommended that therapists become familiar with a variety of interventions, including distracting techniques and formal hypnotic inductions. Storytelling with appropriate metaphors has been recommended by Zeltzer and colleagues and by Kuttner. An image of a cool, moist wind such as that associated with skiing, tobogganing, or walking in gentle rain is one that may counteract the feeling of nausea.

Videotapes are available that demonstrate many of these approaches. (The American Society of Clinical Hypnosis can be of help; the Canadian Cancer Society offers a videotape entitled *No Fears . . . No Tears* [Kuttner,

1986] for $54.00. Contact Promotional Services, Canadian Cancer Society, 955 West Broadway, Vancouver, BC V5Z 3X8.) Video games have also been used successfully to induce self-hypnosis for treatment of pediatric oncology patients experiencing acute psychological and physical reactions to chemotherapy, including nausea and vomiting (Kolko & Rickard-Figueroa, 1985). This access to video games resulted in a reduction of the number of anticipatory symptoms and a diminution in the adverse nature of the side effects.

Parents may be of great help in reinforcing self-hypnosis practice for children who have nausea and vomiting. The following vignette illustrates the need to spend time in getting to know the child. Andrew, age 5 years, had experienced bone marrow transplantation and had not retained food for more than a month. He vomited whenever food was brought to his room. Prior to his illness, he had enjoyed tricycle riding, playing with Transformers, and drawing. He had once lived in Florida and enjoyed seeing oranges on trees. He also liked Michael Jackson's music. During the first visit, the therapist played with Transformers and emphasized changes in Transformers and changes in people. She also asked that hospital staff obtain a Walkman-type tape recorder and arrange for Michael Jackson's songs to be played through the headphones beginning a few minutes before meals were brought in. During the second visit, she asked Andrew to image a story of himself and his mother (he had often expressed fear that she would not return) going for a tricycle ride, going wherever they wished, enjoying what they were seeing, feeling, and hearing. They rode past orange groves. They became hot and thirsty; they stopped to eat a big juicy orange. One hour after this session, Andrew ate a whole orange; he did not vomit thereafter. His mother retold him the story of the trike ride many times.

Cyclic Vomiting

We are unable to find any reports in the literature of hypnotherapy for cyclic vomiting. We have worked with 20 of these patients, each of whom achieved some degree of symptom relief through hypnotherapy. In each case, however, we referred the patient to medical subspecialists for further evaluation, and eventually organic explanations for the vomiting were found. This is a reminder, especially in difficult and uncertain areas, that one should be wary of the grab-bag diagnosis of "psychogenic."

Karen I., age 10 years, was referred for hypnotherapy after 60 hospitalizations for rehydration necessitated by cyclic vomiting. She had previously undergone extensive evaluations and 1 year of psychotherapy. Shortly before the onset of the vomiting, 3 years earlier, she had been frightened by a description of the movie *The Exorcist*. Karen had been informed by one group of consultants that the symptom would resolve at the time of puberty and that there was no cure. In the initial hypnotherapy session, Karen was taught progressive relaxation and given general ego-strengthening suggestions. In subsequent sessions, she was given suggestions to counter nausea. Although she managed to abort her attacks when the therapist was present, she could not use self-hypnosis for this purpose, and the frequency of hospitalizations did not decrease. The therapist asked that she be evaluated by a pediatric neurologist and endocrinologist who, after 1 year of intricate testing, defined a urea cycle abnormality and found that the patient could eliminate the attacks by controlling her intake of protein. They later tested the hypothesis by giving her a protein load and following the rise in her blood ammonia levels. Subsequently, she did well. Although self-hypnosis helped her symptomatically while the cause was being elucidated, it did not substitute for a thorough medical evaluation.

Neurologically Mediated Intractable Reflexes

Both intractable hiccoughs and sneezing may be treated successfully with hypnotherapy. Patients may be taught progressive relaxation and given diagrams of the involved reflex with suggestions to control the "switch" between the brain and the reflex. Daily reinforcement through self-hypnosis is recommended.

Cerebral Palsy

Lazar (1977) described her treatment of a 12-year-old boy with athetoid cerebral palsy and mild mental retardation. After induction using imaginary television, treatment included observation of the self with relaxed and controlled hands, recall of previous relaxing experiences, suggestions designed to increase hand function, and focus on feelings about independence and anger. Sessions were reinforced with cassette tapes. While the boy reached only a light hypnotic state, he nonetheless achieved good results. His teachers noted improvement in his handwriting and in his ability to work in shop class. Lazar postulated that teaching such a patient self-hypnosis encourages independence and a sense of accomplishment, so important in people with disabilities. She suggested that hypnotherapy might be most effective with these children if begun at an early age when there is the best chance of minimizing secondary emotional problems and maximizing motivation for optimal motor functioning.

Secter and Gelberd (1964) also advocated hypnosis as a relaxant for patients with cerebral palsy. In a brief study of 12 children with cerebral palsy, they found that 8 responded to hypnotic induction; intelligence levels ranged from "subnormal" to normal.

The successful use of hypnotherapy in maximizing performance of athletes encourages its trial in any problem involving muscle function. Rehearsal of correct movements mentally is associated with measurable changes in catecholamine responses (Landsberg & Young, 1978). The adjunct use of hypnosis would seem reasonable in rehabilitation following injuries and muscle disease.

Reflex Sympathetic Dystrophy

One of our colleagues (Lewenstein, 1981) shared with us the following case history; so far as we know, it is the first report of successful hypnotherapy with reflex sympathetic dystrophy.

A 15-year-old girl "felt something snap" in her right knee while standing still on a basketball court. Subsequently, she developed pain in her right lower leg distal to the knee and involving the entire lower leg. The pain was described as maximal behind her leg and on the right sole. The entire lower leg distal to the midthigh turned purple.

She obtained several medical consultations. Diagnoses of torn ligaments and/or thrombophlebitis were made. She was hospitalized and given anticoagulants. When X-rays and a venogram were normal, and she did not improve, she was transferred to another hospital for further evaluation and treatment.

On admission she was found to have a mottled, cool, right leg from the midthigh down, and was unable or unwilling to bear weight on the right leg because of intense pain. There was circumferential hyperesthesia with pain on light touch in the lower leg and an area of numbness over the right thigh. In spite of aggressive physical therapy with hydrotherapy, the patient did not improve. She was referred for hypnotherapy 2 weeks after admission.

During the first hypnotherapy session, she was asked to imagine a tree, with multiple branches, growing and blossoming in the spring sunlight. She was told that she could imagine the blood vessels in her legs as similar to the branches of the tree.

She was told that the nerves and blood vessels to her legs had been confused at the time she injured her knee and that she could correct this problem by focusing on the imagery of the healthy tree in her self-hypnosis practice. Since she recognized that she had injured her right arm a number of years ago and it had healed completely, it was likely that her right leg would also heal completely.

The patient noted subjective improvement by the following day and walked without crutches 2 days later. The patient was seen every 2 to 3 days for an additional 10 days and was encouraged to continue self-hypnosis practice. She was discharged to home and was doing well 5 months later.

Successful hypnotherapeutic treatment of eight children with reflex sympathetic dystrophy was later reported by one of us (Olness, 1990a).

Rehabilitation Following Central Nervous System Injury

Crasilneck and Hall (1970) reported the successful use of adjunctive hypnotherapy in the treatment of a 10-year-old boy who suffered cerebral contusion, concussion, and edema following a 15-foot fall. Three and one-half months after the fall, he was discharged to home in a fetal position, with a fixed stare, no evidence of recognition, and no speech. He was also incontinent. The mother then requested a trial of hypnotherapy. In the first session, the therapist told the patient that he could be helped if he could cooperate and then asked him to close his eyes. When the boy did not respond, the therapist gently closed his lids manually and gave him repeated suggestions that he could achieve deep hypnosis. When he was thought to be in trance, he was told that he could get well and that he could communicate by blinking his eyes, once for "no" and twice for "yes." He immediately responded to questions with appropriate eye blinks. He was seen for hypnotherapy once weekly for 1 year. Each time, suggestions were made for return of essential functions. Gradually the patient improved, eventually redeveloping normal speech, ability to walk assisted, and ability to read normally. The authors postulated that the therapist's attitude and persistence, combined with the structured hypnotherapy situation, led to a changed expectation for recovery by the family and facilitated positive motivation and behavior change in the boy. This case also points out the importance of speaking to noncommunicating patients as if they are hearing and as if response is expected.

Tourette Syndrome

In a 1987 report (Kohen & Botts), four children with Tourette syndrome were referred for self-hypnosis training. Three were on haloperidol, and all were experiencing frequent tics, which were socially embarrassing and caused other children to avoid them. Three of the patients learned relaxation/mental imagery exercises on the first visit and demonstrated increased facility with home practice. Diminished frequency of tics was noticed almost immediately by both patients and their families. Improvement was sustained over time, with substantial reduction of medication in one child, cessation of medication in another, and no initiation of medication in the third. (Later, an additional four children with Tourette syndrome were taught self-hypnosis and demonstrated sustained success analogous to the patients described in the report.) In each patient, the focus of hypnotherapeutic suggestion with imagery and relaxation was on the development of metaphors for control of tic behavior. Individualized to the favorite activities of each of the child patients, these included, for example, the imagery of one child as quarterback of the football team (and his brain as quarterback of the muscles of his body) and another as playing the cello (i.e., making all the right movements at the right time in the right way, as the metaphor for control of muscles).

Young and Montano (1988) described a hypnobehavioral approach in which three children were taught to utilize habit reversal and response prevention along with training in self-hypnosis for control of their tic behaviors. Prior to training in tic control, patients were taught increased awareness of tic behavior to help identify the tic(s) that were most troubling to them and also to discriminate tic from other motoric behavior. This would also appear to be of value in helping children with this disorder to overcome the denial (of awareness) of the tic behavior commonly noted in Tourette syndrome. Self-hypnosis training was provided at the same time, utilizing muscle relaxation and favorite activity imagery. Children were asked to notice in imagination the subjective urge or feeling that preceded their tic behaviors and to focus on this. The therapist determined the muscle response that competed with the tic behavior, and then, in trance, children were asked to select and apply either symptom prevention or habit reversal. Training in self-hypnosis and suggestions for daily practice and relapse-prevention training were also provided. The authors believe that self-hypnosis played multiple roles in their patients, including (1) increasing self-awareness, motivation, and concentration, (2) promoting self-confidence through self-selection of habit reversal or response prevention, (3) facilitating decreased tic behaviors, (4) modifying perceptions of tics and allowing the conceptualization of tics as within their control, and (5) reducing symptoms and development of mastery.

Culbertson (1989) described a four-step treatment model of hypnotherapy that helped an adolescent male with Tourette syndrome help himself over the course of nine treatment sessions in 6 months. In addition to classical Jacobsonian relaxation training, this adolescent was also taught finger-temperature biofeedback as a measure of degree of relaxation and as a metaphor for his own ability to create physiological control. Self-hypnosis training, favorite personal imagery, and use of audiotapes for reinforcement of practice are described as integral ingredients in management.

Most recently Kohen (1995b) has described in detail the successful application of indirect, Ericksonian strategies for more than 35 patients with Tourette syndrome and the use of self-hypnosis as a coping strategy in Tourette syndrome (Kohen, 1995d). These and the aforementioned work of Young and Montano (1988), Kohen and Botts (1987), Culbertson (1989), and Zahm (1990) all provide narratives of hypnotic suggestions and verbalizations that were effective with their patients.

The mechanism of these apparent positive results of self-hypnosis on Tourette syndrome remains unknown, as is the precise biological nature of the disorder, which continues to be characterized as a complex neurobehavioral disorder. Is it successful solely because of the therapeutic value of relaxation techniques as an effective coping strategy? Does the attention of a sensitive therapist contribute to its success? Or do these techniques act in a similar way to haloperidol, improving and altering associated behaviors by evoking mediators that stimulate the blockage of dopamine receptors? As research proceeds on this problem, it seems prudent to consider self-hypnosis as a potentially useful adjunct early in the comprehensive evaluation and management of children with this disorder.

PELVIC EXAMINATIONS IN ADOLESCENT GIRLS

Kohen (1980b) reported the successful use of hypnotherapy to assist adolescent girls through their first pelvic examinations. The anxiety of this event can be reduced by gentle, sensitive physicians. The use of hypnotherapy can foster a sense of competency and control in the teen-ager undergoing her first pelvic examination as well as reduction of anxiety prior to future similar examinations.

Prior to the pelvic examination, the physician should allow the patient time to acknowledge her concerns and then express his or her willingness to help the patient be comfortable through the examination. It is explained to the patient that she can use her imagination to facilitate comfort. If she has previously stated that she enjoys skiing, for example, the physician suggests, "Go ahead and let yourself imagine that you're skiing" and continues to give suggestions for progressive relaxation. The physician must explain each part of the procedure as he or she also reinforces the suggestions of relaxation and comfort. A posthypnotic suggestion is given to relax even more easily and quickly during future pelvic examinations.

If patients have negative expectations based on uncomfortable previous examinations, the physician may ask, "Would it be okay if it doesn't bother you this time?" This question may represent the beginning of an indirect hypnotic induction, causing the patient to pause and reflect on the idea that there is a choice in this matter. It is important that the therapist understand how the patient believes things will be different or better because of hypnotherapy. The teen-ager must be reminded of her own skills and responsibility for success in achieving comfort and control. Time spent in adding hypnotherapy as an adjunct to pelvic examinations makes it possible to do better examinations more quickly, thus saving time in the long run.

SPORTS MEDICINE

W. P. Morgan (1980) reviewed potential applications of hypnosis in sports medicine research and practice. Appropriate uses of hypnosis in this area include management of excessive precompetition anxiety and analysis of factors involved in "slumps," long periods when athletes inexplicably perform well below previous levels. Athletes may become aware of errors in body movement that they do not recognize in their usual cognitive state. In some cases, hypnosis may properly be used to help an injured athlete perform, but the therapist must be keenly aware of the signal value of pain and must not put the athlete in a situation where he or she is likely to become further disabled. Facilitation of performance by hypnosis should be attempted only when such an approach is not contraindicated at a medical, physiological, or psychological level.

W. P. Morgan (1980) concluded that evidence for positive effects of hypnosis on muscle strength and endurance is equivocal, although negative hypnotic suggestions often result in performance decrement. These findings lead us to question the validity of the many popular books that state that imagery and relaxation exercises — possibly involving hypnosis — can enhance performance in individual sports such as tennis and skiing (Gallwey, 1974; Gallwey & Kriegel, 1977). Certainly, attempts to "psych up" an athlete to perform at record-breaking levels are not likely to be helpful and may be dangerous.

Morgan further reported that hypnotically suggested exercise alters cardiac rate, respiration rate, total ventilation, oxygen consumption, and cardiac output in the nonexercise state. Observed metabolic changes often approximate responses reported for actual exercise. The application of this finding to actual performance, however, is unclear.

Our clinical experience in using hypnotherapy for sports problems has been limited to its use for pre-performance anxiety.

Jane P., age 11 years, was referred because she had severe anxiety for several days prior to solo ice-skating competition, and this was adversely affecting her performances. She has been skating since the age of 4 and had been in competition many times with no difficulty until 6 months prior to referral. After discussion of her interests, likes, and dislikes, she entered a hypnotic state easily by imagining herself reading a favorite story. She was taught ideomotor signals and asked if she would be willing to review past skating competitions. When she readily agreed, the therapist asked her to regress to competitions at age 8, age 9, and age 10 years. She had positive recollections of the earlier competitions, but recalled an unpleasant comment from a peer at the latest competition, after which her excessive anxiety began. While still in hypnosis, she was asked if she would be willing to get rid of this comment, which was still bothering her. When she agreed, she was given the option of sending the comment off in the distance via pony express, airplane, or train. She chose the pony express and let the horse gallop into the distance until she could no longer see it. Following this, she was asked to focus on the image of herself successfully completing the next competition, doing well, and feeling pleased with her performance and her control. She then practiced self-hypnosis once daily until the next competition. She was calm and happy thereafter, did well in her next public performance, and called the therapist to express her pleasure.

Elaine, age 13 years, was regarded by her tennis coach and family as an exceptional tennis player. She first learned to hold a racket at the age of 4 and had progressed to competition on a national level. She said that she enjoyed tennis and competition until she had an experience that was followed by hyperventilation. It happened on a practice day; she had been playing well, and many players, including adults, had asked to play with her. The temperature was 90 degrees, and the humidity, 30%. She became so absorbed in play that she forgot to eat lunch and had only a few drinks during the day. Not surprisingly, she developed signs of heat exhaustion, including rapid breathing. By the time her parents realized that she had overdone it, she was hyperventilating and required medical attention. Subsequently, she began to hyperventilate before every tennis game; she found that she was playing poorly and did not enjoy playing. She was referred for evaluation and possible hypnotherapy.

Elaine chatted openly with the therapist about whether or not this symptom might keep her out of a game she no longer enjoyed. Her parents had asked the same question. Elaine said that she enjoyed many activities but that tennis had been her favorite. Following a discussion of body response to stress, she learned a progressive relaxation exercise, which she practiced twice daily. A week later, I asked her to add a focus on a favorite safe place. I then asked her questions to which she responded with ideomotor signals, most of them non sequiturs, but including a few questions probing her wish to play tennis. Her responses were immediate and positive. I added a rehearsal of a tennis game while she was relaxed and asked her to review this twice daily. She returned to tennis a week later; she experienced no hyperventilation. Six months later, she won her divisional championship.

In his book *Peak Performance* (1984/1985), Garfield has reviewed Russian approaches to improving the performance of athletes by training them in self-hypnosis. In assessing steps involved in this approach, Garfield has emphasized voluntary relaxation, mental rehearsal, disciplined imagination, poise, and letting go. These steps are entirely consistent with hypnotherapeutic approaches in focusing intensely on imagination and feeling. It is essential that the athlete establish a mental picture of the desired outcome, rehearse the feeling of attaining that outcome, and, at the time of performance, "let it happen."

Although there are no research data in the English literature to document that children can actually improve their proficiency in specific sports by means of self-hypnosis, this seems a reasonable proposition. In the meantime, until this area is studied further, it is appropriate to teach self-hypnosis for reduction of performance anxiety.

GENERAL RECOMMENDATIONS

In a paper on hypnotherapy with pediatric cancer patients, Olness (1981b) made several recommendations to therapists who work in this area. Since these recommendations are applicable to many pediatric medical problems, we have adapted them here.

• Child health care professionals should be encouraged to learn and use self-hypnosis for themselves. Proper use of this modality can lead to reduction of personal stress, which is an inevitable factor in working with children who have medical problems. The heightened ego receptivity of the hypnotic state (Fromm, 1977) may also facilitate creativity in considering diagnostic issues and developing treatment plans. In some cases, health care professionals can participate in group sessions with patients and their families (e.g., groups for children with cancer, hemophilia, asthma). The shared experiences may be of benefit to all.

• Hypnotherapists must be willing to spend time with child patients, getting to know them as individuals and planning treatment accordingly. Standardized or "canned" approaches are likely to fail, given the fact that there is no such thing as a standardized or "canned" patient.

• When hypnotherapy may be appropriate for a medical problem, children should be exposed to this possibility as soon after diagnosis as possible. Progress is slower among children who have developed secondary emotional problems or who have well-established negative conditioned reflexes from months or years of accumulated fears of procedures and drugs.

• Hypnotherapy teaching and reinforcement sessions should occur frequently during the first weeks of diagnosis, and children should be encouraged to practice on their own. Children with chronic illnesses should be invited to attend group practice sessions on a monthly or twice-monthly basis in order to avoid loss of hypnotic skills during long symptom-free or medication-free periods.

• Every hypnotherapy session should enhance the child's sense of mastery and should be conducted at the child's speed. Practice efforts of children should be facilitated, not forced.

• The effects of parental attitudes and mental health status on the evolution of childhood diseases must be considered carefully, and techniques must be developed to meet parental mental health needs. Parents and siblings can be encouraged to learn self-hypnosis and to participate in group sessions.

• For children who are discouraged or uncertain of their hypnotic skills, the use of thermal biofeedback—with its visual proof of control over physiological processes—should be considered as an adjunct.

CONCLUSIONS

Hypnotherapy is useful as a primary or adjunctive tool in the management of a wide range of childhood medical problems. It is of particular value in the enhancement of mastery in children who have chronic diseases, especially if the focus is on early intervention and prevention.

For many medical problems, several different hypnotherapeutic approaches have been reported to be successful. Prospective studies are needed to determine which approaches are most successful and to assess the particular value of hypnotherapy in relation to other kinds of treatment. Long-term follow-up studies of children with hypnotic skills will allow us to note enhancement or waning of those skills as well as possible relationships to ability to cope with medical problems in adulthood.

CHAPTER TWELVE

Hypnotherapy for Pediatric Surgery and Emergencies

The use of hypnosis as the sole anesthetic in major surgery is quite rare, probably because of the relative safety and convenience of chemical anesthetics. Hypnosis has been used infrequently for this purpose with adults (Kroger & DeLee, 1957; Levitan & Harbaugh, 1992; Wangensteen, 1962; Winkelstein & Levinson, 1959; see also Chapter 10, this volume). We know of no similar published accounts with children since the 19th century work of Braid and Elliotson in England.

Hypnotherapy is useful in pediatric surgery to facilitate emergency room procedures, preoperative comfort, induction of anesthesia, and postoperative comfort and cooperation. It is also used for a variety of minor surgical procedures in such areas as burn therapy and dentistry.

We know of no instances in which pediatric surgical patients have used hypnosis inapprorpiately to mask symptoms, such as pain, when awareness is necessary for prompt diagnosis and treatment, although we have heard fears to the contrary. We remind our patients to give themselves suggestions that are in the best interests of their body and good health in order to offset the possibility that the signal value of symptoms will be ignored. The following case history is an example of a child's ability to use judgment in applying hypnotic skills.

Joe T., age 10 years, came into the emergency room with severe periumbilical pain and a history of preceding nausea and vomiting. He also had a history of migraine headaches for which he had successfully learned to use self-hypnosis. While in the emergency room, awaiting the surgery consultant, he was clearly uncomfortable. Nursing staff reassured him, saying he could probably have a medication for pain following the surgeon's visit. The surgeon made the diagnosis of appendicitis and scheduled the patient for sur-

262

gery within the hour. When offered preoperative analgesics, the patient refused, saying, "It's going to be fixed, now I can turn off my switch." He visibly relaxed and was comfortable until induction of general anesthesia. Following surgery, the patient used self-hypnosis to counteract pain and nausea and to facilitate healing.

EMERGENCY SITUATIONS

Modifying Attitudes

If hypnotherapy is going to be successful during pediatric emergency room procedures, one must realize that children bring more to the situation than a laceration or fracture. They bring their own feelings, mixed in unknown ways with attitudes of parents, teachers, and others who have witnessed the current crisis or discussed previous crises with them. Kelly (1976) has pointed out that fear, pain, and guilt are characteristic of virtually every emergency situation. There is the fear of the process of the accident or problem and its outcome, fear of losing control. Pain may include recall of past pain coupled with whatever the present sensation is and anticipation of future pain. Guilt may be real or conditioned by family or friends. In a study of children's emergency room visits, Alpert (1975) concluded that the majority had psychogenic antecedents, for example, a death in the family, a family quarrel, a move, or a serious illness in a parent. Emergency room staff should consider such possibilities, even though the reason for admission is, on the surface, clearly an accident.

Successful hypnotherapy is also dependent on the attitudes of the emergency room staff. That is, if the staff expects a negative experience for all concerned, then negative suggestions will almost guarantee fulfillment of those expectations. For example, the spontaneous immediate use of a mummy or papoose board or other restraints conveys an expectation that the child is going to resist. Likewise, requiring parents to leave the scene of repair conveys an expectation that they cannot be of help to the child. When properly prepared, many parents can reinforce suggestions not only in the emergency room but also later at home. Allowing them to observe the induction of hypnosis and the procedure may be relaxing, desensitizing, and a good learning experience for them. There are exceptions, but most parents can be helpful in emergencies that involve children. Therapists gain more by expecting parents to be helpful and supportive than by expecting them to hamper procedures.

Modifying the Child's Experience

A hypnotherapist usually does not have much time to get to know a child who comes to the emergency room. The situation often precludes opportunities to explain hypnosis and to determine the value of several different induction techniques. However, these circumstances do not rule out the use of hypnosis or of hypnotic language, strategies, and techniques without any formal induction. Precisely because of the emergency, children are often highly motivated to respond to positive suggestions.

Occasionally, direct or indirect hypnotic suggestions can be given before a child even reaches the emergency room. If a parent makes a preliminary telephone call, the doctor can suggest specific phrases that might be helpful. One of us (KO) found such techniques helpful when her daughter cut her forehead while being chased through the house by her sister. When the child felt the blood on her face, she started screaming. Her mother's first comment was, "What beautiful, healthy red blood you have. Let's go into the bathroom to get a better look at it." The child immediately stopped screaming. As she left for the emergency room, she leaned out the car window and yelled at her sister, "And I have strong, healthy blood. Mama said so."

When the physician first greets the child in the emergency room it is important to convey understanding of the situation and its attendant feelings. One might say, "It's scary to be in a new place like this and to have that cut. It's bleeding a lot, and it might bleed some more." When the doctor acknowledges the child's reality, the child is more ready to believe other statements and follow other suggestions. When the clinician acknowledges (to him- or herself) that in an emergency situation (acute injury, pain, anxiety) people are often in a spontaneous altered state of awareness, analogous if not identical to a spontaneous hypnotic state, this allows the clinician to proceed to approach the child hypnotically, offering at once acknowledgment of the reality, reassurances of comfort, and positive expectancy suggestions for improvement. Thus, in addition to "It's bleeding a lot, and it might bleed some more," the physician might also add the very positive and Ericksonian suggestion "and it will keep right on bleeding until it stops . . . soon."

M. H. Erickson (1958b) has pointed out the value of commenting on certain aspects of the child's reality in order to turn apparently negative behavior to advantage. For example, one can comment that a child's tears are beautiful or that loud yelling reveals very healthy lungs.

The child needs reassurance, but vague statements that everything is going to be all right are usually of little value. A clearer, more specific comment may allow the child to be more hopeful that the present situation will change. The doctor who says, "I wonder if it will stop bleeding in 1 minute or 2 or 4" not only suggests hope but also arouses curiosity that modifies anxiety and enhances cooperation. Compare this approach with the negative implications of "I've got to try to stop this bleeding. Now you just have to be still."

After gaining rapport, the physician must explain what will happen to the child, and how and when it will happen. Here again, current approaches are often at variance with successful use of hypnotic techniques. For example, in the name of disclosure, it is very common to hear people tell a child, "It is going to hurt." For two reasons, we believe that physicians may have become dishonest in their efforts to be honest with children. First, it is difficult to predict the extent to which a child will experience the sensory and suffering components of pain. Second, children—as much or more so than adults—can use various techniques to reduce their pain, and so-called honest statements about feeling pain may limit the child's creativity by imposing negative expectations. At the same time, one should not tell a child, "It won't hurt," for such a remark can undermine credibility and trust, both now and in the future. M. H. Erickson (1958b) found the middle ground with comments such as "Now, this could hurt a lot, but I think maybe you can stop a lot of the hurt or maybe all of it." Or, one might say, "This might hurt some, but it just may not bother you very much. Some people say this feels like pressure, some like a kitty scratching, some like a baby chick pecking, some like buzzing. I wonder what it will feel like for you." Here the child's curiosity is again aroused and willingness to cooperate is enhanced.

A pediatric intern at Johns Hopkins Hospital had the following experience, which demonstrates how hypnotherapy can be used in emergency situations (K. A. Torjesen, personal communication, 1994). A 12-year-old girl was referred to the emergency room by her pediatrician for X-rays of her neck because she had not eaten solid foods for 3 weeks. She had choked while eating a strawberry and thereafter was convinced that she would choke and die if she ate any solids. She had lost 15 pounds. She was able to take clear liquids but, during the past few days, even this had become difficult. She had no previous similar episodes, and her general health had been excellent. Detailed family history suggested that her home life was normal and that she was a happy child. Physical examination revealed no abnormalities except that she appeared thin. Lateral neck X-rays revealed no abnormalities.

Following the examination, the intern discussed the history and findings with the emergency room physician who recommended that the family make an appointment with psychiatry. The intern, who had taken courses in pediatric hypnotherapy and who had used self-hypnosis herself, spoke with the family about the psychiatry appointment. They agreed, but she noticed that the girl looked disappointed. She proceeded to draw diagrams for the girl of the esophagus, trachea, and epiglottis in order to explain to her that they were separate tubes and that normally choking did not occur. On impulse she said, "I have something you can practice before you go to bed tonight and tomorrow morning that may help you help yourself. It is easy to understand why you have this problem, because you became very frightened when you choked. You then worried about swallowing solid foods. As the days went by you developed a habit of not being able to swallow solids. You can reverse the habit by using your imagination. Would you like to learn how?" The girl was enthusiastic. The intern told her to imagine herself in a comfortable, favorite place. She was instructed that when she felt very comfortable and relaxed she should imagine she was eating her favorite foods and that swallowing was easy and smooth and comfortable. The parents immediately noted that the intern had given a hypnotic suggestion but said they agreed with this approach. On the following day, the pediatric intern was busy in the clinic when her beeper went off. She was told that a family was waiting in the emergency room to see her. She found her patient eagerly waiting for her and the parents beaming. The patient threw her arms around the intern and said she had been able to eat solids the very next morning. The family had returned to keep the appointment with psychiatry, but there seemed little need for an additional consultation at that time. It is noteworthy that part of the treatment included demystification, in this case, an explanation of the swallowing process (see also Chapter 11). Puskar and Mumford (1990) described the value of cognitive mastery along with hypnotherapy in a 16-year-old boy whose treatment included looking in a mirror (at a scalp laceration) as part of the process of hypnotherapy easing the emergency room experience

We have found that such explanations and demystification are often important, integral parts of the hypnotherapeutic process.

Some children benefit from distraction. Others, for whom cognitive mastery is a major coping mechanism, prefer to watch every detail of a procedure. The physician can ask whether the child wants to learn about how doctors treat injuries or prefers to engage in some other enjoyable activity. Either way, the child achieves dissociation from pain. For example, Gardner (1978b) reported a case in which a 4-year-old chose to play with his cat and cheerfully described his play while the pediatrician placed four sutures in a thigh laceration without any anesthetic. In such cases, the physician might say, "Thank you for telling me what you would like to be doing. Go ahead and imagine you're doing it. I'll fix this while you're doing your favorite thing. You can help me by telling me what you're doing now." Many children readily accept these indirect suggestions for control and cooperation.

For the child who wants careful descriptions of the treatment, one can use relatively soothing words. Injection of local anesthetic is "a squeezing feeling." Antiseptic solution is "cool or cold." A fractured arm or leg may be "like a block of wood." Burns can feel "more and more cool and comfortable." Children can be asked to time the procedure, to count stitches, to estimate blood loss, to hold bandages or instruments—generally to provide assistance in such a way as to enhance mastery, minimize anxiety, and indirectly reduce pain.

Distraction may be used in the context of cognitive mastery by asking the child to observe body parts that are not involved in the injury. For example, if the injury involves the left knee, the physician might also check the right knee carefully and say, "How does your right knee feel? Is it warm? Is there pressure here? Keep feeling that. I need to know if the feeling changes." Direct techniques for pain control, as described in Chapter 10, may also be used. It may also be helpful to include suggestions to stop bleeding (e.g., "It's bled enough. It would be okay to stop bleeding now"), to send "fighter cells" to take away germs, and to start healing immediately. Post-procedure suggestions should focus on ego strengthening, comfort, easy cooperation with future procedures (e.g., bandage changes, suture removal), and rapid healing.

Andolsek and Novik (1980) reported successful use of hypnotherapy for emergency treatment of two 3-year-old and two 4-year-old children. Procedures included suturing lacerations, treatment of a hematoma underneath a fingernail, and incision and drainage of a thumb abscess. Trance states were induced by encouraging the child to pick a topic of conversation and to focus on the most vivid sensory details of the chosen topic. Goals were to direct attention away from fears and to give the children a feeling of control over a potentially traumatic situation. Parents were encouraged to reinforce the positive suggestions. Following the procedures, the children and parents were encouraged to express their feelings about the experience.

Santer (1990) conducted a randomized controlled study of "formal communication techniques," including mental imagery instructions as an adjunct to injected local anesthetic in a pediatric emergency room. Fifteen experimental and 10 control children and their guardians did not differ in scores of behavioral distress, subjective pain, or anxiety. Children ranged from 6 to 16 years. Ten children in the experimental and three in the control group reported using mental imagery during the procedure. Children who used imagery were significantly younger than those who did not ($p < 0.05$). Guardians were with children throughout the procedures. Five, including two parents of control children, were especially helpful to their children, suggesting focus on imagery and encouraging their children with words and touch. One mother of a 7-year-old in the experimental group, when the child decompensated and the suturer insisted upon forcibly restraining the child, offered the child a trip to McDonald's on the way home and then started chanting, "Two all-beef patties. . . . " The child joined in and repeated the chant, held still, and the repair was completed quickly. Three guardians were known to have bribed their children, and two yelled at their children. Santer concludes that the attitude and communications of guardians are important variables in these types of studies, and that some guardians communicated in a way that was the equivalent of a hypnotic induction, whereas others counteracted the therapist's communication efforts.

Kohen (1986b) has reported six cases in which hypnotherapeutic techniques were helpful to children in an emergency room; in five of the cases, the children had no prior knowledge either of the therapist or of hypnosis. Kohen facilitated relaxation and comfort for these children by allowing them to use their inherent imagery skills. Two of the children, grade school-age boys, imagined that they were playing football during suturing procedures. A teen-age girl imagined herself dancing during the diagnostic procedures prior to an appendectomy. In the case of a 12-year-old boy who was having a severe gastrointestinal hemorrhage, Kohen was asked to help when the boy resisted insertion of a nasogastric tube. The boy appeared to go into a spontaneous trance and responded quickly to explanation of the diagnostic and treatment procedures, assurance that the blood was "running in to replace what you threw up," a request to breathe in good feelings and breathe out bad feelings, and the suggestion to turn off the switch to the nose and mouth in order to let the tube "slide easily into the food tube." The tube slid in easily. Two boys, in the emergency room with acute asthma, achieved comfort by focusing on the images of what they would like to be doing rather than being in the emergency room. One imagined himself riding his bike, and the other imagined himself playing basketball.

Bierman (1989) similarly described 3 children who came to the emergency department: a 7-year-old boy with multiple abrasions after a bicycle accident, a 12-year-old girl with a scalp laceration, and a 9-year-old boy with asthma and needle phobia. In each case the quick establishment of rapport, suggestions for favorite activity imagery for distraction and trance, and both direct and indirect hypnotic suggestions were successful in alleviating discomfort and allowing treatment to proceed easily.

Kohen (1986b) notes that physicians are challenged to establish rapport quickly with a stranger (the child), while at the same time they must rapidly conduct diagnostic and treatment procedures — no small task! In such situations, Kohen says, "it seems most prudent and efficient to simply 'do' hypnosis, rather than to engage in lengthy explanatory discussions which in another setting might be appropriate."

PRE-OPERATIVE VISITS

When a child is admitted to the hospital for surgery, a hypnotherapist usually has time to get to know the patient and, it is hoped, to help coordinate attitudes and approaches of the family and the various hospital staff involved in the case. It is indeed unfortunate when a hypnotherapist helps a child develop positive attitudes toward surgery only to be sabotaged by the negative suggestions of someone else who may have had a previous unpleasant surgical experience. It is sometimes helpful to warn children of this possibility and to suggest that they can remember positive images even if someone else suggests something to the contrary. If possible, all members of the treatment team should focus on mastery, reinforcing the concept that the child can be an active participant in the treatment process.

In many hospitals, children and families may take a tour of the operating and recovery rooms, or are encouraged to see short movies or engage in puppet plays describing events that will occur before, during, and after surgery. A hypnotherapist may use imagery techniques to facilitate good adaptation through rehearsal in fantasy. Since hypnotherapy does not involve any standardized equipment, it may be especially useful in dealing with individual surgical problems and psychological needs. For example, amputation of a limb is one kind of experience following an accident and another kind of experience following the discovery of a malignant tumor.

In general, hypnotherapeutic suggestions may focus on comfort and calm, easy return of normal body functions, and rapid healing. Since many children fear death as a result either of anesthesia or of surgery, imagery concerning the immediate and long-term future is important. A sample set of hypnotherapeutic suggestions follows:

> "You know the nurses who get food for you and fix your bed. You know the doctor who will do the operation. He is helping too. I'd like to teach you a way of helping us and helping you. You can help yourself get better faster, and no one else can do that as well as you. You can learn how to help yourself faster than grown-ups can. . . . You have learned many ways to control your body. You know how to use your muscles to walk, to write, to eat, to ride a bicycle. Now you can ride a bicycle without thinking about how you do it. You taught yourself, so it became automatic. You keep many parts of your body running automatically. Your food enters blood and goes to all parts of your body. Your heart beats strongly to push that food around. You breathe in good pure oxygen that your body needs. You're doing it right now. Hardly without even thinking about it much, you just keep all those automatic systems moving smoothly and easily, the same way you ride your bicycle or the same way you write your name, You can do the same things after your operation. Your body can automatically remember nice hungry feelings, and you can enjoy your favorite foods. What is the first thing you will want to eat? And your body can remember how to feel comfortable . . . how to move and walk . . . how to relax your bowel and bladder when you need to go to the bathroom . . . how to enjoy playing with toys and games. The doctors and nurses can help you as much as you need, and you can help yourself. Soon you will be well enough to go home. What is the first thing you want to do when you get home? Good. Think about that now."

Mary was born with sacral agenesis. When she was quite young her legs—which were nonfunctional—were amputated so that the bone could be put in a bone bank, later to be harvested periodically to be used in successive orthopedic operative spine-lengthening procedures. As she would explain to others, in this way Mary could suddenly "grow" 5 to 6 inches all at once (in surgery) every couple of years. Having learned hypnotherapy for pain control when she was a young child, Mary called when she was about 13 with a special request for help. She explained that in a month or two she would be having her next spine-lengthening operation. While she was a little nervous in general, she was most concerned from previous surgery about being "so hungry" post-operatively and not being permitted to eat until her intestinal tract had "started working again" after the operation. She knew that the use of morphine for post-operative pain control contributed to slowing down her intestinal motility, and she had already decided that she'd be able to eat sooner if she had no morphine. She asked me to lobby on her behalf with her spine surgeon and the nursing staff that she not have to have morphine or codeine unless she asked for it. She asked to review hypnotherapeutic suggestions for pain control, hunger, and return of normal gastrointestinal function. She assured me, her parents, her surgeon, and the nursing staff that she would take care of her discomfort (with hypnosis), and that they should simply make sure they had some food available for her to eat! After two hypnotherapy review sessions a month apart (the second a week before surgery), Mary had an uneventful 5- to 6-hour operative lengthening of her spine. Post-operatively she used self-hypnosis and acetaminophen (Tylenol) for control of discomfort and ate supper 4 hours after her operation. She was very proud.

Although the focus is on positive suggestions, we are careful not to suggest that the child must deny appropriate feelings of anxiety, depression, or anger. In the course of therapeutic interviews, we listen carefully for evidence of these feelings in conversation, play, hypnotic fantasy, and reports of dreams. Then we help the child recognize and integrate the feelings, both in the context of supportive counseling and hypnotherapeutically.

ANESTHESIA

It is well known that patients who approach surgery with a high degree of fear and agitation require larger amounts of chemical anesthesia, thus increasing the risks of complications. Their post-operative course is also likely to be more difficult from both a surgical and a psychological perspective.

As anesthesiologists have appreciated the significance of the pre-operative psychological state in pediatric surgical patients, they have made efforts to allay fears of general anesthesia by use of such techniques as stroking, storytelling, or rubbing a pleasant scent of strawberries, perfume, or bubble gum inside the inhalation mask. Although many anesthesiologists have had no formal training in hypnosis, they may use the analogy of a space trip, talking to the child about a space mask and about breathing special air like astronauts.

Since the 1950s, there have been several reports of use of hypnosis with children as an adjunct to chemical anesthesia (Antitch, 1967; Betcher, 1960; Cullen, 1958; Daniels, 1962; Marmer, 1959; Scott, 1969; Hopayian, 1984). These reports describe several advantages of hypnotherapy and of the resulting alliance between the child and the anesthesiologist. By becoming more active participants, children cope better with the psychological trauma of surgery. They adjust more easily to the hospital environment and formulate more positive attitudes about the hospital experience. Pre-operative sedation can be reduced or omitted altogether; this is particularly valuable for children who respond to partial clouding of consciousness by becoming more agitated rather than less so. With the child in hypnosis, it is easier to induce general anesthesia, and it is often possible to reduce the amount given. Many anesthesiologists note a smoother course both during surgery and in the postoperative phase.

The techniques of hypnotic induction used by anesthesiologists vary with the age of the child. With infants and very young children, a soothing voice is sufficient even if the child does not understand the words (Cullen, 1958). Techniques reported for older children include storytelling, television games, suggestions for eye heaviness and sleep, eye fixation, and progressive relaxation.

Some anesthesiologists give suggestions for post-operative comfort and return of normal body functions during the operative procedure. Simple suggestions may encourage the child to shift from negative to positive attitudes about the healing process. For example, one might say, "The sensations you have in the area of the incision are reminders that healing is taking place in that area." These suggestions may be aided if the child has, pre-operatively, seen a drawing or diagram that explains the procedure. Some authors (e.g., Cheek, 1959) believe that anesthetized patients may hear comments in the operating room and respond accordingly to intended or unintended suggestions. Others (e.g., Trustman, Dubovsky, & Titley, 1977) have found methodological flaws in studies on this topic and have questioned the validity of the conclusions. In any case, it seems reasonable to be guided by the dictum that operating room staff members should not say anything they do not want the patient to hear.

Bensen (1971) reported the use of post-anesthetic hypnosis in surgical patients in the recovery room. This report included 30 children and adolescents post-tonsillectomy and one 11-year-old boy post-circumcision. Among 16 children, ages 5 to 12 years, only one child needed pain medication during the first day post-tonsillectomy. Of 14 older patients, ages 12 to 18 years, three required one dose of analgesic prescription a few hours post-operatively. The author pointed out the need for a reliable and accurate laboratory method to assess and measure the effectiveness of post-hypnotic suggestion.

It is unfortunate that anesthesiologists often do not continue their post-operative visits beyond the recovery room. A child can benefit from frequent reinforcement of positive suggestions following surgery. A cassette tape can be helpful in this regard, as can reinforcement by well-trained nurses or parents (Olness, 1977c).

Gaal, Goldsmith, and Needs (1980) reported a controlled pilot study of the effect of hypnotic suggestion on expressions of anxiety and pain in a group of 10 children, ages 5 to 10 years, undergoing tonsillectomy. No child had previous experience with either hospitalization or surgery. Each child met with the experimenter before surgery, at which time the experimenter answered questions truthfully and engaged in pleasant conversation designed to put the child at ease. In the 10 minutes immediately prior to surgery, the experimenter continued in the same way with the control group, asking about interests, hobbies, favorite TV programs, and so on. For the experimental group, this 10-minute period was devoted to a hypnotic induction using a television game/visual-imagery technique with suggestions for strenuous activity followed by fatigue, relaxation, and desire to sleep. After induction of anesthesia, the experimental group received tape-recorded suggestions for post-operative feelings of calm, comfort, ease of swallowing, and trust; the control group heard a tape-recorded nonsense story.

Assessment of anxiety and pain was made by independent observers who did not know to which group each child belonged. Anxiety was rated by behavioral indicators such as level of motor activity, tearfulness, verbalization of fear, and physical resistance. There were no differences between experimentals and controls prior to the pre-induction conversation; both groups were relatively calm and cooperative. After surgery was completed, the control group was significantly more anxious ($p = .05$). The experimental group was as calm as at the first measure of anxiety. Post-surgical intergroup comparisons showed the controls to be significantly more anxious and uncooperative than the experimentals ($p = .01$).

Assessment of post-operative pain was based on the children's own reports and on their needs for chemical analgesics. Both measures showed significant differences between the two groups. That is, children in the experimental group complained less frequently and of less severe pain, and they required only one-fifth as much analgesic medication as the controls. The authors planned to extend the study to include 60 children.

As we review these reports, we are not certain whether it is best to utilize hypnotic suggestions with pediatric surgical patients before, during, or after surgery or at all of these times. Further, one cannot be certain if the patient responds to deliberate positive suggestions or to the absence of negative suggestions such as "I'll bet this kid is going to vomit a lot." Controlled studies could clarify these issues.

PLASTIC SURGERY

Few articles can be found in the literature that deal specifically with the use of hypnosis in plastic surgery. There have been many reports on the value of hypnosis in conditions encountered by plastic surgeons, who are concerned (as are all surgeons) with pain and the anxiety generated by it. Studies by Wiggins and Brown (1968) and Kelsey and Barron (1958) reported on induction of a cataleptic state to aid in immobilization of the patient or of extremities during pedicle graft procedures. Scott and Holbrook (1981) used hypnosis to aid in selection of patients for cosmetic surgery. Many studies have been made on the use of hypnotherapy in treating pain, but hypnotic techniques have not been studied extensively as a routine adjunct to the use of local anesthesia.

A study by Tucker and Virnelli (1985) states that "hypnosis can usually produce effective relaxation and frequently allow actual enjoyment of the experience of undergoing a surgical procedure" (p. 141). They have used hypnosis since 1976 with both their pediatric and adult plastic surgery patients. Both formal induction and informal or indirect techniques have been employed; the latter have become part of the routine daily management of these patients. "Formal induction is used on hundreds of patients as an adjunct to local anesthesia; it has also been used to obtain hypnoanesthesia for removal of lesions without chemical anesthesia" (p. 142). Hypnosis sessions have also been found to be useful in decreasing anxiety and apprehension about an upcoming procedure.

BURNS

Children who are severely burned face multiple problems: pain, fear and depression, anorexia, insomnia, physical disability, itching, and cold. They also have to deal with significant changes in body image and with reactions from other people in the hospital and at home. These problems can interact in a vicious circle of pain, anxiety, depression, anorexia, and poor healing secondary to another circle of inadequate nutrition, more grafting, and more pain.

Bernstein (1963, 1965) and LaBaw (1973) have published anecdotal reports describing successful use of hypnotherapy for several of these problems, especially pain, anxiety, and anorexia.

Wakeman and Kaplan (1978) reported a controlled prospective study in which patients, ages 7 to 70 years, who learned hypnosis used significantly lower percentages of maximum allowable analgesics as compared to controls who received supportive psychotherapy. Among the patients who used

hypnosis, the youngest group, ages 7 to 18 years, used significantly less analgesics than did two adult groups, ages 19 to 30 and 31 to 70 years. In addition to suggestions for pain control, these patients were also given suggestions
for general ego strengthening, improved body image, and ability to cope effectively after discharge from the hospital.

In our work with burned patients, we prefer to begin hypnotherapy on
the first day of admission, before the patient has been negatively sensitized
to whirlpool therapy or debridements or is lethargic from narcotics. It is especially true with burned patients that suggestions must be individualized
and revised from day to day in order to keep pace with the child's changing
condition and perceptions. We explain our approach to other members of
the burn team and encourage them to reinforce specific hypnotic suggestions.
In addition to suggestions for symptom relief, we sometimes give suggestions
that the child can use hypnotherapy to facilitate healing directly. As yet, there
are no data to support this hypothesis, but we think it a reasonable one in
light of other indications that children can successfully use hypnotherapy for
treatment of dermatological problems (Mirvish, 1978; Tasini & Hackett,
1977) and that they can control their peripheral temperatures and, presumably, blood flow to extremities (Dikel & Olness, 1980).

The following case report is an example of our approach with burned
patients. In this case, the problem was relatively circumscribed, namely, pain
and poor cooperation during whirlpool therapy.

Tammy S., age 4, was hospitalized with second-degree burns on her
chest, sustained when a pot of coffee overturned on her at home. One week
later, she was referred for hypnotherapy to control her discomfort during
whirlpool therapy. She was a bright, active child who related well to hospital staff except at the moment of whirlpool baths.

Initially, the hypnotherapist sat by Tammy's bed and looked at drawings she had made that morning. She explained the figures in the drawings,
including a girl with a bandaged chest. That provided the entry for discussion of her burns. She seemed relieved when the therapist said her burns were
getting better every day and wondered if she had decided what she would
do first when she got home. Then the therapist said she knew Tammy did
not like whirlpool baths, and she could teach her what to do so they would
not bother her. She added that she knew Tammy could learn easily and that
she would need to practice her skills regularly. Leaving the decision to the
child, the therapist played a game with her and then left with the comment
that she would return when Tammy asked to learn these new skills. As she
walked down the hospital corridor, Tammy came running after: "When will
you teach me?" "Whenever you're ready." "Now."

In the office visit that immediately followed, trance was induced using
eye fixation on a coin. The therapist then explained about nerves, how they
carry feelings of cold, wet, warm, burning, sticky, soft, and many other feel-

ings to her head. She was then taught the switch-off technique for pain control. She seemed very pleased at the conclusion of the session. When the therapist asked if she could go with Tammy for her whirlpool therapy the next day, the child agreed. She reviewed the hypnotic procedures and turned off the "switch" for her chest until the whirlpool therapy was over. In complete contrast to the previous day, she did not struggle, kick, scream, or cry. The nurse's notes said, "She tolerated the whirlpool therapy well." On the following day, Tammy said she did not need the therapist to show her how to "turn off her switches," and she did well. On the third day, she was discharged.

In a pilot study of hypnosis and pain in patients with severe burns, Van der Does, Van Dyck, and Spijker (1988) included two adolescents in their group of eight patients. Both successfully applied self-hypnosis for pain control, finding distraction and relaxation particularly important components of their (self-) hypnotic procedure.

It is often inappropriate to use tape-recorded hypnotic suggestions for burned children in the early phases of treatment when problems are changing from day to day and even from hour to hour. However, a tape may be very useful in the later stages of treatment when the child's condition is stable and problems are more predictable, at least for a few days at a time. The following material is a typescript of a tape recording made for one of our 11-year-old burned patients several years ago when the therapist was going to be out of town for 4 days. Suggestions covered a variety of problems on which the child was then working. Wording was quite flexible as it was expected that the child might use the tape at any time of day or night, with or without other patients present. We have made no changes from the original transcript except to alter the child's name. If we were to make such a tape today, we would omit the word "try" in the suggestions, since this suggests the possibility of failure. The patient, however, reported no problems, saying she listened to the tape nine times during the therapist's absence and found it helpful in a variety of ways.

> "Hi, Sherry. This is the tape recording that I told you I would make, and while you're getting ready to listen to it, try to get yourself in as comfortable a position as you can. Just fix your bed or wherever you are so that you are as comfortable as you can be. And then just as we have done before think about the ways and the many, many times we have helped you get more and more relaxed. That's what we are going to do on this tape. We are going to think about helping you relax more and more. And we are going to think about the many positive things, the many things you can do now that you couldn't do before. How much better you are now, than you were before, knowing that you are getting better and better. You are getting well.
>
> "So try to make yourself just as comfortable as you possibly can and

just listen to my voice on this tape. You can put the earphone, the ear plugs in your ears if you like, or you can just listen without them, whichever feels more comfortable. And just try to imagine me there with you, imagine me sitting close to you. If you close your eyes and think very hard you can almost see a picture of me in your mind. You can hear my voice more and more clearly, almost as if I were really there. And it will be almost as if I am there. Even though I am away for a little while, you know I am thinking of you. You know I still want you to get well. You know how very much I like you. You and I are pretty good friends. Sometimes we can get mad at each other, but we both know that's okay, and we can still be very good friends.

"And now as you have this picture of me in your mind, more and more clear, just let your whole body begin to relax, listening to everything I say. First, think about your head relaxing and your face, beginning at the very top of your head, and your forehead relaxing, and your eyes feeling very relaxed and maybe a little heavy, and if you feel like closing your eyes, you can do that. And your whole face feeling very relaxed and very comfortable. And think of your neck feeling very relaxed and very comfortable; your neck is going to get well. You have had grafting on your neck, and it is going to get better and better. So any worries you have about it, you can just let them go, knowing it's going to get better. And your shoulders can become more and more relaxed, and your arms and hands. Put your hands in a nice comfortable position. Your right hand and left hand. And think a minute about your hands, how much better they are, how much more you can do with your hands. Opening your mail, feeding yourself, making pizza in OT. So very many things—writing; and each day there will be more and more things you can do. More and more, so that your hands can feel very comfortable now and very relaxed, and you can feel more and more good. And let those very nice feelings go down and down deeper and deeper through your whole body. And down and down through your legs, and all the way down through your feet, knowing that your legs and your feet are getting better too.

"All of you is getting well little by little. And I want you to think of that thought that you are getting better. And every time that thought begins to slip away from you, you can catch it with your mind and bring it back, bring it back. Just like we focus a camera, you can focus your mind on that idea. Focus that thought. You are getting better, more and more safe, more and more deeply relaxed, through your whole body now.

"And we know that there are times when you have some pain or some itching somewhere. And we don't like that, but we know that it is going to happen from time to time. But we also know that more and more you can control the pain and the itching, because you can let the pain or itching, whenever it begins, be like a signal for you to relax deeper and deeper down and down until comfortable feelings fill you up more and more. And there is no room left for bad feelings or scary feelings, or painful feelings. Whenever there is any pain or itching, it will be like a signal for you to focus and bring into your mind those nice relaxed feelings, immediately and completely until you are deeper and deeper relaxed, and comfortable feelings fill your whole body and your whole mind. And you know that more and more you can control any kind of feeling. Letting the scary feelings and the pain and the itching drift away, and letting the comfortable feelings fill you more and more. Fill you more and more with comfortable feelings, until there is no room left for any other kind of feelings.

"And you know that this is getting to be more and more automatic; it happens without your even thinking about it. So that more and more you are able to sleep, you are able to sleep as much as you need to. And you may find that when it's time to go to sleep at night, you just let those relaxed and comfortable feelings just come to you closer and closer. Filling you more and more, because you know you are getting better. So you will have a good night's sleep, when it's time to go to sleep. And just as you will be able to sleep as much as you need to, you will also have nice hungry feelings and enjoy the things you eat. And just as you will find that more and more you're interested in getting up and doing things. All the activities on the ward, you will like those activities more and more. Because you will be able to do them more and more. So you can sleep, you can eat, you can do all the activities, but most important, you can let yourself know you are getting better, because you deserve to get better. You're a good person, Sherry. You have worked very hard to get well.

"And we will continue to work. When I see you, we will work more, as much as you need. And you will listen to this tape, Sherry, as much as you need to, as much as you want to. It will be just up to you how much you listen to it. But when you do, you may find more and more each time that you can let yourself become very relaxed. Just as if I'm there talking to you. Feeling very safe, and very good. Knowing that if you need any medication for pain or itching, you can ask the nurses for it. But knowing that more and more you are getting to be able to control these problems yourself. And each time you listen to this tape, just as we practiced together, you will be more and more able to relax deeper and deeper. So that the pain and the itching and all the scary feelings will drift away and you will have comfortable feelings, more and more.

"Now I am going to count up to five, and as I count, you can get just as awake as you would like to. If you want to, you can get very wide awake, and then you can do whatever would be good to do. Whether it's getting up, or eating or doing some activity, or just drifting off to sleep. Whatever would be good for you to do now, you can do. You can wake up as much as you like, as much as you need to as I count to five. So that if there are activities you want to do, or things like eating, or getting up, you'll be very wide awake. But if you want to go to sleep, you can be nice and relaxed, and drift off to sleep. Even if you wake up, you can stay nice and relaxed, but you'll be wide awake. I'm going to count now, and when I get up to five, you can turn off the tape recorder, by pushing where the little square is, and that will turn off the tape recorder. Now I am going to count one . . . two . . . three . . . four . . . five . . . feeling very good, feeling very good, and I'll see you soon. Turn off the tape now."

Because burned patients have extensive practice in using hypnotherapeutic techniques, they often develop considerable confidence in their abilities. Betcher (1960) capitalized on this confidence in his work with a 10-year-old girl who had suffered third-degree burns and had used hypnosis successfully for dressing changes. Six months later, the child was readmitted for surgery in order to release severe flexion contractures of her neck that had forced the chin onto the sternum with complete inability to extend the head. Initially it was planned to do the operation under general anesthesia. However, the position of the child's head combined with the depressive effect of the chemical agent had compromised her respiration to such an extent that she rapidly became cyanotic. The surgery was canceled, and it was decided to reschedule it later using hypnosis as the major anesthetic agent until the contractures were released. Betcher (1960) gave the following account of the second surgical attempt:

Two weeks later the child was readmitted a few days before surgery. The patient and her parents were given an explanation of the method of anesthesia and since they were familiar with its use for the changing of the painful dressings during her first admission, they agreed readily. Two rehearsal sessions were performed on the days prior to surgery. Suggestions were given that her left arm was becoming numb. When the numbness was complete, she was to place it across her neck for transference of the numbness. Complete analgesia to pinprick was achieved at each session. The operation was rehearsed step by step using a blunt instrument and demonstrating how the surgeon would do the procedure. No pre-medication was given to the patient. On the operative day, the patient was again hypnotized in her room and taken to the operating room. After the patient was placed on the operating table, the hypnosis was deepened. Numbness was achieved in her left hand and was transferred to her neck.

During the preparation by the surgeon, constant reassurances were given to reinforce the numbness in the region of the neck. Although analgesia to pinprick was complete, the patient began to whimper softly at the incision of the scalpel. The face had been covered by the sterile drapes since the operative area was from the mandible to the sternum. This draping was utilized to fashion a tent over the face and an anesthetic tube was placed in this area to allow the gases to flow over her face. The analgesia proved sufficient to allow the surgeon to proceed without any objection from the child. As soon as the neck was opened wide, the anesthetic mask was attached to the tubing and was applied to the face. Total chemical anesthesia was then produced. It was simple to introduce an endotracheal tube with the head now fully extended. The surgeon then completed the necessary surgery including skin grafting in two and a half hours. Only small increments of cyclopropane anesthesia were necessary for the smooth conduct of the anesthesia. Since posthypnotic suggestions had been given, the postoperative period was completely without discomfort even though the child was placed in a plaster of Paris shell from the head to the waist. (pp. 818–819)*

DENTISTRY

Bernick (1972) reported a variety of applications of hypnotherapy in children's dentistry including (1) raising the pain threshold, (2) reducing the resistance to local anesthesia, (3) assisting in the adaptation to orthodontic appliances, (4) reduction of the gag impulse during the taking of impressions or X-rays and during general operative dentistry, (5) relieving general apprehension, (6) breaking habit patterns for thumb sucking and myofunctional problems, (7) motivating the child and parents to accept treatment and to improve oral hygiene, (8) relaxation of facial muscles, (9) control of saliva and capillary hemorrhage, (10) maintenance of patient comfort in long procedures, and (11) as a premedication for general anesthesia.

Both Bernick (1972) and Shaw (1959) emphasized the importance of using nonhypnotic suggestion to help the child perceive the dental experience in a positive way. They suggest positive and pleasant communications from parents and dental office staff, getting to know the child's interests, allowing the child to experiment with various instruments, modeling behavior, behavior shaping, and giving careful explanations at a level the child can understand.

Pediatric dental patients respond to a variety of hypnotic techniques to achieve pain control. Bernick (1972) used glove anesthesia with a 13-year-old boy who had developed a morbid fear of injections. This child used hypnosis as the sole anesthetic agent for several dental visits. In later visits, he used hypnosis to facilitate acceptance of injections of local anesthetic for more extensive work. Shaw (1959) reported his use of the "switch technique" in which the child is asked in hypnosis to turn off pain "switches" to various parts of the mouth. He also described other methods, including glove anesthesia and direct suggestions for numbness. All these methods may be used with or without additional local anesthesia, depending on the child's needs.

Neiburger (1976, 1978) reviewed patient reactions to dental prophylaxis for 150 children, ages 3 to 12 years, with and without waking suggestions that they would experience a tickling feeling and would want to laugh during the procedure. He found that the children were more cooperative when these "sensory confusion" suggestions were used than when no suggestions were given.

---

*From Betcher (1960). With permission.

Hypnotherapy has been particularly helpful in controlling bleeding in patients with hemophilia who require dental work (Lucas, 1965). The mechanism by which bleeding is controlled is not yet understood, although Lucas emphasized the factor of emotional stress.

Crasilneck and Hall (1975) used hypnotherapy to help a 10-year-old boy overcome extreme apprehension about dentistry. Therapeutic procedures included abreaction of past dental trauma and post-hypnotic suggestions for feelings of relaxation and well-being during future dental work. The boy subsequently remained calm and cooperative during several visits for extensive dental work.

Thompson (1963) reported use of hypnotherapy with a 12-year-old girl who had a hysterical fear of dentistry. Suggestions focused on this child's ability to let go of fears that belonged to earlier experiences. Thompson heightened motivation for treatment with the "three crystal balls technique" in which the child was asked to imagine her teeth (1) in their present state, (2) in the future without dental correction, and (3) in the future with dental correction. She then focused on the third image. Although the child achieved only a light hypnotic state, she did become sufficiently cooperative for dental work to be accomplished.

Recently Heitkemper, Layne, and Sullivan (1993) reported a study of 45 children 8 to 11 years old about to undergo local anesthesia and either restoration or extraction of teeth. After obtaining three measures of anxiety while children waited in the waiting room, children were randomly assigned to one of three audiotaped treatment groups: (1) "paced respiration," (2) "cognitive coping," and (3) "a placebo tape controlled for expectations and experimenter contact." In the paced respiration tape, subjects were told that the tape helps children relax and then given suggestions for imagery of walking down steps and becoming progressively relaxed while rhythmically slowing respirations to eight times per minute. In the so-called cognitive coping tape, children were told that the tape helps reduce discomfort associated with dentistry by allowing thinking different things and by imagining an injection as pressure, numbness, or tickling. In the third condition, the authors present this as a placebo control but describe yet another version of imagery and relaxation noting that the children listened to: "This story may be an interesting way to pass the time while waiting for the dentist and might help your discomfort and also may help you relax and feel more at ease in the dentist's chair." On a measure of expected discomfort, the "placebo" or story with no particular guidance for how to use positive suggestions was significantly less believable. Both treatment conditions (both hypnotherapeutic in our opinion) showed reduction of anxiety on two measures, but the children's experience of pain was not affected by either of the approaches. The authors speculate that this was a function of excellent local anesthesia which "left little pain to reduce." Although the authors do not identify their interventions as hypnotherapeutic per se, their descriptions clearly depict hypnotic suggestions. We wonder if the inclusion or addition of specific pain reduction or pain control hypnotic suggestions in one of the conditions might have provided better discrimination between the techniques described. Such distinction may be particularly important since the authors conclude that "expected discomfort may be the most important part of dental pain, so expectations might well be the focus of such treatments."

We have taught self-hypnosis to, and prepared audiotapes for, many children with dental anxiety in whom such described "expected discomfort" seemed to be the most important consideration. As in most children and circumstances, the imagery, relaxation, and pain control strategies for these children seem to be most effective when constructed and offered in the context of their individual experiences, personal style, and desired outcome.

As this brief review indicates, there has been an awareness of the positive value of hypnosis in pediatric dentistry for over 35 years. In spite of this, however, a recent survey (McKnight-Hanes, Myers, Dushku, & Davis, 1993) of dental practice reported that only 2% of general dentists and 6% of pediatric dentists said that they utilized hypnosis in their dental practices. The survey included responses from 663 general dentists and 475 pediatric dentists, a response rate of 39% to a once-mailed random survey to 3,000 dentists. By contrast, all pediatric dentists and 96% of general dentists reported using "tell–show–do" techniques and "voice control" strategies as behavioral management approaches with children. These behavioral strategies, which may well contain elements of hypnotherapeutic approaches, are not described in further detail. We speculate that in view of these dentists' awareness and acknowledgment of these other behavioral strategies, that their use of hypnotic techniques is probably higher than their self-reported 2% and 6% as noted. Nonetheless, we hope that more dentists and their assistants will seek out training in hypnotherapy for the benefit of their patients.

OPHTHALMOLOGY

Browning, Quinn, and Crasilneck (1958) compared 9 children treated with hypnotherapy for suppression amblyopia with 10 children who did not receive hypnotherapy. In hypnosis, the nine children were told that they would be able to see clearly with the amblyopic eye. Immediately following the hypnotherapy sessions, eight of the nine experimental subjects improved in near vision compared with only one of the control group who received "nonhypnotic persuasion techniques." Distance vision was unchanged in both groups. A few days following hypnotherapy, some of the experimental subjects regressed in near vision. This led the authors to question whether emotional factors might play a role in suppression amblyopia. At a 3-year follow-up (G. G. Smith, Crasilneck, & Browning, 1961), eight of the nine experimental subjects showed regression, although not always to the original prehypnotic level. A second hypnotherapy session produced improvement in near vision in six of these subjects, again suggesting a functional component in suppression amblyopia.

Look, Choy, and Kelly (1965) published a case report of a girl who had undergone unsuccessful surgery for strabismus at age 22 months. In spite of orthoptic training for several years, at age 12 the patient had no binocular fusion. Hypnotherapy was then begun. Over the next 5 months, her visual acuity without glasses became normal, and binocular fusion was developed. Orthoptic training and hypnotherapy continued regularly, and her gains were maintained over 3 years. This success suggests that long-term hypnotherapy is necessary to maintain gains as is generally true of all methods used to treat suppression amblyopia.

Williams and Singh (1976) reported use of hypnotherapy in an 8-year-old girl with hysterical amblyopia. Two hypnotherapy sessions over a 3-day period resulted in full restoration of vision with no recurrence of symptoms in 14 months of follow-up.

Olness and Gardner (1978) reported the successful use of hypnotherapy to facilitate comfortable insertion of contact lenses in a 2-year-old boy. When this patient developed bilateral cataracts, he and his mother were faced with two surgical procedures, followed by having to adjust to contact lenses in addition to glasses. The patient's mother sought anticipatory hypnotherapy for herself and her son to allow them to cooperate with each other when she inserted the contact lenses. In two sessions of hypnotherapy, the mother and child learned imagery techniques in which they associated the contact lenses with feelings of quietness, gentleness, and mastery. The boy participated in the imagery exercise and, although he sometimes engaged in anticipatory fretting, he never had to be held down. His participation in this experience allowed him the opportunity to make a positive growth experience out of a potentially traumatic situation.

Lewenstein (1978) used hypnotherapy as the sole anesthetic with two children, ages 6 and 11 years, for post-operative evaluation and adjustment of sutures placed in the extraocular muscles during strabismus operations. Accurate adjustment is possible only when the patient is fully alert and cooperative. In one child, measurement of ocular alignment in hypnosis revealed that no further adjustments were necessary after initial surgery. In the other child, examination aided by hypnosis revealed that the initial correction was inadequate; adjustment was made while the child remained in hypnosis, thus obviating the need for reoperation under general anesthesia.

NEUROSURGERY

In some neurosurgical procedures it is important to have the patient conscious and cooperative so that the surgeon can make decisions concerning ablative procedures. Crasilneck, McCranie, and Jenkins (1956) reported the use of hypnotherapy, combined only with local anesthesia in a 14-year-old girl who was having an epileptogenic focus removed from her cortex. The patient had two or three seizures daily, in spite of anticonvulsant medications, since a head injury 4½ years earlier. She underwent four hypnotherapy sessions prior to surgery before undergoing a 9-hour neurosurgical procedure. She remained cooperative and was comfortable throughout except for mild pain while the dura was separated from bone. Of special interest is the fact that she alerted from trance twice when the hippocampal region was stimulated.

ORTHOPEDICS

C. W. Jones (1977) reported the use of hypnosis as an adjunct to the anesthetic protocol in 23 children, ages 11 to 16 years, having the Harrington procedure for idiopathic scoliosis. This procedure necessitates the operative placement of one or two metal rods for correction of the spinal curve. A risk of paraplegia exists. If the patient can be awakened during the surgery to demonstrate voluntary motor ability, the surgical team can check for the complication of paralysis and achieve immediate decompression if necessary. Patients in this study were seen by the anesthesiologist on a daily basis for 1 week prior to surgery. Hypnosis was explained and induced several times. The sequence of events in the operating room was rehearsed in hypnosis, and the patients were also taught self-hypnosis for relief of post-operative symptoms, especially secondary muscle spasm. About 4 hours after the beginning of surgery, the depth of chemical anesthesia was lightened to the point where the patients could blink their eyes on command. The patients were then asked to bend their toes and ankles. If they did so easily, they were reassured and reanesthetized. Post-operatively, the pre-arranged signals for relaxation were begun as soon as the patients began to awaken. A general decrease in the need for post-operative analgesics, increased cast tolerance, and decreased nausea were observed post-operatively.

Hypnotherapy can be useful both before application of splints and casts and during the recovery period for relief of muscle spasm and for preparation for cast removal and reestablishment of normal movement. It can also be useful in the post-operative period following amputation. Two representative case histories follow.

Mark C., an obese 8-year-old boy, suffered a fractured femur while playing football in a neighborhood lot. Following operative reduction, he was placed on oral codeine for treatment of the pain associated with quadriceps spasm. Three days later, he had developed nausea as a side effect from codeine, and his frequent vomiting episodes necessitated complicated bed changes (he was in traction) and more discomfort. He had also developed constipation as a side effect of the codeine, and defecation in his bed-ridden position became exceedingly difficult. At this point, he was referred for hypnotherapy.

We asked Mark if he would be willing to make himself feel better without the medicine, and he agreed immediately. When asked what he would like to be doing rather than being in the hospital bed, he said he would like to be riding a bicycle down a hill. We asked him to imagine himself doing that, and he quickly entered a trance. We taught him the concept of nerves and central "switches" and encouraged him to find his own switches and turn them off for the area of the femur. We also gave suggestions for rapid healing and restoration of normal body functions. These suggestions were reinforced daily for 1 week. He had no further complaints, no further requirement for codeine, and was very pleased with his personal success. Following discharge we asked Mark to practice visualizing normal leg motion in walking and running in preparation for removal of his cast. Rehabilitation was accomplished rapidly, and the patient again was pleased with his participation in therapy.

Nancy S., age 11 years, developed pain in her right leg. Bone biopsy revealed a Ewing's sarcoma and amputation above the knee was performed. She was first seen by the hypnotherapist in the recovery room where suggestions were given for comfort and normal sensations of hunger. Following return to her room, she experienced no vomiting and requested only oral medication for pain. On the first post-operative day, she was somewhat depressed. She asked to be hypnotized before attempting to move from her bed to a chair. She said she wanted to imagine taking a nap at home. After the therapist assisted her with this imagery, she moved to the chair and then back to bed with only minimal discomfort. The next morning, she was markedly depressed and expressed fear of pain during a physical therapy session scheduled later in the day. She consented to using hypnotic imagery to facilitate ambulation but involved herself only half-heartedly. In physical therapy, she was markedly anxious and cooperated poorly. However, the therapist continued to give informal suggestions for easy return of ambulation. The third day Nancy was in better spirits and stood up with the aid of parallel bars. The staff gave much praise for each bit of improvement. By the fifth post-operative day, she was walking easily with crutches, clearly proud of her independence. The surgery and physical therapy staffs were very impressed with her progress. She was discharged 2 days later. This patient demonstrates the fact that significant depression and anxiety may interfere with optimal response to hypnotherapy but that, nonetheless, hypnotic suggestion may have a positive delayed effect, especially if other staff members approach the patient positively.

OTOLARYNGOLOGY

There are few reports of specific applications of hypnotherapy to otolaryngological problems in children. Edel (1959) reported the case of a severe nosebleed controlled by hypnosis (see Chapter 11), and Bensen (1971) has noted the successful use of hypnotherapy in children and adolescents following tonsillectomy. The following reports describe successful hypnotherapy used to overcome otolaryngological problems.

Susan, age 10 years, had been unable to swallow solid foods for 6 months. She had lost approximately 5 pounds. The parents and patient recognized that the problem began when the patient witnessed her grandmother choke at the dinner table. The grandmother had no untoward sequelae, but the child was frightened of swallowing solids thereafter. Results of otolaryngological evaluation were normal. We told Susan that she could learn a method to solve the problem herself if she wished. Trance was achieved via the coin induction method, and the patient appeared very comfortable while focusing on a favorite place where she could enjoy being happy, comfortable, and safe. We taught her ideomotor signals, and she was asked, while still in trance, if she would like to solve her problem of eating. When her response was immediately positive, we proceeded to ask her to recall a happy meal prior to the frightening event, to remember her favorite foods, how good they tasted, how easy it was to swallow them. When the patient seemed comfortable with this, we suggested she imagine the same menu in a future meal, enjoying eating, tasting, swallowing, knowing she was in control of swallowing, and that she had solved the problem herself. General suggestions were given for relaxation, feeling better than before, and finding it easy to review the exercise at home. The patient went home and ate her first complete dinner in 6 months without difficulty. One-year follow-up revealed no recurrences.

Charlie Y., age 24 months, had a history of chronic ear infections. During many ENT visits, he had been restrained on a mummy board for examination and treatment. Hypnotherapy was requested when his anxiety increased to the point that he began crying as soon as he walked through the clinic door. He was seen for three hypnotherapy sessions during which suggestions for comfort and ease were given as he played with toys and participated in mock ear examinations, alternately taking the role of doctor and patient. Clinic staff agreed to discontinue use of the mummy board. At the end of 3 weeks, his anxiety was markedly reduced, and he cooperated easily with subsequent ear examinations. This little boy's mother was a nurse who prompted the referral by insisting that "there had to be a better way." Many parents are not as assertive. We hope to see surgical staff members make increasing use of techniques that minimize anxiety in their young patients. We also hope to see decreasing use of such methods as mummy boards, which are bound to increase anxiety.

Recently Kohen (1994) reported the use of hypnosis by an adolescent with cystic fibrosis (CF) who had developed the common complication of nasal polyps. Laura, a 16-year-old young woman with relatively minor lung disease did not have lung problems from her CF until she was 11 or 12 years old. She was referred by her mother, a clinical psychologist who had recently attended a hypnosis workshop and had asked if hypnosis might help her daughter with "mild CF with tremendous anxiety about needles." She was quite confident that the techniques *she* had just learned would be useful for her daughter and equally certain that she was *not* the right one to teach her daughter hypnosis. We agreed.

At the first visit Laura presented as a bright, engaging young woman excited about the potential for hypnosis to help her. Her clear focus was her needle phobia, heightened by the prospect of forthcoming surgery to remove nasal polyps. Almost as an afterthought, she wondered if it was possible to "get rid of the polyps with hypnosis." Clearly well "programmed" by her mother's positive expectations, Laura told me "I think hypnosis might help with my health. I think it's like someone talks to you and you take in information while you are relaxed, and you feel more relaxed and then you help yourself." We agreed she would learn hypnosis at the second visit, at which time we reviewed a videotape of other teen-agers learning and talking about hypnosis. A decision had been made to have her nasal polyps removed in 4 weeks. Laura's mother wondered if I believed hypnosis could help make the polyps shrink or disappear, and I said I thought that was possible, but not predictable. Multisensory imagery and progressive relaxation served to intensify a trance that was initiated easily with favorite place imagery. Self-hypnosis was taught, and she agreed to practice 10 to 15 minutes twice a day. At a subsequent visit she explained to a pediatric resident:

> I'm here to get rid of my polyps that used to be there and to use hypnosis to not be afraid of IVs anymore. . . . I do hypnosis while I'm sleeping. I start with a tape, then I fall asleep, and I also do it two times a day myself in the daytime. First you go to an area where you're comfortable, then sit down and then shut your eyes, and go where you wanna be in your imagination—. . . sit wherever you like and relax, slowly but surely, your whole body and then put a message in the corner of your mind, whatever you want to give yourself, in my mind my dog eats my polyps. . . .

At the third visit specific suggestions were added to enjoy breathing, and "switch" imagery was taught for pain control.

Laura returned for her third hypnosis session 5 days before scheduled surgery. She shared her intuition that the "polyps are gone"; but her doctor declined to do a follow-up CT scan before surgery. Five days later, the patient's mother called to tell me that the ENT surgeon had found "no polyps at surgery for the first time ever" (though they had been there on X-ray before treatment with hypnosis). Two weeks after the scheduled surgery, at the fifth visit, she told me the ENT doctor reported that what had previously been polyps large enough "to hang down forward, out of the nose" were now "hardly only little buds"; he had observed marked regression "for reasons not very clear to him. . . . " I asked Laura if she would write down her ideas about what had occurred as well as a description of the imagery she had used in hypnosis:

> As you've already heard, the polyps in my sinuses were almost totally gone! There were just a few buds. Unfortunately, I still had the surgery, due to the X-ray show[ing] that my sinuses were totally occluded. It wasn't until Dr. B_____ performed the surgery that it was found otherwise. The last few hypnosis sessions I gave myself before my surgery were unreal. As I have been having my dog Spanky, a Blue and Gold macaw, and a Bangle [sic] Tiger eat my polyps, a rush of brown stuff like a river came rushing threw [sic] my sinuses! This is I think when my polyps were pretty much abolished! I then was doing my hypnosis with the same animals as before, and all of a sudden the entire jungle was in my sinuses eating the polyps. Then all the jungle animals rushed down into my lungs and started eating. And [a] rush of brown came again threw [sic] my sinuses! I was in shock along with my Mom! Thank-you.

A subsequent conversation with a CF expert (W. Warwick, personal communication, 1994) indicated the likelihood of spontaneous regression of nasal polyps to be "next to zero."

UROLOGY

Hinman and Baumann (1976) have reported the use of suggestion and hypnotherapy in seven of eight boys with complications after corrective surgical procedures for dysfunction of the voiding mechanism. Four of these patients improved. It was pointed out that operation or reoperation in five of these children might have been unnecessary if bladder coordination had been established earlier.

These patients had been referred to the urologist because of incontinence, recurrent infections of the urinary tract, or both. Two children had posterior urethral valves, one had an imperforate anus, three had bilateral reflux without demonstrable anatomical abnormality in the lower tract, and two had large bladders with upper tract changes. All patients were diagnosed as having voiding incoordination on a psychological basis. The authors pointed out the hazards of complex urological procedures, such as reimplantation of ureters, if the problem of bladder incoordination is not solved. In the case of these patients, hypnotherapy was associated with achievement of bladder coordination as demonstrated by urodynamic assessment.

CONCLUSIONS

Hypnotherapy can be a useful adjunct in many surgical situations and can often be used as the sole anesthetic for minor surgical procedures. Children who use hypnotherapy successfully can be more cooperative with surgical care and may experience fewer complications and more rapid recovery.

CHAPTER THIRTEEN

Hypnotherapy for Grief and Mourning and with the Terminally Ill Child

Reports of hypnotherapy with terminally ill patients have focused on three areas: (1) modification of pain, anxiety, and other symptoms and by-products of the disease and its treatment; (2) modification of the disease process itself; and (3) modification of the patient's ability to respond with mastery in the dying process.

We will review published reports and our own clinical experience with children in these areas and in the more general area of grief and bereavement management. To illustrate the ways in which hypnotherapy can facilitate mastery, integration, and even creativity in the dying child and his family, we also reprint portions of the previously published report of David, a 12-year-old boy who died of leukemia on Christmas day (Gardner, 1976b).*

CHILDHOOD GRIEF AND MOURNING: APPLICATIONS OF HYPNOTHERAPY

Much has been learned and written about the process of grief and bereavement in children since Kübler-Ross first described the stages of grief and the mourning process in 1969 (Kübler-Ross, 1969, 1974). To even note the

---

*Although many of our examples concern children who die of leukemia, it is important to remember that about 70% of children with leukemia now achieve full recovery from their disease. The outlook for childhood leukemia has improved considerably since 1960.

myriad of references available for parents, clinicians, and especially for children to help with the navigation of the grief and bereavement process is well beyond the scope of this book. We refer, therefore, to some of our favorite books and stories that have been helpful to children and families (Grollman, 1991; Miles, 1971; Viorst, 1971; White, 1952).

It seems clear that grief in its many forms is ubiquitous; and, therefore, that child health clinicians must be mindful of when to consider that a diagnosis of grief (bereavement) response may be appropriate in a child or adolescent. Any change in a child's behavior may be a reflection of the sadness, anger, helplessness, fear (of the future, of his or her own safety), sense of responsibility (guilt), or confusion the child feels over some loss, whether that loss represents the death of a loved one, or the symbolic, and almost equally profound loss felt in the common experiences of divorce of parents, death of a pet, move to a new home (and/or school), move of a best friend, loss or disappointment of an expected outcome.

In the experience of their grief, children, like adults, respond in a highly individualized fashion, as well as according to their level of development and concomitant degree of understanding of death. Their reactions are also to some degree, but not always, reflections of the way in which those in their lives and families experience grief. Symptoms, therefore, may include:

- Somatic complaints (headache, abdominal pain, limb pain, vomiting, recurrence or exacerbation of existing problems, e.g., enuresis, encopresis, asthma, etc.)
- Sleep disturbances (inability or fear of going to sleep, nightmares, trouble staying asleep, exacerbation of existing parasomnias such as night terrors, sleepwalking)
- Eating disturbances (increase or decrease in appetite, exacerbation of existing problems)
- Disruptive behaviors (tantrums, oppositional behavior, angry outbursts)
- Sad behaviors (withdrawal, weepiness, etc.)
- School problems (disinterest, school refusal, avoidance or phobia, deterioration in performance)
- Anxiety (increase in separation anxiety, performance anxiety, etc.)
- Habit problems (e.g., development or exacerbation of tics or twitches, other habits)

Approaches That Work

In the context of rapport and review of the history, clinicians must acknowledge and validate the helplessness, emptiness, anger, and whatever other feelings are expressed in order to help the child and family begin to themselves acknowledge, and then move toward understanding, the nature of their grief and bereavement, particularly as a process extending over time. This allows for the setting of a tone in which one can offer and teach strategies both to children and their families that they may use to help themselves in accepting the sadness and associated feelings, as well as the intensity of those feelings—however normal such feelings are.

Naturalistic Uses of Hypnotic Language and Hypnotherapeutic Strategies Work Well

Not unlike children or adults in an emergency situation (see Chapter 12) people who are grieving, and especially in the early, acute stages of grief and mourning, are often in a spontaneously altered state of awareness, a spontaneous hypnotic trance, narrowly focused on the loved one (or other loss) who is gone, and/or on their own sadness, worry, aloneness, and confusion. Also as with patients in emergencies with acute, severe pain, the spontaneous trance of acute grief is, in a sense, a "negative" trance as it commonly is narrowly focused and cycling negatively on the feelings of sadness, helplessness, self-recriminations, and, in turn, on the anticipated continued sense of sadness, loneliness, and helplessness. Awareness of these states as analogous to spontaneous trance behavior will allow the clinician to not only observe other characteristics of trance in children who are grieving—such as spontaneous regression—but also to approach helping such children through the application of hypnotherapeutic suggestions and self-hypnosis strategies.

We find it useful to invite the patient to talk about how his or her grief is experienced now as compared to when the loss occurred. Such inquiry is framed hypnotically to convey the expectancy that, in fact, the grief feelings *now* are not quite the same as they were *then,* even if the *then* is very recent. This sets the tone, and implies that in a future *now* (e.g., next week, next month), further change, comfort, acclimation, accommodation can and will come. This approach seems to be effective both to normalize and validate grief, and to begin to move from that posture to one that is better, easier, and ultimately healthier as needed. This naturalistic, hypnotherapeutic communication is often easily accomplished by following M. H. Erickson's (1958b) dictum to "follow the child." Such "joining" may occur by saying something like "What have you noticed about how you have been feeling since your [friend, grandmother, brother, uncle, cousin] died?" Hypnotic characteristics of such an inquiry include the compliment to the patient that the therapist believes that she or he has been able to *notice* feelings and the expectancy and comfort in the invitation to share those feelings.

Recognition of the spontaneous hypnotic state might allow for simple history taking to take place through invitations for spontaneous "waking" hypnotic regression; for example, "Would you tell me about the funeral please—where was it, what was it like, what was going through your mind during that time? Just take yourself back there *now* . . . that's right . . . just be there for a few moments and take a look at how you are." With the expression, or revivification of the affect of the moment, the therapist can, again, offer suggestions for progress through implication; for example, "And, since then, notice now how things have *changed?*" Such invitations for reframing help people to acknowledge that, as awful as they feel, things are, in fact, moving forward, and they are coping okay. If they happen to be "stuck" and do not feel as though they are moving forward, the hypnotic strategy of future projection may be useful. Thus:

> "*Now,* take a look in your mind a month or two or three into the future, see a calendar in the side of your inner mind . . . notice when it is . . . that's good . . . and notice how things are starting to be different, and to improve, I don't know how much, maybe a lot, or a little, or in between, but you can *notice,* and the more you notice it the way it can be, then it will, when you're ready, because you can create it this way using the strength of your inner mind and memories."

As noted, integration of education and information about the normalcy, length, and see–saw nature of the bereavement process with hypnotherapeutic approaches and suggestions will often serve the child and family very well. These also set the tone for offering additional suggestions about how to cope even more with time.

It may be useful to invite the grieving child or adolescent, in his or her spontaneous trance behavior, to consider "What can you say to that person right now in your imagination—because you know he (she) will always be with you within your mind . . . and you can talk to him (her) right now?" The therapist can help the patient protect his or her privacy and reinforce the patient's sense of control by adding a permissive suggestion to choose to keep these images confidential. Thus:

> " . . . and you can have a conversation *now* in your inside mind . . . take your time . . . hear yourself and hear them . . . as long and as short as you need . . . and *notice* the feelings . . . and you can tell me what you *noticed* in this conversation, or you can keep it private because you know you are *in charge* of your imagination. . . . "

In addition to the ego strengthening presented, this is another way of offering "permission" for people to do what they may have already been doing in their mind and may even have been thinking was wrong, bad, morbid, or confusing. As such, what had been potentially a disturbing, confusing, or recurrent thought, can be reframed in this manner as something that is not only normal but also useful and "a good way that you are taking care of yourself, and allowing yourself to remember _____ the way you want."

Shifting the same concept to focus on future orientation, the therapist might then add that "it's good to know that you can *always* talk to grandma [or whoever has died] in your imagination this way—because you know her so well and you both love each other [present tense] so much you'll probably even be able to hear her voice and her love in your inner mind when you do it this way. That's really a good thing to know."

Sometimes children or adolescents may get caught in "I can't get _____ out of my mind" and confused by the ambivalence of wanting the images of the person to stay and yet wanting the sadness and helplessness to go away. Direct permission to have both of these feelings and some guidelines for how to do that hypnotically may be useful; for example:

> "Each hour [or 2 hours or 4 hours, or bedtime] it would really be good to *really picture* _____ in your mind for about—how long do *you* think would be good?—1 or 5 or 10 minutes, and *when* you do that, really enjoy reviewing a conversation you had, a place you went, something you did together, and just notice all the wonderful things about them and you and that time—the sounds, the smells, the tastes, feelings—and then, before it's over for this time [this puts definitive closure on it hypnotically], remind him/her and yourself that you'll be together again in your mind again tomorrow [or in a few hours, etc.] at the same time, for a similar or different and special time together in your mind. As time goes on you may both discover that you want to have more time in between such connections, but for, now every _____ is just right. . . . "

Recently a 13-year-old boy, Jay L., was referred to one of us (DPK) by a family therapist for medical evaluation and hypnotherapy for the problem of "panic attacks" that had been occurring nightly for 4 months, beginning the night before school began in the fall (Kohen, 1995a). As the history unfolded at the first visit, a sad story of multiple grief experiences was revealed. The family had recently moved to the city from their home of many years, 4 hours away. Jay was angry and sad about leaving his home and especially missed his friends. The added stress of starting a new school seemed at first to explain the timing of the "panic attacks." A closer examination of the symptoms, however, indicated that the "panic attacks" were occurring as he was "awakening" with these "spells" within an hour of going to sleep, "in a panic," confused, running around angrily and frightened, and with subsequent amnesia. A more likely diagnosis seemed to be night-terror disorder with the stress of change, grief, and loss seemingly a trigger to the night-terror behavior. (See also Chapter 7.) It was then noted in the history that the reason for moving was for the family to be able to be physically closer to Jay's father who had recently completed a prison term for sexually abusing Jay's step-sister, and was now completing his therapy living in a group home in the city. Jay's sense of loss of—and ambivalence toward—his father, and loss of his sister (now out of the home), were obvious. These added to the rapidly growing list of reasons for Jay to be grieving.

With three-quarters of the first hour visit gone, Jay's mother abruptly became sad, and explained, through emerging tears, that Jay had been very close with his maternal grandmother who had died 5 years before and that he missed her very much. As Jay's mother spoke of this, Jay too began to cry quietly; and his father noted that Jay always preferred to stay in the car when they visited the grandmother's grave. Jay's spontaneous trance behavior was evident, with stillness in his chair, slowing of his respiratory rate, tears, and a "far away" look in his eyes. Acknowledging his sadness and his love for his grandmother, I asked him if he had a picture of her. He said he did not. At my request the mother agreed to give Jay a picture of his grandmother that day. When Jay returned for follow-up 5 days later, he reported, and his family confirmed, that the nightly "panic attacks"/night terrors had abruptly stopped the night after our first visit. Again in a spontaneous trance, Jay observed curiously, "Isn't it odd that my panicky stuff stopped the very same night I got my picture of grandma?" Jay's grief therapy, with hypnotherapy as one integral component, is continuing.

THE USES OF HYPNOTHERAPY WITH DYING CHILDREN

It is virtually impossible to be certain that hypnotherapy per se is the source of positive clinical results. However, especially in cases of dying children, it has often been demonstrated that ordinary forms of reassurance and counseling, medications, and other traditional therapies have failed. Therefore, even in the complete absence of controlled studies, and usually in the absence of any formal measures of ability to enter the hypnotic state, we are inclined to believe that hypnotherapy is indeed valuable for many who suffer terminal illness.

Modification of Symptoms and By-Products of the Disease and Treatment

Reports from several centers agree that hypnotherapy can be valuable—sometimes in dramatic ways—for a vast array of physical and psychological problems that arise in children with terminal illness (LeBaron & Zeltzer, 1985b; Olness & Hall, 1985; Olness & Singher, 1989; Reaney, 1994).

Crasilneck and Hall (1973, 1975) described their work with two boys, 4 and 8 years old, one with inoperable brain cancer and the other with leukemia. The specific problems treated included severe pain, poor tolerance of medical procedures, generalized anxiety, fear of dying, depression, insomnia, anorexia, and behavioral difficulties. Each of the boys went into deep hypnosis and responded very well to direct suggestions for symptom relief after one session. The younger boy was seen daily the first month, then three times weekly until his death the first week of the third month of hypnotherapy. The older child achieved rapid remission of his leukemia and was to be seen when necessary for further hypnotherapy. At the time of the report, this boy was successfully using self-hypnosis for therapeutic procedures. O'Connell (1985) described the use of hypnosis in several cases of terminal illness in which patients were taught self-hypnosis to ease pain and remain able to function with minds unclouded by medication. The hypnotic state was described as "a natural state, similar if not identical to the mental state of artists during creative periods and students during boring lectures" (p. 122).

Anecdotal reports of this kind are now common, as hypnotherapy becomes widely used with children who have cancer. Three research studies have reported results for a series of patients, both adding to our understanding and bringing out some of the complex issues not yet understood in the area of symptom relief.

LaBaw, Holton, Tewell, and Eccles (1975) utilized adjunctive hypnotherapy, in both group and individual sessions, with 27 pediatric cancer patients, ages 4 to 20 years. In addition to the specific problems treated by Crasilneck and Hall (1975), this study reported successful modification of nosebleeds and of vomiting associated with chemotherapy. The results were presented in the form of brief clinical vignettes for 12 of the children, said to be representative of the group as a whole. Based on these 12 descriptions, we have classified the response to hypnotherapy as follows—none or minimal: three; moderate: three; good: six. The authors did not draw conclusions as to which types of symptoms were most amenable to treatment. In this small group of 12, successful response to hypnotherapy did not appear to be clearly related to age or sex, though there was a tendency for girls to respond better than boys (Table 13.1).

The authors noted that reasons for difficulty in using hypnosis and/or self-hypnosis included excessive dependency needs, extreme anxiety or pain, defensive passivity, and lack of parental support.

J. R. Hilgard and Morgan (1978) reported their use of hypnotherapy for modification of specific problems—chiefly pain and anxiety—in 34 pediatric cancer patients, ages 4 to 19 years. Seven other children were offered hypnotherapy but refused this treatment modality. The children's ability to use hypnotherapy for symptom relief was associated with age, score on the

TABLE 13.1.   **Response to Hypnotherapy by Sex and Age**

Age (years)	Minimal		Moderate		Good	
	M	F	M	F	M	F
5–6	1	–	1	–	–	–
7–8	–	–	–	–	2	–
9–10	1	–	1	1	–	1
11–12	–	–	–	–	–	–
13–14	1	–	–	–	1	–
15–18	–	–	–	–	–	–
19–20	–	–	–	–	–	2
Total	3	0	2	1	3	3

Note. Adapted from LaBaw et al. (1975).

Stanford Hypnotic Clinical Scale for Children (SHCS-C), anxiety level, and the nature of the problem. The data are summarized in Table 13.2.

Olness (1981b) taught self-hypnosis for symptom relief to 21 pediatric cancer patients from a group of 25 consecutive referrals; three children and one set of parents refused this treatment modality. The age range at referral was 3 to 18 years. Symptom relief was defined as a reduction in pain associated with procedures, such as intravenous injections, spinal taps, and

TABLE 13.2.   **Response to Hypnotherapy for 34 Pediatric Cancer Patients**

Problem	Age range (years)	Number of patients	Degree of symptom relief[a]	
			Poor or partial	Substantial or excellent
Ancillary symptoms[b]	14–19	10	2(2)	8(2)
Poor tolerance of short procedures[c]	9–16	5	1	4
Continuous pain	13–19	3	3(1)	0
Poor tolerance of bone marrow aspirates or lumbar punctures[d, e]	7–13	6	2	4
Totals		34	18	16

Note. Adapted from J. R. Hilgard and Morgan (1978).

[a]The numbers in parenthesis refer to the number in each group obtaining a low score on the Stanford Hypnotic Clinical Scale for Children. For these subjects, significant symptom relief cannot be attributed to the use of hypnosis and is probably related to anxiety reduction by other means.

[b]Includes diffuse anxiety reactions, depression, insomnia, nausea, and high blood pressure.

[c]Includes intravenous injections and bandage changes; does not include bone marrow aspirates and lumbar punctures.

[d]Data grouped separately for younger and older children.

[e]Children in this group manifested the most severe anxiety.

bone marrow aspirates, and/or a reduction in anorexia, nausea, or vomiting associated with radiation or chemotherapy. Specific indicators of improvement included reduction in analgesic or antinausea medication.

Of the 21 patients taught self-hypnosis, 12 were referred at the time of initial diagnosis. These 12 all demonstrated substantial symptom relief. Of the nine patients first trained during relapse, seven demonstrated substantial symptom relief. Of the other two, a 3-year-old had only one practice session, and a 4-year-old was referred on the day of his death. Children who practiced most regularly obtained the most consistent relief. Benefits accrued about equally to both younger (5 to 11) and older (12 to 18) children, but the younger children achieved symptom control more quickly, in an average of two sessions as compared to four sessions for the older children.

It is difficult to make meaningful comparison of these three studies. In the first two, about half of the patients achieved significant symptom relief following hypnotherapy; in Olness's study, the success rate was 90%. In the LaBaw et al. study (1975), girls seemed to fare better than boys; the other two studies did not report sex differences. Hilgard and Morgan found that children 4 to 6 years old responded poorly as compared to older children; Olness found no such difference. Hilgard and Morgan noted that the younger children had the most severe anxiety about major medical procedures, a finding similar to that of Katz, Kellerman, and Siegel (1980). It is not clear whether Olness treated anxiety in her young patients differently or whether they were less anxious. Hilgard and Morgan found different success rates according to the nature of the problem; Olness's report does not permit this kind of comparison. Olness stressed the value of regular practice and early referral; the other studies did not comment on these issues. In two studies, the patients were trained from the beginning to use self-hypnotic techniques; Hilgard and Morgan encouraged self-hypnosis but apparently not to the same extent. Only Hilgard and Morgan used any formal measure of ability to achieve hypnosis and found two patients whose low scores on the SHCS-C suggested that their symptom improvement was due to factors other than hypnosis; we do not know how many similar cases were included in the other studies.

In all three studies, we do not know whether or how the results are related to the fact that the patients all suffered from cancer. Would the results be different for children suffering chronic illnesses that are not life threatening? Or, are these data representative of pediatric patients as a whole? In short, we are unable to explain the available data in any truly satisfactory way. Now that three independent studies have demonstrated the possibility of moving from anecdotal reports to studies including a series of patients, we urge researchers to move a step further to controlled clinical trials in which identical research protocols are used simultaneously at several medical centers.

Modification of the Disease Process

The idea that physiological and psychological processes are intertwined goes back many centuries. More recently, there have been reports of the association of psychological factors with a variety of children's diseases, including cancer (W. A. Greene & Miller, 1958; T. J. Jacobs & Charles, 1980). Since these are retrospective studies, the data are very difficult to interpret. For example, T. J. Jacobs and Charles (1980) emphasized that their review of life-stress events for children with cancer and with other illnesses must be interpreted only as contextual and not as causal. They also noted that a given event, such as parental divorce or change of residence might be very stressful for one child, whereas it might have little impact on another. Other important variables cited included the availability of social supports and the child's habitual coping skills. None of these factors has been adequately studied.

Although we agree with the T. J. Jacobs and Charles (1980) conclusion that the role of psychological factors as antecedents of childhood cancer remains a matter of conjecture, we also agree with their conclusion that there is a possibility that childhood cancer is a psychobiological phenomenon.

If psychological factors play a role in the development of cancer, then it is conceivable that psychological treatment might also affect the course and ultimate outcome of the disease. Recently, there has been a great deal of interest, especially in the press, in the possibility of using certain imagery techniques—which we would put in the general category of self-hypnosis— to affect the course of potentially terminal disease, especially cancer. Basically, the technique consists of asking a patient to visualize some process in which cancer cells are destroyed and to focus on images of physical health and general well-being. The process is both appealing and benign to cancer patients, and some who have used it have gone on to make a good recovery from their disease, with the aid of more traditional forms of treatment. The data consist mainly of anecdotal reports, and there exist no reports of prospective studies documenting causal relationships between these imagery techniques and positive therapeutic outcomes. Yet, despite the lack of any supporting scientific data, desperate cancer patients are increasingly asking their physicians for treatment by imagery techniques. These requests come not only from adult patients but also from pediatric cancer patients and their families.

We respond to requests for imagery therapy in the same way we respond to requests for other experimental forms of treatment. We tell our patients the nature of the available data, noting that, while there is also no good evidence that the method can affect the course of cancer, there is also no good evidence that it cannot do so. We say that the treatment has no known harmful effects, provided patients continue with other prescribed treatment such as radiation or chemotherapy. Further, although the treatment may have no effect on tumor growth, its use may have benefit in other ways. Patients who focus on positive ideation may become more hopeful, more motivated to get adequate nourishment and exercise, and more able to relax and get adequate rest. In such instances, patients can improve the quality of their lives even in the face of continued tumor growth.

For these reasons, we have both provided imagery therapy to patients who requested it and who continued to show interest after hearing our cautionary remarks. Some have died; others continue to use the method with enthusiasm. Until further data are available, we will continue to use imagery with patients who request it, always in the context of scientific integrity and modesty.

An example of the imagery method to combat cancer is cited from Olness's (1981b) report of her work with cancer patients. A 13-year-old boy described his cancer cells as black knights lined up for attack, but smaller, weaker, and fewer in number than his healthy, white blood cells, depicted as white knights. The white knights continually chop up the black knights with daggers. The drugs are vicious beasts who support the white knights in their attack. This patient thought about his imagery several times daily for 6 years. He is alive and well 15 years later.

Another of our patients was a 17-year-old boy who requested imagery therapy 4 years after losing an arm to cancer. He was well for 3 years after diagnosis and had achieved national ranking as a disabled downhill skier. When he then developed multiple lung metastases, he underwent vigorous chemotherapy; he began imagery therapy several months later. He visualized himself in a downhill slalom race, increasing his feelings of love, safety, strength, health, and competence as he passed each flag on the course. Then he visualized feelings of physical, mental, and spiritual well-being held tightly in his hand and absorbed into his entire body. He enthusiastically practiced these and related techniques at least twice daily. His metastases disappeared, but he later suffered another relapse. He died about 1 year after beginning imagery therapy, having survived more than 5 years since initial diagnosis.

Modification of Patient's Ability to Respond with Mastery in the Dying Process

There comes a time in the lives of some terminally ill children when it is clear to them that they will inevitably die as a result of their disease. The possibility and even the probability of dying have been stated directly by several of our young patients. One 4-year-old leukemic boy said to his therapist, "Leukemia is a bad disease and you could die from it. [Die?] Yes, you just lie there and never wake up and you can't do anything any more and then you are just bones." Another 4-year-old boy, who was losing his life-long battle against chronic granulomatous disease, said simply to his mother, "Mommy, I'm going to die."

Although denial is a common and frequently adaptive defense mechanism for children with life-threatening illness, as well as for their families and their doctors (LaBaw et al., 1975), it is also true that most of these children have quite an accurate understanding of their chances for survival. Families and doctors — more often than they would like to admit — are tempted to impose their own need for denial on the child, creating a maladaptive conspiracy of silence in which the child must bear the burden of dying alone. For example, a 12-year-old girl with a recently diagnosed inoperable brainstem tumor told her psychologist that she knew she would eventually die. When asked if she had talked about dying with her parents, she replied, "Oh no, it would upset them too much!"

Gardner (1977b) outlined four basic rights of dying children. First is the right to know the truth about the probable outcome of their illness. Actually, since most children have already figured it out for themselves, it would be more accurate to say affirm the truth rather than to imply that these children are learning it for the first time. Second is the right to share thoughts about dying — not just the probability of death, but the many questions that follow. Does it hurt to die? Are your parents with you when they bury you? What do you wear when you get buried? If they bury you down in the ground, how do you get up to heaven? Third is the right to live as full and normal a life as possible, truly to live until they die. Fourth is the right to participate in the process of dying, to have input concerning whether treatment should be continued or stopped, to state a preference for dying in the hospital or at home, and so on. Not all children choose to exercise these rights, but we believe the option of choosing should be available to them.

We have found that hypnotherapy can sometimes facilitate the process in which dying children exercise their rights. The mechanisms are occasionally direct: that is, interviewing the dying child in hypnosis concerning his or her problems. Much more often, hypnotherapy facilitates these goals indirectly. In such cases, the terminally ill child is usually first referred for hypnotherapy for some sort of specific symptomatic relief. A positive transference develops between the child and the therapist. In the context of a safe and trusting alliance, the child becomes more able to exercise his or her rights, usually with full parental support. After achieving initial symptom relief with the aid of hypnotherapy, much of the work toward the larger goals of solving problems rather than enduring them may be done in the waking state, with hypnotherapy used adjunctively as needed. Several case vignettes illustrate these direct and indirect processes.

D. M. Markowitz (personal communication, 1980) described to us his hypnotherapeutic work with an intelligent adolescent boy, on the day of his death from leukemia. In a waking interview the previous day, the boy had said he wanted to "write a will." That is, he wanted to state what he would like done with some of his personal belongings, and he wanted to give some advice to his parents concerning how they should deal with their lives after his death. Unfortunately, he went into a coma before making the will. The following day, the therapist went to the boy's home, where he lay unconscious, and repeated a hypnotic induction that he had used successfully on earlier occasions. He reminded the boy of his previously stated wish and told him that, if making a will was still important to him, he could become more alert, open his eyes and dictate his thoughts to the therapist. In 90 seconds, the boy opened his eyes, and he then dictated to the therapist for nearly 2 hours, giving his skis to his father, his guitar to his sister, and so on. He then talked with his family for another 45 minutes, following which he relapsed into coma and died 3 hours later.

Becky S. was a 7-year-old girl in the end stages of cystic fibrosis, who was initially referred to us for hypnotherapy to improve her tolerance of painful medical procedures such as fingersticks and tests of arterial blood gases. She achieved better pain control after one hypnotherapy session and proudly told the therapist the next day that she had pricked her own finger. Some weeks later, during her terminal hospitalization, she complained to the therapist of diffuse anxiety, dizziness, and double vision. Recognizing the symptoms of hypoxia, and noting the results of a recent blood-gas evaluation, the therapist asked the ward nurse whether the child could be given higher levels of oxygen. The nurse replied that the child was getting maximal oxygen through the nasal prongs she was using. She could get additional oxygen if she would use an oxygen mask instead of the nasal prongs, but she had refused suggestions from nurses and doctors that she wear a mask, apparently because she was afraid to have her face covered. The therapist returned to Becky's room and offered the same explanation and suggestion previously given by others. Becky immediately accepted the mask. The increased oxygen eliminated her hypoxic symptoms and allowed her to spend the evening cheerfully talking and playing with her family. It seemed that the context of the hypnotherapeutic relationship allowed this child to make more constructive decisions about her own treatment.

LaClave and Blix (1989) described a case history of a 6-year-old girl with malignant astrocytoma who had severe vomiting. Hypnotherapy was successful in resolving the vomiting, thus allowing chemotherapy to continue; and hypnotherapy was also utilized for pain and anxiety. In spite of significant neurological problems, the patient used audiotapes of hypnotherapy sessions and was able to use visual imagery very effectively to create drawings reflecting her awareness and acceptance of dying. She used hypnotherapy tapes effectively until she lapsed into a coma and later died.

Reaney (1994) described the inspiring story of Tommy, a young boy with immune deficiency and an overwhelming fungal infection, and the creative applications of hypnotherapeutic techniques he and his family learned and used to ease their experience of Tommy's dying. Kinesthetic hypnotherapeutic images were especially important for Tommy. His favorite was the flying "home-bed" that allowed him to dissociate from the intensive care unit, and to provide safety and reduce anxiety that had increased as illness led to blindness in the last weeks of life. In addition to teaching pain and anxiety control with "switches" imagery and rocking, the therapist integrated his own and the family's strong spiritual and religious beliefs into hypnotherapy, by preparing audiotapes of personalized spiritual songs and hymns for Tommy. This sensitive and creative use of auditory imagery was a source of comfort and strength for Tommy and his family before, during, and after his death.

Joanne, 17 years old, was in end-stage respiratory failure from cystic fibrosis when her family arranged the trip to Europe that she had always wanted. Though the trip was shortened by increasing respiratory difficulty, she was able to enjoy more than a week of sightseeing that she and her family thought was exhilarating. When the trip was cut short, she was immediately rehospitalized. Within a few days she expressed the decision that she have no further treatment and was ready to die. Even though some members of the health care team thought she might benefit from "resting" on a ventilator for a few days, she declined, and her family respected her wishes. She did not wish to suffer, however, and, though we had never previously met her, we were asked to consult to see if hypnosis could help her relax during her last days and hours.

When I (DPK) came to see her, the room was dark except for slight backlighting at the head of Joanne's bed. Her sister and mother sat quietly in chairs at the side and foot of the bed, reading. When I introduced myself, they indicated they knew I'd be coming and said that I should just proceed as though they weren't there. As I approached the right side of Joanne's bed, she seemed oblivious to me as she lay motionless in her bed, severely air hungry with an oxygen hood over her head, face puffy and with an expression that exuded stress, fatigue, sadness, and helplessness. I touched her right hand gently as I said her name and told her mine. She turned so she could see me and opened her eyes. I asked if she knew I was coming, and she said she did. Her shortness of breath permitted no more than two or three words per breath. I told her that I needed to know one or two things and that after that she didn't need to talk except in her imagination, and I would do the talking. She smiled. I told her I heard she'd just been to Europe. At first she smiled and said yes, and then tears appeared as she told me the trip had

had to be cut short. This was quickly reframed to at once acknowledge that and to shift to asking what had been her favorite part of the trip. Slowly she told me of the beauty of the mountains of Switzerland. Recognizing her spontaneous state of hypnosis, I asked her if it would be okay to just be there in Switzerland and not be here. She smiled and closed her eyes. Multisensory imagery suggestions were offered to deepen the trance, and suggestions were given for being able to be totally there, knowing that everything here was being taken care of by her doctors and nurses and family and friends. Assurances of safety and comfort and not being alone were given as she was given explicit suggestions to be there as long and as much as she needed and wanted to. Her respiratory rate slowed and breathing became less labored. Over Joanne's next and final 2 days, the family did not permit any further hypnotherapy visits as they gathered to say good-bye. Though there had only been this single official hypnotherapy session, Joanne's nurses reported that they reinforced suggestions of dissociation and comfort and that her last hours seemed easier as a result.

Steven T., a 10-year-old boy, also in the end stages of cystic fibrosis, was referred to us for hypnotherapy because of depression and decreased tolerance of medical procedures, including postural drainage and intravenous infusions. He would resist and cry, asking the medical staff members why they continued these painful treatments when they knew as well as he did that he was going to die anyway. In the first hypnotherapeutic session, Steven quickly learned self-hypnosis to control pain and to decrease his anxiety about being unable to get enough air during postural drainage treatments that resulted in prolonged and violent coughing. He was also able to clarify that he really did want continued treatment, since he wanted to live as long as possible, and he asked that the nurses ignore his pleas when his frustration resulted in "temper-tantrum" behavior. He immediately developed a strong positive alliance with the therapist. His mother concurrently responded well to brief counseling from the therapist and to more extensive therapy from her social worker.

In a later, nonhypnotic psychotherapy session, Steven openly discussed his concerns about dying, especially his awareness that vigorous antibiotic therapy was no longer producing significant improvement in his pulmonary status. The therapist introduced a "life and death game" in an effort to modify the boy's increasing obsession with dying. Outlining a "life circle" and a "death circle" on a sheet of white paper, the therapist showed Steven two crayons, red and green, stating that life was to be represented by the color green and death by the color red. She then affirmed that treatment was of decreasing value and sometime soon would be of no value at all. She stressed that some day the doctors would have no more "life" (treatment) to give Steven and could offer him only a relatively comfortable death, with medications as needed for pain and/or anxiety. She then removed the green crayon, illustrating the problem. Steven said he still wanted life, and he asked for the green crayon so that he could color the life circle green. The therapist reminded him that she had no more green to give him, and she challenged him to create green by himself. Steven quickly saw that his only option at this point in the game was to color the death circle red. As he worked at the task, the therapist encouraged him to look at death, to acknowledge death. Then, using the principle of complementary colors, the therapist asked Steven to look again at the life circle. It turned green before his eyes.*

Both amazed and amused, Steven saw conceptually as well as graphically, that he could take some responsibility for his own experience, acknowledging death, then setting it aside and creating a more enjoyable life. For example, he proceeded to arrange a pre-birthday party for himself in the hospital, instead of continuing to worry that he might not live another month until his 11th birthday. This being successful, he arranged a second pre-birthday party when he went to visit relatives. Then, on his actual birthday, he enjoyed still a third party.

In many other ways, Steven created life for himself. Shortly before he died, he made a new contract with hospital staff to the effect that he could refuse postural drainage if he wished and have narcotic medication when he requested it, all knowing that this was now his terminal hospitalization. Supported by his family, he spent his last days relating to them and to the hospital staff members, for many of whom he had become a favorite patient. On the night before he died he requested and fully enjoyed a special dinner sent in from a local restaurant. For Steven, the initial use of hypnotherapy seemed to facilitate this dying child's ability to exercise all four of his basic rights. To a large extent he shifted his approach to the task of dying from helpless frustration to mastery and control.

Hypnotherapy in the Broadest Context of Experience

Recent developments in holistic medicine are rapidly changing the way we treat children with life-threatening illness. Rather than directing efforts only at the disease process, we now emphasize the need for simultaneous attention to the physical, psychological, and spiritual needs of the patient and the family and the involved community (Whittam, 1993).

As compared with the more narrow area of symptom relief, it is even more difficult to assess the value of hypnotherapy in holistic medicine. We

---

*For readers unfamiliar with this phenomenon, a similar effect can be produced by staring for 30 to 60 seconds at a red piece of paper and then immediately staring at an adjacent blank white area.

can speculate that hypnotherapy may have an impact on several interrelated areas. For the child, it can provide (1) symptom relief; (2) decreased anxiety, depression, passivity, helplessness; (3) enhanced ego functions, especially feelings of safety, trust, hope, autonomy, competence, initiative, humor, reality testing, self-esteem, dignity, and grace; and (4) increased ability to relate positively to others in age-appropriate ways. For the family, it can provide (1) decreased feelings of anxiety and impotence; (2) increased ability to relate to the child and to offer comfort and reassurance rather than to engage in defensive withdrawal; (3) increased ability to make constructive use of community resources such as friends and clergy; and (4) increased ability to deal creatively with loss of a child, using the grief process in the service of personal growth. For the community, it can instill (1) increased responsiveness to the greater receptivity of the child and the family; and (2) increased awareness of the value of such responsiveness.

Every one of these areas affects all others, each making its own contribution, perhaps including enhancing the child's ability to use hypnotherapy, thus coming full circle in a complex set of causal relationships. Thus, although the formal use of hypnotherapy may appear to serve limited functions, it can interact with other resources in the child, the family, and the community to facilitate growth and mastery, thus utilizing emotional upheaval in the service of attaining higher levels of ego integration.

We do not mean to overvalue the role of hypnotherapy but, rather, to recognize the whole spectrum of possible actions and reactions in the total experience of a dying child who uses this treatment modality. In the context of perceiving hypnotherapy as one resource among many, each affecting the others in the broadest context of experience, we present a previously published account (Gardner, 1976b) of the child David.*

The authors would like to express their appreciation to David's parents for their assistance in the preparation of this material and especially for their permission to include excerpts of a family tape recording.

The Child David

A Brief History

David was the second of four boys born to intelligent, capable middle-class parents. The family valued religious commitment and, at the time of David's illness, were members of an Episcopal church. Outgoing and sociable, they frequently spent time both with personal friends and with the father's business associates. The father especially enjoyed the challenge of hiking, back-

*From Gardner (1976b). With permission.

packing, and skiing—activities that demand and develop physical and mental stamina, independence, and persistence in the face of difficulty. He encouraged the children in these and other rigorous pursuits such as baseball, football, and swimming. The mother, through her qualities of gentleness, tenderness, and obvious pleasure both in sharing laughter and in relieving distress, complemented the father in conveying to the children that sense of security and involvement in living that is the foundation for personal growth. Of course, there were differences of opinion and periods of significant tension and strain, but, more than most, this family found real reward in doing things together. Birthdays and holidays were special family "happenings," so much so that every year each child had two birthday celebrations, a party with his friends and a separate birthday dinner for the family alone.

Up to the age of 11, David was healthy. He often lacked enthusiasm at school, annually causing enough concern that his teacher requested a conference with his parents; yet his schoolwork was satisfactory. He excelled in outdoor activities with family and peers, while at the same time he was able to enjoy himself when alone. A bright child, he shared his parents' good sense of humor and enjoyed playing jokes on people. Though capable of anger, he also expressed love and tenderness to his family and especially to his dog. He tended not to worry about things and to take life as it came, proud of his past, secure in the present, and not giving a great deal of thought to the future.

Then, soon after his 11th birthday, a routine blood test showed abnormalities that led to hospitalization and to a diagnosis of acute lymphatic leukemia. The parents were stunned but found hope in the knowledge of many potentially helpful drugs. David reacted characteristically, without much concern, even enjoying the new experiences of his first hospitalization, yet very happy to return home to his family and his dog. Having achieved remission, David perceived his disease primarily as a nuisance and joined his parents in their developing denial that it was really a serious threat. Life routines returned essentially to normal. He completed the school year successfully, went on a family backpacking trip, and pitched his Little League baseball team to a first-place win.

The Introduction of Hypnotherapy

In early fall, 10 months after the initial diagnosis, relapses began, and inexorably the periods of remission became progressively shorter. The parents faced the truth all over again, this time more realistically and more painfully. They counseled with their priest and with a few very close friends, trying to make some sense theologically out of their predicament and to begin planning a funeral that could properly reflect their evolving feelings about the meaning of death. Fundamentally, knowing they might not function very well if they had to face the situation alone, they began building a support system, both interpersonally and philosophically. Active planning replaced denial as a coping mechanism.

Though David's outlook remained essentially positive, he too was more often confronted with the devastating consequences of his illness. Soon after he began sixth grade, he was told he could no longer play football. On Halloween, he began to revel in neighborhood fun but became too tired and returned home after he had visited only three houses. On his 12th birthday, he was again sick and spent much of the day sleeping. In these difficult times, he was frustrated and depressed, sometimes in tears, but he responded well to overtures from others; on Halloween, his little brothers shared their candy with him, and, on his birthday, a high school choral group came to the house to sing him show tunes for an hour. He was also sustained by his own resources, especially his undaunted desire to enjoy living. Important as it was that his family and friends never deserted him, it was more important that he never deserted himself.

Then, during a hospitalization in November, David developed vomiting that did not respond to medication. Both for him and his parents, frustration quickly mounted into anxiety and then into depression and despair. It was Michael, a nurse, who, sharing in the frustration, first discussed the problem with the author (G. Gail Gardner), a psychologist experienced in using hypnotherapy with pediatric patients. We agreed that hypnosis might alleviate David's vomiting and, after discussing the situation with the medical staff, proposed the idea to David and to his mother, who was staying with him at the time. They both voiced immediate enthusiasm, ready to grasp at anything that might help. David's positive response was further enhanced by his curiosity about hypnosis, which he put in the same category of intrigue as black magic, and his anticipated pleasure in experiencing it. Thus, there were no problems with initial motivation and cooperation.

Selecting Induction Techniques. The selection of appropriate induction and deepening techniques was based on several factors. First, because David now feared he had lost control of his disease, it was important to use techniques that would enhance his sense of control and mastery. He needed to feel that hypnosis was not something done to him by some other powerful person but rather a state he could achieve for himself after proper training. Thus, hypnosis was described as analogous to learning to write or ride a bike, and techniques were avoided that involved any sort of gadgetry or emphasis on cues from the hypnotherapist.

Second, the induction techniques needed to be consistent with David's capabilities and interests, especially in the case of visual imagery. Through interviews with David and his mother, the therapist obtained the relevant information, including knowledge about David's enjoyment of new experiences and his love of imaginative activities. For example, his mother described how he and his brother enjoyed creating an imaginary house from pine shrubs on a recent backpacking trip.

Third, because it seemed likely that David would be taught self-hypnosis, the most preferable induction techniques were those he could use himself or with only minimal aid from his mother. As a corollary to this, the induction techniques needed to be easily mastered by the mother, as her interest in the method suggested that she could become a hypnotherapeutic ally, assisting her son in hypnosis when the therapist was not available. Parents have been taught to be effective therapists for children's behavior problems (Stabler, Gibson, & Cutting, 1973), and this author (Gardner) has had successful experiences in teaching parents to assist with hypnotherapy.

Based on this initial information, the therapist decided to begin with suggestions for progressive relaxation and guided visual imagery related to David's interests and experiences. The boy was first given some elementary facts about hypnosis (e.g., that it was not the same as black magic and that he would be awake and able to remember what happened) in order to minimize confusion and develop a concept of active partnership in the therapeutic alliance. After this brief teaching session, the induction was carried out as planned, and David went into hypnosis without difficulty.

Early Goals. The immediate goal was, of course, to try to reduce the nausea and vomiting. The therapist first reminded David of his own wish to work on this problem and added her agreement that the vomiting served no useful purpose and therefore should be eliminated. She then asked David to recall specific foods that he particularly enjoyed and to bring these vividly to mind, together with sensations of mild hunger and gustatory pleasure. As he enhanced these images, he was told that these good feelings could fill his entire body and mind more and more, until there was just no room left for the unpleasant feelings that had plagued him. Generally, the idea was to create a positive state that would be antithetical to nausea. As David indicated that he was immersed in the good feelings, and the bad ones had disappeared, he was given posthypnotic suggestions that he could maintain the good feelings after returning to the normal waking state, could actually enjoy food and fluids, and could take medication without difficulty. After he was aroused, the therapist remained with him while he ate a small meal. He was both astonished and proud to find that the problem was resolved after this one session.

Toward the larger goal of mastery, the therapist suggested during the hypnotic session that, just as David was now able to achieve physical relaxation and visual imagery when he wished, he could look forward to using this method for other purposes such as pain control, knowing that he had more control over his physical and emotional state than he realized previously. This sense of control could make him more relaxed and less anxious, and then he would be even more able to reach his goals. He was asked to recall earlier experiences of mastery, such as winning at baseball, and then to bring these feelings into the present, with post-hypnotic suggestions that they could carry over into the future. Thus, the therapist created the growth cycle that seems so often to be at the root of successful hypnotherapy.

David was indeed pleased with his new skill and readily found that, in addition to achieving control of the nausea, he could respond to hypnotherapy for control of pain and of marked anxiety related to the start of an intravenous infusion. Here the therapist used the same paradigm as for control of nausea, namely, creating an antithetical feeling state. David was asked to recall his arm feeling very comfortable, to bring that comfort into the present so thoroughly that there was simply no room for pain.

Extensions of Mastery

Self-Hypnosis. It was David himself who asked to learn self-hypnosis so that he could better control problems of nausea, pain, or anxiety that might arise at home. Accordingly, prior to discharge from the hospital, and after careful discussion with him and his mother about the nature and use of hypnosis, David was taught self-hypnosis. He was cautioned regarding its abuse by being told that it was so easy to learn hypnotic induction that he could probably hypnotize his friends or other people, but that he should not do this because, though it is easy to learn *how* to hypnotize, it takes special training to learn *when* and *why* to use hypnosis and what suggestions to give people. He was reminded that, just as special training is needed to know when and why to use medications, the same is true for hypnosis. He and his mother agreed that he could be responsible in this regard. There were no particular limitations put on his using hypnosis for himself, except to emphasize that it was not to be done "just for fun" and to suggest that he talk with his mother or the therapist before using it for any new problem.

Some interesting difficulties arose at this point that are illustrative of the need to be alert to idiosyncratic responses to hypnosis, to be skilled in a variety of induction methods, and to be ready to modify therapeutic techniques on short notice. The first problem concerned induction in self-hypnosis. Most patients, including children, can readily adapt the induction methods of heterohypnosis to autohypnosis, providing the therapist has not structured the situation otherwise. Thus, in David's case, he was asked simply to close his eyes and allow himself to enter the state of physical relaxation now familiar to him while focusing his attention on pleasant visual imagery. As he began to respond, he became curiously anxious. When asked what troubled him, he said that he could achieve the relaxation and imagery but was worried because, without any comments from the therapist, he didn't know whether or not he was "really in hypnosis." That is, he wanted some sort of clear external cue that hypnosis had been achieved, and did not feel comfortable or confident having to rely solely on his experiential state. It was easy enough to give him the needed cue by adding reverse arm levitation to the induction procedure. He was asked to raise one arm and then to notice how it would begin to feel heavy and drift downward as he relaxed. He was told that the arm would drift lower and lower and that, when it reached his lap or the bed or chair, he could be sure he was in hypnosis. David accepted this suggestion without question, and used this technique successfully until 3 days before his death.

The second problem that arose in teaching David self-hypnosis concerned anxiety when he was asked to do something in self-hypnosis that he had not done in any previous heterohypnosis session, namely, to talk. He had never been required to give any verbal response because simple motor responses such as nodding or shaking his head were sufficient for communication around the problems at hand. Now, however, it seemed desirable to demonstrate to him and his mother that he could respond to her verbally or initiate verbalization while in hypnosis, should the need arise.

When this was first proposed, David expressed his fear that he would "come out of hypnosis and wake up" if he talked. Despite reassurance, he maintained this anxiety during the hypnotic induction and avoided the problem of having to talk by soon drifting off to sleep. The therapist took the opportunity to note to the mother this example of ego control in the hypnotic state, with David finding a way to avoid the feared unwanted self-arousal that would have impaired his confidence that he could use hypnosis alone. The therapist also used this incident to demonstrate to the mother that, if David were to fall asleep while using hypnosis, it was quite easy to awaken him gently, just as one might awaken any sleeping child. Once David was awake, the therapist provided further reassurance and explanation. Following this, David again induced self-hypnosis and, this time, gave appropriate verbal responses to questions and commands from his mother as well as from the therapist. It is important to note here that the therapist did not respond to the unexpected events with anxiety but turned the situation into an opportunity for teaching and further development of skills. If hypnosis has been initially presented as a technique that may have to be modified to fit individual needs, then it is not a disaster when problems of this sort occur.

The third problem in teaching David self-hypnosis was related to his mother. Both she and the therapist agreed that it might be useful for her to experience a hypnotic induction herself because she wanted to know "what it feels like," and first-hand knowledge of the state might enhance her effectiveness in helping David use hypnosis. When this was suggested, David expressed interest in seeing his mother in hypnosis. She was willing, and it was convenient to have her go into hypnosis in David's room because the therapist's office was in another part of the hospital, and only a brief experience of induction and dehypnotization was anticipated. The mother went into hypnosis without difficulty but soon became spontaneously alert, commenting briefly that she felt a bit silly. She later told the therapist, "Really I was getting so relaxed and my defenses were breaking down; I was near tears and I didn't want to cry in front of David." It seems that sharing the hypnotic experience with her dying child brought out feelings of sadness and anticipatory grief that she did not want David to have to bear in addition to his already heavy burden. More than the other two problems, in retrospect, it seems this one could have been anticipated. It would have been better to have insisted on David not being present when his mother experienced hypnosis. Then, perhaps she could have made constructive use of the emergence of her feelings of grief.

In spite of these difficulties, both David and his mother gained confidence that he could use hypnosis himself and that she could assist him as needed. As with induction, the method of dehypnotization was simple, merely counting silently to five. David never abused the privilege of learning self-hypnosis. With characteristic responsibility and humor, he later told the therapist that he had resisted the temptation to talk in detail about hypnosis to his friends, but he confessed that he had tried to hypnotize his dog.

The Eagle Dream. In chronic and terminal illness, one sees extended hope and relief when the patient and the family learn that hypnosis can be useful not only for the treatment of painful or negative experiences but also for enhancement of positive experiences such as safety and joy. This idea was introduced to David by suggesting that he might have a pleasant hypnotic dream that he could repeat as often as he liked. He dreamed that he was an eagle who enjoyed flying from one safe and peaceful place to another; whenever anything disturbed him, he could simply fly off to another, even safer and happier place. At home, when David was in distress, he successfully combined reverse hand levitation with the eagle dream to achieve quietness and calm enjoyment, sometimes at his own initiation and sometimes following his mother's suggesting, "David, just find your peaceful place." Family friends, who were unaware of what was happening, were astonished at the rapidity and ease with which he could shift from a negative to a positive feeling state.

For David and his family it became more possible to tolerate gradual physical deterioration and to avert the threat of psychological disintegration by learning to achieve a feeling of emotional ease and dignity. The sense of threat gradually gave way to a sense of challenge and then to task accomplishment and general mastery. That is, David expressed and at the same time enhanced his growing trust in himself and turned his attention to solving problems rather than enduring them. The therapist took this opportunity to remind him and his mother that they could consider using hypnosis for new problems as they arose, feeling free to contact the therapist for consultation and assistance as needed.

An Example of Contraindication. On Thanksgiving Day, just before being discharged from the hospital, David suddenly asked a doctor if having leukemia meant that he was going to die. To his horror he learned that he would die "in a month at the least and a year at the most." Despite his size, he sat in his mother's lap and wept bitterly in the car driving home; then, as if to indicate his beginning acceptance, he began parceling out his belongings, emphasizing that he wanted his dog "to be for the whole family." By the time he got home, less than an hour later, he had somehow regained his sense of trust, hope, and integrity. He shared the news with this older brother, again with tears, though only briefly, and then told a few friends who immediately came to the house. After talking about his problems, they resumed normal activities, as if to say there was no great reason for concern or for deviating from their usual habit of enjoying life and taking things as they came. The hospital staff reported the incident to the therapist by telephone, but by the time she telephoned the family, everything was under control and no special intervention was needed.

During the next couple of weeks, when David did not talk any more about his impending death, both his family and his doctors wondered if he had questions or ideas he wanted to share but was reluctant to do so. It was hard to believe that he had either denied the truth, which had been put to him so plainly, or integrated it successfully into his general life style. At the next outpatient visit, his mother asked if it might be valuable to question him about these issues in a hypnotic session and then to create amnesia for the session so that he would not be upset by the content of the interview. She was told that it is extremely difficult to predict how a person will react to this type of hypnotic interview and that it is especially difficult to be sure of obtaining amnesia. Therefore, the plan was abandoned, not only because of the uncertainty of success but also because we did not want to take the risk of having a distressing hypnotic experience interfere with David's successful use of hypnosis in other areas.

Because a hypnotic approach seemed contraindicated in this instance, the mother asked for other ideas and accepted the suggestion that we ask David quite straightforwardly if he had any questions about his illness or about death. She feared that she might upset him if she herself wept during the interview, but she overcame her fear when reminded that we had solved difficult problems before and could surely trust in our resourcefulness now. We agreed to terminate the interview by observing David's response and following his lead. In response to questions, David said calmly that he knew he was going to die but was not worried and had no questions. Like many dying children, his only stated concern was that he did not want his parents to be sad or upset because of him. Though assured that he could bring up the subject at any time in the future, he never raised it again.

An Example of Creative Use of Hypnosis. Glad to have a treatment technique that was both painless and portable, David and his family went to visit relatives in Texas in mid-December. The therapist taught David to go into hypnosis by telephone, demonstrating this with him during a clinic visit. Putting a hypnotic induction on tape was considered but not carried out because, with David's condition now likely to change in unknown ways almost from day to day, there was little chance that suggestions on prerecorded tape would be useful.

Once in Texas, David developed a ravenous appetite associated with high-dose steroids that had recently been prescribed. When it reached the point that he woke two or three times a night to have his mother fix eggs and toast, they decided to try hypnotherapy for appetite control. David was assisted by his uncle, who is a psychotherapist, and, after one session, his appetite returned to normal levels.

After a week, David was again in relapse. His parents conferred with their doctor and agreed to return home, not to attempt further treatment, and to keep David as comfortable as possible so that he might die in dignity and peace.

The Last 3 Days

Early Saturday, December 23, David entered the hospital for the last time. He had vomited blood several times during the night, and neither he nor his parents had had much sleep. He had recurring sharp pain in his leg, which he could no longer control with hypnosis. He was admitted to a private room and intravenous morphine was begun. Though in such poor condition, David once again spontaneously raised his arm and lowered himself into hypnotic comfort before the needle was put into his vein. Even the therapist now marveled at his continuing ability to maintain some degree of control of experience.

In the hallway, both parents wept. The father was angered that there seemed to be no way to hold off this inexorable march toward death until David had had one last Christmas. The mother feared that she would "fall apart" and be unable to support David now, when he most needed her. The therapist decided to stay to try to help the family regain touch with their inner resources so that they could once again express the courage and love and tenderness that had sustained them before. The father went home to arrange for the other three children to be with grandparents. David and his mother slept. By afternoon, the parents were refreshed, and David was comfortable, sleeping most of the time.

On December 24, when David's condition was relatively stable, and when he seemed comfortable in spite of labored breathing, the decision was made to reduce the morphine, which seemed to be controlling his pain and anxiety but only at the expense of his ability to maintain ego functions. It was hoped that a smaller amount of morphine combined with hypnotic suggestions might control the pain and still allow him to be more alert and to spend maximal time relating to his family. Likewise, if he was more alert, his parents could be more active in comforting him, caring for his needs, and sharing conversation, thus again averting passive submission and impotence.

True to himself, David maintained his capacity for trust and hope. Once when his leg hurt, he responded readily to a suggestion that he could "just let the pain go," but he said he feared it might come back. When reassured that he could "just let it go again," he immediately relaxed; further episodes of the leg pain were infrequent and brief. That afternoon he unexpectedly became fully alert and began spontaneously reminiscing about pleasant experiences of the past. Wishing to preserve this precious experience, his mother asked that this conversation be tape recorded. The therapist found a tape recorder and granted the request. In the evening, his older brother brought his Christmas presents, but David was sleepy and showed little interest. Friends and hospital staff brought food and wine, and someone remarked that a new family began to be created, united by some mysterious sense of sharing, freedom, and warmth, enhanced by David's attitude of calm as he began his final approach toward death. Christmas Eve was quiet.

On Christmas Day, again without warning, David became alert and now asked to see his presents. He opened several, making his usual wisecracks, and then gave gifts to his father and mother. He tired easily, and his breathing became increasingly labored. His father helped him to a more comfortable position in bed while his mother spoke softly to him, repeating simple phrases remarkably similar to the rhythm and language of hypnotherapy. Because the tape recorder had been running, this, too, was recorded, and an excerpt follows:

> That's a boy. Find your quiet place and just rest now. There David. There Davey, there Davey, just rest, honey. Just rest. Just rest, honey. Just rest. Just rest. That's a boy. It's all right, honey. Just relax. Just rest. Just relax, honey, Just rest. That's a boy, honey. That's a boy. Just rest, honey. That's a boy. We'll open more presents later, honey. There now. There now, there now, there now. There now. There Davey, just relax, just relax. There. Just relax, honey. That's a boy. That's a boy, find your quiet place. Just

relax. That's a boy. Okay, honey, okay, just relax, honey. Just rest, just find your peaceful place and rest. Just find your peaceful place and rest. Mommy and Daddy are right here and we're going to keep you good and safe. It's okay, honey. It's okay.

Joined by a close family friend, the therapist, and Michael the nurse, both parents continued to comfort their son. Later, on that Christmas afternoon, David died.

Hypnotherapy in the Grieving Process

David's parents had many sources of strength to sustain them through the next months, especially religious faith and strong ties to the community and to the church, in addition to inner courage and creative acceptance. Family and friends participated in a Requiem Mass. In the summer, when the snow melted in the mountains, a priest and a few friends hiked with the family to an alpine lake. Following the Eucharist, they scattered David's ashes amid the pine shrubs where earlier he had joined his brother in imaginative games.

The parents and children each found their individual ways of expressing their grief and integrating David's death into a concept of meaningful life. The children talked with friends and family. The parents returned to the scattering site in early October to experience the beauty of the first snowfall. A family friend drew a sketch of Michael holding David after death, when told that this scene had reminded the therapist of the Michelangelo Pietà in Rome.

The mother, having experienced hypnosis before, now used it again to enhance her capacity for full expression of her feelings, to enjoy fresh and vivid memories of David, to find meaning in her loss, and to allow opportunity for further personal development in the context of her son's death. She said, "Dying was the hardest thing Dave ever had to do, and he did it well." Once, in a letter to the therapist, she wrote, "David is so real to me—not externally but internally—bound up in all that I cherish and wonder at and reflect on, that his reality is very present, very real, very full of meaning. And so I rejoice, mainly, that God should so bless me as to make meaning out of chaos."

CONCLUSIONS

Although hypnotherapy seems to be valuable for many children with life-threatening illness and for their families, there are instances in which it is of limited value or none at all. Some children and parents simply refuse this

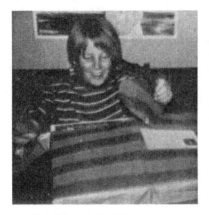

1. Eleventh birthday party.

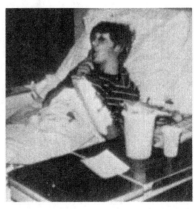

2. First hospitalization.

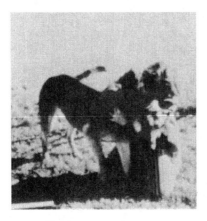

3. First return home.

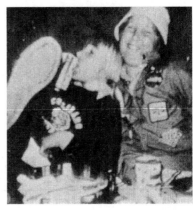

4. Clowning with a friend.

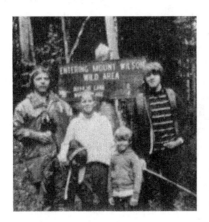

5. Family backpacking trip.

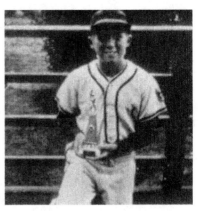

6. Baseball victory.

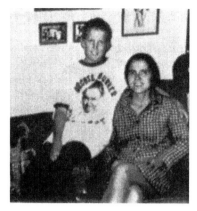

7. David and his mother.

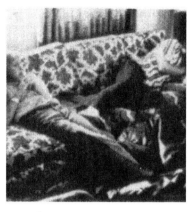

8. The last Thanksgiving.

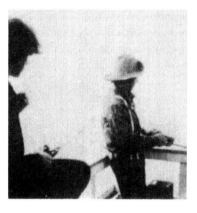

9. Fishing, a week before death.

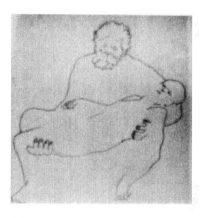

10. Sketch of Michael holding David after death.

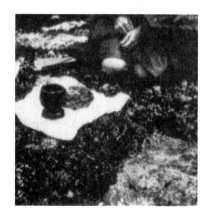

11. Outdoor Mass before scattering ashes.

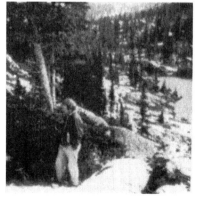

12. Father at the scattering site a month later.

treatment modality. Other children eagerly embark on learning hypnotic skills only to fail, for known and unknown reasons. Still other children respond well to hypnotherapy for one purpose but not for another, or respond well at one time and poorly at another. We still have a great deal to learn about potential uses of hypnotherapy with dying children. How do we help them maximize their use of hypnotic talent? What are the limits of the possible uses of hypnotherapy? How can we best facilitate the interaction of hypnotherapy with many other forms of medical, surgical, and psychological treatment?

Child health professionals who utilize hypnotherapy with dying children must also consider issues related to their own involvement. The hypnotherapeutic relationship is characterized by more intense emotional responses, not only in the patient but also in the therapist. When working with dying children, the hypnotherapist must be able to deal with his or her own reactions to loss and with the emotional stress of personal involvement, combining human caring with professional objectivity in such a way that the end result is positive not only for the child and the family but for the therapist as well.

CHAPTER FOURTEEN

Biofeedback and Child Hypnotherapy

Biofeedback is a useful form of adjunctive therapy for many biobehavioral conditions in children and adolescents. Biofeedback refers to provision of information about specific physiological responses in humans. The child or adolescent can observe this information and practice changing his or her thinking to effect a desired change in the response. A blood pressure monitor, an oral thermometer, or a bathroom scale are examples of biofeedback instruments.

The study of biofeedback really began in 1969 when Miller described operant conditioning of autonomic nervous system functions such as heart rate, blood pressure, intestinal motility, urine production rate, and gastric and peripheral blood flow in the curarized rat. Subsequently, there was a great deal of optimism leading to predictions that humans, via self monitoring devices, would be able to self-regulate many autonomic functions. Hundreds of studies have documented that certain types of biofeedback are useful for certain clinical problems (Brown, 1974; Basmajian, 1989; Olton & Noonberg, 1980). However, several studies using false biofeedback have been associated with positive clinical results (Andrasik & Holroyd, 1980; Mullinix, Norton, Hack, & Fishman, 1978). M. S. Smith (1991) has noted that "The application of biofeedback may be useful in many clinical conditions, although there appear to be few conditions in which biofeedback is demonstrably superior to other behavioral techniques, such as relaxation training, hypnosis, or meditation."

It is noteworthy that manuals provided with biofeedback equipment invariably include relaxation imagery or hypnotic inductions to be used in the training process. Although it is extremely useful in clinical conditions such as Raynaud disease or hypertension to receive immediate feedback of peripheral temperature or blood pressure, long-term improvement related to biofeedback does require home practice of self-hypnosis-type exercises. Although the reduction of costs and computerization of biofeedback devices now makes it possible for many families to purchase the equipment for home use, provision of biofeedback equipment will change nothing unless active, regular mental rehearsals are employed.

There have been a number of prospective, controlled studies with children naive to hypnosis or biofeedback that have documented their ability to intentionally change a number of autonomic responses. We have described the study of Dikel and Olness (1980) that documented the ability of children to increase and decrease peripheral temperature with a few minutes of mental effort. Other studies include documentation that children can intentionally change auditory evoked potentials (Hogan, MacDonald, & Olness, 1985), tissue oxygen measures (Olness & Conroy, 1985), blood pressure (Kohen & Ondich, 1992), electrodermal activity (Olness & Rusin, 1990), and muscle responses including anorectal function (Olness, McParland, & Piper, 1980). Recent work (Lee & Olness, 1995) has demonstrated that intentional changes in imagery are associated with measurable changes in physiological responses such as heart rate, peripheral temperature, and electrodermal activity, although children may not be receiving any direct feedback. This is consistent with the work of Wang and Morgan (1992) who have found that athletes demonstrate changes in physiological measures when they are imagining a sports activity that are equivalent to those when they are actually participating in the sport. The magnitude may relate to genetics or unrecognized conditioning experiences. It may prove to be important clinically to know how children respond physiologically to ordinary changes in thinking. For example, if thinking of something active such as riding a bicycle causes blood pressure to increase, it might be useful to coach a child (with biofeedback) to reverse this response.

CLINICAL APPLICATIONS
WITH CHILDREN

We find that we use biofeedback very often in the course of hypnotherapy. It provides an excellent teaching device to help children understand that, by changing their thinking process, they cause changes in their body and that they can be in control of that. The use of appealing biofeedback can help a child to concentrate attention and focus, to cultivate self-awareness and internal locus of control, and to learn conditioned relaxation. Emphasis on the child's mastery and coping ability is the central theme in hypnotherapy, and this is facilitated with adjunct biofeedback. We use biofeedback often when the clinical problem has no relationship to the specific type of feedback, for example, temperature feedback or electrodermal activity for enuresis. In such situations, the biofeedback response functions—we believe—as a metaphor for the concept that the focused concentration of hypnotherapy can effect physiological changes.

We also find that monitoring of multiple autonomic responses concurrently gives us useful information about the child. Although there are no standards for autonomic measures such as electromyographic, electrodermal, or peripheral temperature changes in children, we note that children seem to have an autonomic "fingerprint" or "stress profile." This is consistent with the work of Kagan (1994) on infants. Some children show extremely labile responses in all measures; some show lability in the heart rate but not in electrodermal activity; others have autonomic measures that are very stable. Children have also been shown to vary in immunological reactivity. Inasmuch as immune cells have numerous receptors for neurotransmitters associated with autonomic responses, it is possible that other autonomic measures may be surrogate measures for immune reactivity. We hope that further studies of the autonomic "fingerprints" will be done because such information may be relevant to diagnosis and treatment procedures in hospitals or clinics, to prevention programs, to the anticipatory guidance provided by pediatricians, to how one prepares a child for a new situation such as the beginning of school, or to coaching and teaching strategies for a given child.

BIOFEEDBACK EQUIPMENT

Believing that it is important for children to have the opportunity to understand that changes in thinking can impact on body responses, we have designed and developed a "mind–body" machine, a biofeedback unit that reflects electrodermal activity and that uses touch-screen methods. The prototype unit is currently used in the Cleveland Health Science Museum as a centerpiece for a special exhibit. Pilot studies with more than 350 children determined that only two could not effect changes in the electrodermal activity during a first attempt of a few minutes. Children enjoy this experience, which allows them choice of a touch-screen animal that will respond to their changes in thinking (either relaxation or excitement), and they usually ask to repeat their effort (see Figure 14.1). Information about this unit is available from Performance Concepts (8250 Tyler Boulevard, Mentor, OH 44050; phone 800-969-9550).

Biofeedback equipment can be very simple. Inexpensive biobands and biodots (Bio-Temp Products Inc., P.O. Box 29099, Indianapolis, IN 46229; phone 317-637-5776) reflect temperature changes. A company from Montreal, Thought Technology, has developed the "Calmpute" system, which includes programs for computers that can then reflect peripheral temperature or electrodermal activity changes. These are appealing to many children and are available for about $100. This company also sells battery-run devices

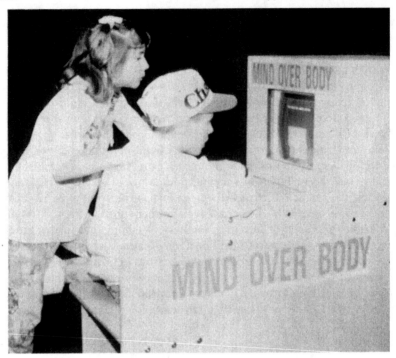

FIGURE 14.1. The "mind-body" machine.

(GSR/TEMP 2 Biofeedback System) that provide sound feedback for electrodermal activity or peripheral temperature and more expensive programs for computers that allow concurrent measurement of heart rate, temperature, and electrodermal activity (Thought Technology, Ltd., Cimetra Industrial Park, 8396 Route 9, West Chazy, NY 12992; phone 514-489-8251; fax 514-489-8255). There are also software programs that allow biofeedback information to be presented in game format. One example is the J&J 1-330 Physiologic Monitoring System that provides feedback in the form of games, "Traffic Light" and "River Rafting." The SRS Orion System provides an appealing "Tortoise and Hare" race; as the child relaxes, the tortoise moves ahead of the hare. We have found that games enhance initial interest but that children will later request "a new game." Some of the computer biofeedback programs provide the option of a print-out that reflects performance. This has appeal for older children who enjoy comparing their performance from one practice session to another.

The Association for Applied Psychophysiology and Biofeedback (10200 West 44th Avenue, Suite 304, Wheat Ridge, CO 80033-2140; phone 303-422-8436; fax 303-422-8894) focuses primarily on adult applications of biofeedback but is the best central source for obtaining more information about the latest in biofeedback equipment.

The following sections provide examples of how biofeedback can be used clinically. They are not intended to be all-inclusive.

MIGRAINE

There are more controlled studies documenting the efficacy of nonpharmacological methods including hypnotherapy and biofeedback in the management of juvenile migraine than there are controlled studies documenting the efficacy of pharmacological methods (Burke & Andrasik, 1989; Olness et al., 1988; Osterhaus et al., 1993; Smith, Womack, & Pertik, 1987). Nonetheless, children continue to receive medications that have not been adequately studied. In offering nonpharmacological methods to children with migraine, we may offer hypnotherapy alone or a combination of hypnotherapy and biofeedback. We are unaware of any specific mechanism by which learning to increase peripheral temperature or electrodermal activity or heart rate will interrupt the cascade of internal events that end with a migraine headache. Nonetheless, many children with migraine enjoy recognizing that they are intentionally changing various autonomic parameters. Inasmuch as migraine is a biological disorder and the triggers for symptoms may be multiple, it is possible that regular practice of self-hypnosis with an emphasis on relaxation may prevent some internal physiological response that sets off the symptom cascade. This may be true for other chronic conditions such as asthma, hemophilia, or sickle-cell disease. Osterhaus and colleagues (1993) reported on "combined behavioral therapy" for school children with migraine. This included relaxation training defined as progressive relaxation, autogenic relaxation, and relaxation based on self-hypnosis. It also included temperature feedback and rational emotive therapy to reduce tension. Each of 32 children was seen eight times, four times in individual and four times in group therapy. They noted a rise in finger temperature during each successive biofeedback session (from 1.3 °C to 2.9 °C). Undoubtedly, this reflected success in relaxation practice, for this phenomenon is evident in children doing self-hypnosis practice regardless of the presenting problem. Because pharmacological prophylaxis of juvenile migraine is not adequately studied and side effects may be significant, we believe that nonpharmaocolgical methods are treatments of choice.

REFLEX SYMPATHETIC DYSTROPHY

This problem provides one of the few medical conditions in which the biofeedback may be essential to therapeutic success. Children and adolescents with this problem often have significant peripheral temperature differentials between the affected and nonaffected extremities. Sympathetic and parasympathetic signals are irregular and/or abnormal causing the uncomfortable symptoms of edema, pain, and sometimes numbness. We have reported eight children and adolescents who responded well to training in self-hypnosis with biofeedback (Olness, 1990b). As is true with many chronic conditions, the time for remission of symptoms is directly related to the length of time they have existed. We recommend that all children with this problem be referred early for a trial of nonpharmacological management.

RAYNAUD DISEASE/PHENOMENON

Raynaud disease is another disorder of imbalance between sympathetic and parasympathetic nervous system tone resulting in vasoconstriction and cold extremities. Again, skin-temperature feedback provides direct proof to the child or adolescent that he or she is succeeding in increasing peripheral temperature. The use of inexpensive, portable monitors such as a Radio Shack thermistor or a Bioband is especially useful as an adjunct to home practice of self-hypnosis for this problem.

SEIZURE DISORDERS

E. Green and Green (1989) at the Menninger Clinic have developed a portable EEG biofeedback unit. This unit provides sound feedback varying with the percentage of alpha, theta, or beta EEG rhythms. This has been used to treat adults with seizures and children with attention-deficit/hyperactivity disorders (ADHD). Lubar (1991) has reported the successful application for ADHD. In our behavioral pediatrics clinics, we have used this unit for children with intractable seizures and also for children with ADHD. We have done no controlled studies. Our clinical impression is that EEG feedback may be helpful to some motivated children who have severe seizure problems or ADHD. B. Camp and J. Ledbetter (personal communication, 1995) at the University of Colorado in Denver are planning a prospective controlled study using EEG feedback with children who have ADHD. This study is funded by the U.S. Department of Education. One of their first tasks has been to establish EEG norms for children with and without ADHD.

MOVEMENT DISORDERS

Electromyographic (EMG) feedback has been used clinically to treat some children with movement disorders. However, we are not aware of any controlled studies in this area. The primary dystonias of childhood (Moskowitz,

1991) improve with relaxation, hypnosis, and rest. However, EMG feedback might also be helpful to children with dystonias. Children with cerebral palsy have benefited from visual feedback of muscle stretch reflex sensitivity and from auditory feedback for gait training (Flodmark, 1986; Nash, Neilson, & O'Dwyer, 1989).

FECAL INCONTINENCE

Anorectal biofeedback training has been used to help children with prolonged severe constipation and associated encopresis, post-repair of imperforate anus and post-myelomeningocele repair. Although initial training systems (Olness et al., 1980) focused on both internal and external anorectal sphincter control, more recently training has involved provision of feedback from the external sphincter only (Loening-Baucke, 1990). Equipment has also become less complex. Twenty years ago we used complex three-balloon devices that were hand constructed by a surgeon colleague. We now use Foley catheters connected via transducer to a simple oscilloscope. We made drawings on plastic cards placed over the oscilloscope screen to represent games such as basketball, kicking field goals, going to the moon, and so forth. As the child contracted the external sphincter correctly, he could watch the pattern on the oscilloscope making a basket, moving over the goal posts, or reaching the moon. Rusin also developed a system of connecting the Foley catheter via a Radio Shack transducer to a tape recorder (Rusin, 1988). When the child contracted the external anorectal sphincter, he or she could hear favorite music or a favorite story via the tape recorder. In working with these children, we also teach them self-hypnosis to use at home while sitting on the toilet. For example:

> "When you sit on the toilet, pretend you are riding your bike, going exactly where you choose to that special place where you would like to be. You can go as quickly or as slowly as you like, enjoying what you are seeing and feeling, and hearing. Tell yourself when you get to that special place, you can slow down, get off the bike, and enjoy your place. And, when you are ready, you can easily pass the bowel movement into the toilet."

HYPERTENSION

Biofeedback and hypnosis have been used to help adults and adolescents increase awareness of the contribution of feelings (e.g., worry, tension, excitement, distress, frustration) to blood pressure recordings. H. Benson (1990) described the ability through the relaxation response that adults have to lower blood pressure, and these methods have been demonstrated to reduce sympathetic nervous system activity, thereby decreasing cardiac output and lowering blood pressure (Ewart et al., 1987). It has also been noted that operant heart rate speeding and slowing are associated with changes in cardiac vagal tone (Hatch, Borcherding, & Norris, 1990).

Self-regulation techniques have been demonstrated to be useful in the nonpharmacological treatment of adolescents and adults with borderline high blood pressure and those with hypertension (Achmon, Granek, Golomb, & Hart, 1989; Barr, Pennebaker, & Watson, 1988; Blanchard, 1990; Crowther, 1983; Ewart et al., 1987; Patel & Marmot, 1987; Southam, Agras, Taylor, & Kraemer, 1982), but there are no studies to date that involve the investigation of self-regulation of heart rate (HR) and blood pressure (BP) with children. A recent assessment of the physiological concomitants of stress and anxiety was completed by observing HR and BP with preschool children who had been assigned stressful tasks. The tasks elicited measureable changes in BP and HR across subjects (Boyce et al., 1990). Increases in BP and cardiac output are viewed as resembling the classical defense reaction, and it has been suggested that this pattern prevails in the early stages of hypertension (Freyschuss, Hjemdahl, Juhlin-Dannfelt, & Linde, 1988). In a recent study examining the BP and HR of 395 healthy children, it was postulated that anxiety reactions may operate as a mechanism in the development of elevated BP (Murphy, Alpert, & Walker, 1991).

Current pediatric hypertension management guidelines include definitive recommendations that "stress reduction techniques involving meditation, relaxation, or biofeedback are part of nonpharmacologic management," which is advised and seen as "often effective in the young" (Jung & Ingelfinger, 1993). It is clear that the control of BP and cardiovascular reactivity in children at risk for hypertension and its cardiovascular sequelae is of major importance.

We recently conducted a study (Kohen & Ondich, 1992) in which normal children with no history of hypertension were divided into four groups. Twenty-five children in one group were previously familiar with relaxation/mental imagery (self-hypnosis) for some clinical problem and were instructed to use that skill to lower their BP to a healthy level. Seventy-five additional children were randomly assigned to one of three groups: (1) children in the experimental group listened to an audiotape of a hypnotic induction with specific instructions to lower their BP; (2) children in the "waking suggestion" control group listened to a tape that gave them similar suggestions to lower their BP but without a hypnotic induction; and (3) those in the control group listened to a tape that asked them to rest quietly during the experiment/measurement time. All children had BP measurements during three 10-minute trial periods at week 1 and again at week 2. None of the children had hypertension or were at risk for hypertension. Children did not see their BP recordings.

In each group there were some children who were able to change their BP, but no group demonstrated significantly more subjects with this skill. Distinguishing characteristics of those individuals from each group who were most able to alter their BP voluntarily in this experiment have yet to be defined. The individual differences provide a focus for future investigation and understanding of voluntary BP control.

We have clinical experience with many adolescents who came to a teen medical clinic to undergo physical examinations, mandated by a variety of circumstances. For many, the circumstances were stressful; that is, they were brought from a crisis center after running away from home, or came in for a first pelvic examination, or for a pre-participation sports physical examination. In such situations, the initial BP was often elevated, and a simple relaxation/imagery exercise resulted in decreased blood pressure. An example of the spontaneous intervention follows:

> "You'll probably be surprised to discover how easy it is for this kind of slight increase in blood pressure to get lower by just using your imagination. So, just let your eyes close . . . that's right . . . take a deep breath. When you let it out, notice the relaxation that automatically begins at your shoulders naturally as they go down . . . and, as the relaxation moves down your arms and chest gradually or quickly — either is okay — let your mind's imagination drift off to somewhere where you are very comfortable and happy, because when your mind is relaxed, imagining being somewhere that's just right, the body listens. When you are very comfortable and can notice the sights and sounds and what you are doing in your imagined place, then let me know, and I'll check the blood pressure again while you remain very comfortably relaxed."

Often such an approach results in a reduction in the BP that was elevated in association with anxiety in the clinic environment. In such situations, the patient is well aware of the BP cuff and often watches the recording of the follow-up measurement (visual biofeedback) at the end of the hypnotherapeutic suggestions as described.

It is well known that the reaction to stressful circumstances can also raise BP and HR to unhealthy levels (Chesney et al., 1987; Crowther, 1983; Ewart et al., 1987; Menkes et al., 1989). It is appropriate not only to consider preventive management by avoidance of the stressors but also by the development of skills to manage the physiological sequelae of stressors that are unavoidable. Although the best ways to accomplish this are not yet clear, it seems appropriate to learn intentional modulation of autonomic functions such as HR and BP and to practice these skills, especially during distressing times. This may be of lifelong significance with respect to cardiovascular health (Jung & Ingelfinger, 1993). We believe that it may be prudent to train children from hypertension-prone families in the self-regulation of BP.

BIOFEEDBACK RESEARCH WITH CHILDREN

There is a great need for further research in these areas. Advances in computer technology make it not unreasonable that biofeedback equipment will soon be inexpensive enough for general home use. Miniature telemetry devices may make it possible to provide biofeedback to children in school and on the playground. With respect to biofeedback of autonomic responses as a general adjunct to hypnotherapy, we believe that individual differences should dictate which type of feedback is chosen. However, research data does not yet allow us to do that. Personality types, learning styles, interests, likes, and dislikes of children must also be significant factors in whether or not biofeedback is used and what type of equipment is most likely to interest a given child.

CHAPTER FIFTEEN

Self-Hypnosis
A Tool for Prevention and Prophylaxis

Prevention has long been intrinsic to pediatric research and practice. Immunization programs, anticipatory guidance in pediatric clinics, nutrition programs, laws related to phenylketonuria (PKU), thyroid testing and other newborn screening, and many school programs are designed to prevent diseases (Christopherson, Finney, & Friman, 1986; Miller, 1985). Recently, child health programs have been focusing more closely on prevention of behavioral problems. A collaborative multidisciplinary approach is essential to a successful prevention program (Bass et al., 1993; Creer, Stein, Rappaport, & Lewis, 1992; Irwin et al., 1993). Where does self-hypnosis fit into such an approach?

INFANCY

The application of self-hypnosis for prevention of infant morbidity can begin in pregnancy and continue through the life of the child. A number of authors have noted that the use of self-hypnotic techniques for relaxation during pregnancy, labor, and delivery has been found to be helpful to both mother and child (Vadurro & Butts, 1982; Cooper, Shafter, & Tyndall, 1986). Mothers who practice self-hypnotic strategies often require less medication during labor and delivery, thus reducing potential harmful effects on the infant. Self-hypnosis has also been helpful in facilitating breastfeeding, which has many benefits for the child.

Prolonged infant crying due to presumed colic triggers much stress in families. Although the cause of colic is not clear, both parents and infants may benefit from hypnotic strategies to reduce the anxiety of parents.

TODDLER STAGE

Anticipatory guidance might well include training of parents to use phrases that encourage a young child to use his or her natural gift of imagery in positive ways. By means of simple games, young children can become aware of sensory imagery (auditory, visual, gustatory, or olfactory), which they can learn to apply as distracters during procedures such as diaper changing and dressing. By 3 or 4 years of age, a young child can learn that, by thinking in certain ways, he or she can change peripheral temperature or galvanic skin resistance by means of simple feedback (a bioband) or can even alter breathing patterns associated with illness such as asthma (Kohen & Wynne, 1988). Complex feedback (a computer game) has also been used (Kolko & Rickard-Figueroa, 1985). Prospective studies will be needed to determine whether or not this skill facilitates maintenance or enhancement of physiological self-regulation in adulthood.

Pediatricians and other child health professionals might teach young children prophylactic pain control, which the child can apply in unexpected emergency room visits, during dental procedures, and in other stressful situations. Although this possibility has not yet been studied, there are numerous anecdotal reports of preschool-age children taught pain control who were subsequently able to use this skill in emergencies and during medical procedures (Olness, 1989).

Compliance with Medical Regimens

Existing studies of chronic illnesses, such as hemophilia, diabetes, juvenile migraine, and malignancies, provide data to support the recommendation that children so diagnosed should learn self-regulation strategies as soon as possible in order to reduce morbidity, lessen symptoms, and enhance mastery and comfort (Agle, 1975; J. R. Hilgard & LeBaron, 1982; Kohen et al., 1984; Kuttner, 1989; Olness et al., 1987).

Self-hypnosis is helpful in facilitating compliance with injections (e.g., for diabetes or allergy), special diets, nebulizer or inhaler regimens, frequent oral medications or nutritional supplements, special exercises, and other procedures

SCHOOL AGE

Stress

The following book list will be useful to parents and therapists concerned with helping children cope with stressful situations, whether caused by disorders or by various pressures at school.

S. Bedford: *Tiger Juice: A Book about Stress for Kids*
B. Brown: *Between Health and Illness*
L. Chandler: *Children under Stress*
N. Garmezy and M. Rutter (Eds.): *Stress Coping and Development in Children*
G. Hendricks: *The Centering Book*
J. Humphrey: *Controlling Stress in Children*
J. Humphrey: *Stress in Childhood*
B. Kuczen: *Childhood Stress*
B. Phillips: *School Stress and Anxiety*
B. Samples: *The Wholeschool Book*
A. Saunders: *The Stress-Proof Child*

We believe that the use of such resources is maximized by parental consultation with child health professionals who can provide informed support, reinforcement, and guidance in the most appropriate utilization of such materials.

Performance Anxiety

All children must perform in the course of family, school, religious, creative, and sports events. Many overcome performance anxiety by means of self-hypnosis training. Prophylactic training in this skill is recommended for all children who perform in some way. Books such as Garfield's *Peak Performance* (1984/1985) emphasize the successes of adult athletes in using self-regulation to improve performance. School children may also learn these techniques to maximize their athletic potential. Presently, children in grade schools in Sweden are taught self-regulation techniques in physical education classes as part of the regular school program. With the increased social awareness, popularity, and success of sports psychologist consultants for Olympic and professional athletes and entire teams, universities and even some high school athletic teams similarly have engaged various health professionals to consult with and coach young athletes in self-hypnosis-like techniques. Minimally the expectation with such training is to reduce, eliminate, or prevent performance-interfering stress. Optimally, such strategies might also promote improved performance through, for example, focused imagery of desired outcomes occurring through mechanisms yet to be defined or understood.

Prophylaxis against Drugs and Alcohol Abuse

Studies indicate that children who take prescribed drugs such as aspirin or acetaminophen are more apt to start taking mood-altering or nonmedicinal drugs as adolescents (Olness et al., 1987). Training in self-regulation for pain control and relaxation can not only reduce the requirement for pain medications in young children but can also provide a method of relaxation and stress reduction that may reduce the attraction of mood-altering drugs later on. As one 11-year-old girl said after successfully applying self-hypnosis for elimination of chronic headaches, "It works. It's like *I'm* the medicine. I don't have to take any pills, 'cause the medicine is me" (Kohen, 1987b).

Prophylaxis against Cardiovascular Diseases

In families prone to cardiovascular diseases such as hypertension, it may be prudent to train children in blood pressure regulation early in life. Prospective studies in this area are needed (Porges, Matthews, & Pauls, 1992).

Reduction of Morbidity from Allergies

There are clinical reports and prospective intervention studies that indicate that self-regulation training in children can reduce morbidity with respect to asthma, hives, and eczema (Kohen, 1986c; Kohen & Wynne, 1988). Current research may allow therapists to be more precise in setting up appropriate times and strategies for self-hypnosis practice for children who have allergies.

COST REDUCTION

Existing studies in clinical applications of hypnotherapy in children suggest that one can anticipate a significant reduction in overall health care costs for children who learn and use these techniques (Kohen et al., 1984). The average number of visits for treatment of habit problems is four, and long-term follow-up indicates that relapses are rare. Children with chronic problems such as asthma require fewer emergency room visits. Overall, children who use self-regulation strategies can be expected to require fewer medications, to miss fewer school days, and to make fewer demands on parental time for clinic and hospital visits.

COPING AND HAPPINESS

People who practice self-hypnosis in order to regulate body processes learn that directing one's own thoughts not only brings about rapid physiological responses, but also affects feelings, emotions, attitudes, expectations, and overall perceptions of comfort and satisfaction. Images produce feelings; feelings are preceded by specific thinking patterns. Humans can change their feelings by changing their thoughts. In the past, American children have been taught that a feeling simply "is," that it is good "to express feelings" whether they are angry or happy or sad. This concept can lead to frustration and feelings of helplessness. If children are taught early that feelings can respond to changes in thinking and that they can be controlled, or at least modulated, this provides them with a basic tool for coping and mastery. Indeed, if we can master our thoughts, life becomes easier and happier.

CHAPTER SIXTEEN

Psychoneuroimmunology

In 1979, before the term "psychoneuroimmunology" had appeared in print, we conducted a pilot study of voluntary control of white cell function in five children and six adults. Three of these children, who had prior experience in self-hypnosis, demonstrated changes in neutrophil chemoluminescence in the requested direction. This pilot study stimulated us to continue the difficult research in this area. Because studies of voluntary regulation of other autonomic processes indicate that children achieve such control more quickly than adults, we believe that it is reasonable and important to study voluntary immunoregulation in children. The developing immune system of the child may be particularly responsive to behavioral effects. Early conditioning of the immune system, whether intentional or not, may have profound long-term effects on immune capacity (Schleifer, Scott, Stein, & Keller, 1986).

The number of studies in psychoneuroimmunology, involving both animals and humans, have skyrocketed in the past 5 years. Nonetheless, we still lack a precise definition for the term.

In the first edition of his book *Psychoneuroimmunology,* Dr. Robert Ader did not provide a definition for the title. The nearest he came to a definition was with this sentence: "There is a growing awareness of an intimate and relatively unexplored relationship between the immune system and the central nervous sytem, and an analysis of this relationship might reveal much about the operation of the immune system and the brain" (1981, p. xxi).

Others produced definitions, usually those that implied the existence of intentional immunomodulation by humans, something that was not yet proved. The majority of Ader's first and second editions of *Psychoneuroimmunology* (Ader, 1981, 1991) is devoted to animal experiments. However, in the second edition Ader became a little bolder and more assertive with respect to the relationship between the immune and central nervous systems:

There [are] now abundant data documenting neuroanatomical, neuroendocrine, and neurochemical links to the immune system. . . . The existence of bidirectional pathways of communication between nervous and immune systems provides an experimental foundation for the observation of behavioral and stress-induced influences on immune function and, conversely, the effects of immune processes on behavior. (Ader, 1991, p. xxvi)

CONDITIONING OF IMMUNOSUPPRESSION AND IMMUNOENHANCEMENT

The essence of Ader's exciting discovery was that the linking of a taste stimulus to an immunosuppressive drug, cyclophosphamide, led, after relatively few pairings, to conditioning of the physiological effects of that drug, including immunosuppression. This was a serendipitous discovery in rats. Ader was actually studying a model for conditioned taste aversion that might be relevant for humans who developed taste aversions while undergoing treatment for cancer. There have now been dozens of animal studies that confirm Ader's observations.

Immunoenhancement has also been conditioned in animals. A most impressive study (MacQueen, Marshall, Perdue, Siegel, & Bienenstock, 1989) conditioned rats to effect an immune response—the secretion of rat cell protease II by mucosal mast cells. The original unconditioned stimulus was the injection of egg albumin, which is known to elicit a mast-cell response. The stimuli to be conditioned were flashing lights and the sounds of fans. After only two pairings, the mast-cell response to the flashing lights and sounds of fans was equivalent to that in animals injected with egg albumin on the test trial. Mast cells are recognized as increased and hyperactive in a number of human diseases. It is possible that some mast-cell functions in humans are inadvertently conditioned to environmental stimuli that happen to be concurrent with the presence of an antigen that would ordinarily trigger mast-cell responses. There are numerous reports of urticaria, a mast-cell-mediated phenomonen in humans, that seem conditioned to a sight or sound. Possibly, an inadvertent conditioning occurred in those individuals some time in the past when that sight or sound happened to be paired with an allergen that then triggered mast-cell responses. Shertzer and Lookingbill (1987) reported hypnotherapy as successful in the tretment of urticaria.

I (KO) saw an 11-year-old girl, Cindy, who was unable to participate comfortably in ice skating competition because she developed generalized hives whenever she got on the ice. She had a history of a number of allergies and had previously taken antihistamines but was afraid they might interfere with her ability to skate. Several members of her family had used self-hypnosis successfully for various problems, and she asked about this for herself. I began by teaching Cindy a progressive relaxation exercise while I monitored her peripheral temperature. She was pleased to note that her temperature increased as she became more comfortable. I explained to her the mechanism of hives and told her that mast cells were much less likely to release substances causing hives under conditions of relaxation. I also asked her to think about a control system in her brain that she could use to shut down the mast-cell response when necessary. She thought of a joystick that would move in "on" and "off" directions. I also asked her to imagine skating a favorite routine and enjoying knowledge that her brain sent directions for skating that her muscles and nerves followed perfectly. I asked her to imagine that she had finished a performance, was feeling very comfortable, very pleased with how well she did and delighted that the problem of hives had disappeared. I asked her to practice this exercise at home twice daily and saw her once for review 2 weeks later. In a 1-year follow-up, Cindy had no further problems with hives in connection with ice skating. She said that, on one occasion, she felt a few hives appearing and "I quickly moved the joystick to 'off!' "

It has been demonstrated in several human studies that conditioned immune responses are developed quite easily in humans. For example a study in Germany (Buske-Kirschbaum, Kirschbaum, Stierle, Lehnert, & Hellhammer, 1992) demonstrated this phenomonen in 24 university students. A neutral sherbet was paired four times with a subcutaneous injection of 0.2 mg epinephrine. Subsequently, conditioned subjects showed significantly increased natural killer (NK) cell activity after reexposure to the sherbet alone. A control group in which the sherbet was paired with subcutaneous saline showed no similar increases in NK cell activity. A study of conditioning of anticipatory nausea in women receiving cyclic chemotherapy for ovarian cancer found that they not only demonstrated conditioned nausea but also conditioning of cellular immune responses. Inasmuch as hypnotherapy can facilitate the deconditioning of negative physiological responses (e.g., tachycardia associated with the sight of a dog), it seems reasonable that it can be applied to deconditioning of undesirable immune responses such as those of Cindy.

Pharmacological Conditioning

Ader has extended the principle of conditioned immunosuppression to pharmacological conditioning. His work in lupus-prone mice found that animals could be trained, via pairing of a taste such as chocolate milk or saccharin-flavored water with cyclophosphamide, to elicit a life-lengthening immunosuppression (Ader, 1989); that is, the response to the conditioned stimulus was equivalent to that of the drug. There is one clinical report of application of this principle to treatment of an adolescent female suffering from life-threatening lupus eythematosus (Olness & Ader, 1992). The patient had 2 years of prior experience using self-hypnosis for relief of pain and anxiety related to her disease. Cyclophosphamide was paired with the taste of cod liver oil and a pungent rose perfume over a 3-month period. Subsequently, the cod liver oil and pungent rose perfume were used as the conditioned stimuli once monthly. The patient improved clinically but, after 15 months, refused further cod liver oil because it triggered unpleasant nausea, a side effect of cyclophosphamide. However, she said that she continued to imagine a rose and believed that this image had become a conditioned stimulus for the desirable immunosuppressive effects of cyclophosphamide. It is intriguing to consider that the imagined visual image or smell or taste could be the equivalent of a tangible conditioned stimulus in effecting certain physiological responses. This is an important research area to pursue.

Effects of Stress and Relaxation on Immune Responses

Most of the studies in this area have been done with adults. A recent meta-analytic study on the effects of stress and relaxation on the in vitro immune response in man (Van Rood, Bogaards, Goulmy, & van Houwelingen, 1993) reviewed 24 stress studies and 10 relaxation studies. The weakness of the meta-analysis was that it assumed parity among interventions that were, in fact, very different. For example, some studies included in the "relaxation" group asked subjects to focus on changing specific immune parameters; some asked subjects merely to relax. The two requests are very different. Other studies in this meta-analysis included imagery with relaxation. While authors concluded that there were immunological changes in association with either stressors or relaxation, the confusion about interventions makes the changes difficult to interpret.

The first study in the English language medical literature to ponder an association between stress and the clinical expression of an infectious agent in children was published in 1962 (Meyer & Haggerty, 1962). This article found that children in stressful environments were more likely to have clinical symptoms associated with group A streptococcal infection than were children in less stressful environments.

Boyce and colleagues began a study in 1989 to assess immunological changes that might occur at kindergarten entry (Boyce et al., 1993). Their study protocols focused on individual differences that might mediate responses to stress. Twenty children were enrolled, and blood for immune measures was drawn 1 week before they began kindergarten. Two weeks later, these were repeated. At enrollment, mothers completed a variety of psychometric instruments including problem behaviors, stressful life events, child temperament, and family environment. During the 12-week follow-up period, the incidence, severity, and duration of respiratory illnesses was assessed from parent interviews done every 2 weeks. At 6 weeks, the Loma Prieta earthquake struck the San Francisco area where the study was in process. Therefore, data assessment was divided into two periods, before and after the earthquake. Six weeks following the earthquake, the Child Behavior Checklist (CBL) was readministered along with a Child Earthquake Experience Checklist, and a Parent Earthquake Impact Scale.

For the three immune measures — the helper: suppressor ratio, pokeweed mitogenesis, and antibody responses to Pneumovax — there was broad variability in change scores. This was also true for respiratory illness incidence. Up-regulation of either helper: suppressor ratio and pokeweed mitogenesis was associated with increased respiratory illness incidence following the earthquake. Change in behavior problems was significantly related to scores from the Parent Impact Scale and inversely associated with pokeweed mitogenesis, that is, high earthquake-related parental distress and low immune reactivity were predictive of an increase in parent-reported problem behaviors. With low parental distress, neither highly nor minimally reactive children experienced a marked change in respiratory illness incidence. By contrast, under conditions of high parental distress, highly reactive children showed a marked increase in illness while minimally reactive children showed a decrease.

Boyce believes that the health effects of psychologically stressful events are best predicted by an interaction between the intensity of environmental stressors and the biological reactivity of the individual host. Only a subset of children within any given population are truly at risk under environmental stress and adversity. Past studies using hypnotic interventions for a variety of problems have not considered the variables of biological reactivity and intensity of environmental stressors. This failure may explain results that are variable or inconsistent as reflected in existing studies of intentional immunomodulation by humans.

Is There Evidence for Intentional Immunomodulation by Humans?

The short answer to this question is yes, but qualified, because most reported studies are essentially laboratory studies in normal humans. Clinical implications are not yet clear. Although there are more than 30 reported studies in the English language, most are studies of adults (Beahrs, Harris, & Hilgard, 1970; Black, Humphrey, & Niven, 1963; Halley, 1991; Kiecolt-Glaser, Glaser, Stain, & Stout, 1985; Locke et al., 1994; G. R. Smith, McKenzie, Marmer, & Steele, 1985). Many of these studies relate to the impact of hypnotherapy on delayed cutaneous hypersensitivity responses. The recent study by Locke and colleagues (1994) is an example. They studied 24 college students, selected for their high hypnotizability and ability to change skin temperature with hypnotic suggestions. Students were assigned randomly to undergo a pre-determined sequence of four different experimental conditions with each condition including varicella (VZ) skin testing: (1) hypnosis with suggestions to enhance the delayed type hypersensitivity (DTH) response to VZ antigen; (2) hypnosis with suggestions to suppress the DTH response; (3) hypnosis with suggestions for relaxation only; and (4) skin testing without hypnosis. They found no significant effects on the area of the DTH response. Limitations of the study included use of a standardized script and induction technique, hypnotic suggestions given after injection of the antigen, and the assumption that high hypnotizability and skin temperature changes were predictors for success. There were individuals who achieved changes in the suggested directions, and these should be studied carefully to guide experimental methods in future studies of intentional immunomodulation.

Intentional Immunomodulation in Children

In a prospective, controlled study with 57 children, ages 6 to 12 years, children who were assigned randomly to a 30-minute self-hypnosis practice associated with specific instructions to increase salivary immunoglobulin A (SIgA) demonstrated significant increases in SIgA compared to attention controls and to children who practiced the relaxation only (Olness, Culbert, & Uden, 1989). The children were seen twice, once for a baseline collection of saliva and to watch a puppet video that explained the immune system, and once for the experimental intervention. There was no significant increase in immunoglobulin G within or across groups. There was no correlation with outcome and performance on the Stanford Children's Hypnotic Susceptibility Scale.

Barbara Hewson Bower (1995) has replicated our work that demonstrated SIgA increases in children who practiced relaxation and imagery. She has taken this information into the clinical arena in an exceptionally complex and excellent thesis study of children with recurrent upper respiratory infections and a waiting-list control group. She taught one group relaxation and imagery techniques focused on increasing SIgA and a second group relaxation and imagery techniques, problem solving, and coping skills. Both interventions were equally effective in reducing the number of days of upper respiratory illness in children with recurrent infection problems in comparison to the control group.

Hewson Bower then did a follow-up study that combined the two treatments described above. Combination treatment resulted in reduced days of upper respiratory illness in children with a history of recurrent colds and flu (both within subjects compared to a pre-treatment baseline and cross-sectionally with a matched control group). Twelve-month follow-up indicated that treatment gains persisted for days of illness. Hewson Bower included psychometric assessments of subjects and families as well.

We have also conducted controlled prospective studies of intentional modulation of neutrophils in 45 adolescents who were assigned randomly to one of three groups. Group A (the control group) had blood samples taken before and after a rest condition for two sessions spaced 1 week apart. Peripheral temperature and pulse recordings were also taken before and after the rest intervention. Group B (the untrained experimental group) had blood, peripheral temperature, and pulse recordings taken before and after a self-regulation exercise with imagery focused on increasing neutrophil adherence, a measure of white-cell function. Group C was an experimental group that received four training sessions prior to their attempts to increase neutrophil adherence. The immunology results from this study revealed that neither the control group A nor the untrained experimental group B demonstrated increased neutrophil adherence in either session. Only the experimental group that received prior self-hypnosis training demonstrated a statistically significant increase in neutrophil adherence for the second session. These studies were conducted in a clinical research center with controls for time of day, no prior experience with hypnosis, and no immunological disorders. There were no changes in total numbers of neutrophils or chemiluminesence but only in the specific parameter they had been asked to change (Hall et al., 1992). Although practice of a self-hypnosis exercise was associated with success, the most successful subjects did not demonstrate physiological evidence of relaxation, whereas the "resting group" did (Hall, Minnes, & Olness, 1993). This suggests that some cognitive effort is associated with intentional changes in neutrophil adherence. The control group, who simply rested, did demonstrate physiological evidence of relaxation. The amount and type of practice related to outcomes in these studies as is true of other cyberphysiologic studies, especially with adolescents and adults. Young children learn quickly and seem to require less practice to achieve success.

Warts

There are numerous clinical reports about warts remitting in association with nonpharmacological treatments including hypnotherapy (Noll, 1994; Tasini & Hackett, 1977; Spanos, Stenstrom, & Johnston, 1988). We have had many clinical experiences similar to the one we describe here.

Andy, a 10-year-old boy, had a total of 27 warts on both hands, his right arm, and abdomen. They had been present for 2 years, and he had been seen by his pediatrician and dermatologists who had prescribed topical therapy followed by cryotherapy. Some of the warts would get smaller for a period and then grow to a larger size. Andy had no prior experience with hypnosis and was intrigued with the possibility that he could make his warts disappear. He and his mother completed a questionnaire about his likes, interests, skills, fears, and imagery. He was a good student, was taking piano lessons, and enjoyed basketball, his favorite sport.

During the first hypnotherapeutic session, I monitored his peripheral temperature, electrodermal activity, and heart rate in order to document for him that changes in thinking could effect physiological changes. He noted that the lines on the computer screen that reflected his heart rate and electrodermal activity jumped immediately when he thought of something exciting. I suggested he begin his hypnosis training by imagining himself standing at the free-throw line and shooting a free throw with great ease. He could note the connections between his brain and muscles that are involved in throwing the basketball and enjoy imagining the basketball swishing through the net. I asked him to repeat this 10 times and then to imagine himself in a comfortable place, enjoying the feeling of having done so well with the free throws. I asked him to lift a "yes" finger when he was in a comfortable place. Within 2 minutes, Andy lifted his right index finger. I said,

> "You're doing very well. I can tell by the monitor. Your temperature has gone up, and your heart rate has gone down. That means you're comfortable and relaxed. Now when you are so comfortable, it's a good time to program your body to get rid of the warts. So, when you're ready, very easily, just once, tell yourself to stop feeding the warts on your hands, stop feeding the warts on your arm, and stop feeding the warts on your abdomen. And, when you have told yourself that, continue to enjoy your comfortable, pleasant place in your imagination a little while longer, and when you're ready, slowly and easily, you can open your eyes and enjoy the rest of today."

After Andy opened his eyes I asked if he had questions and asked if he would practice this exercise twice a day at home. I reminded him that he could telephone me if he had additional questions and that I would review with him in 2 weeks.

When he returned in 2 weeks there were only 10 warts left, and they were much smaller. He called a month later to report they were gone. There was no recurrence in a 1-year follow-up.

We have recently completed a 4-year consortium study of nonpharmacological management of warts (Felt et al., 1994). This involved collaboration of seven institutions. Children between ages of 6 and 12 years who had warts on their hands and arms were randomized to topical or self-hypnosis or attention-control treatment in management of warts. Each child completed a questionnaire related to likes, dislikes, interests, preferred imagery, and activities. Each child saw a video that explained about warts. Children also chose a "signal" wart that would be photographed and measured over the course of the study. Each child was seen four times over a 3-month period and followed over an additional 6 months. Signal warts were photographed at each visit. Children in the hypnotherapy group were taught a standardized self-hypnosis exercise. Group data analysis found no significant differences among groups, although there was evidence of wart regression in each group. Some children in the hypnotherapy group had dramatic wart regression. Data analysis is continuing to determine whether or not intrinsic skills in mental imagery, and/or frequency of self-hypnosis practice are significant factors in how children responded to treatment. This study was limited by the need to use a standardized method of self-hypnosis and the large amount of attention paid to warts, for example, photographing warts, in all groups.

Lewis Thomas (1979) wrote, "We will understand more about tumors if we could understand what goes away and in what order when warts are hypnotized away." We are still a long way from that ideal.

THE FUTURE IN
PEDIATRIC PSYCHONEUROIMMUNOLOGY

This is an exciting and important area. Although it is too early to make definitive statements about the clinical applications of research described in this chapter, there is merit in encouraging the pure laboratory group, the pure clinical group, and the mixed group of researchers to move forward concurrently. This has happened in other areas of medical science in which medications were used long before their mechnisms of action were clear.

From designing many protocols over the years, we recognize that conventional protocol design does not lend itself easily to cyberphysiologic interventions. Protocol review committees prefer that interventions are "constant and equal" for each child, yet we know that intrinsic thinking processes, imagery preferences, and learning styles vary (Olness, 1990a). As noted in the research of Boyce et al. (1993), there are also intrinsic differences in immunological reactivity. By using the same coaching for each subject in a study, we ensure some failures. Data analysis of the Children's Cancer Study Group (CCSG) assumes that children in the study received the same intervention, that is, medication dictated by the protocol. But clinicians who work with these children are aware that, depending on the personality of the child and the innate persuasion skills of physicians, nurses, or parents, some medications reach the alimentary tract of the child and some go under the mattress or into the toilet bowl. The same principle applies in training for self-hypnosis. Clinically, we observe that coaching that varies according to developmental state, interests, and learning style of a given child results in more predictable receipt of the intervention.

Research protocols should consider:

Quality and quantity of behavioral interventions
Amount and type of self-hypnosis practice if required
Quality and quantity of antigenic stimulation
Temporal relationship between behavioral and antigenic stimulation
Nature of the immune response
Host factors such as age, sex, genes, intrinsic immune reactivity, sleep requirements, diet, and life experiences
Chronobiological factors

It is also important that the possibility of inadvertent conditioning of immune responses be kept in mind and that researchers should follow children over long time periods.

Solomon (1993) has stated his thesis that psychoneuroimmunology represents a conceptual breakthrough that offers the opportunity to approach the body, in health and sickness, from a new theoretical perspective.

It is tempting to speculate about how voluntary immunomodulation might occur in children. Persinger (1987) has noted that any condition that enhances temporal lobe lability will increase recruitment of immune processes. Children have enhanced temporal lobe lability especially during the school-age years (Carey & Diamond, 1980). Of relevance to the voluntary control of immune processes is the interaction between the cerebral cortex and hippocampus. The hippocampus provides access to the imagery of memory presumably stored in the cortex. In children, the typical adult distinction between the imagery of memory and the imagery of experience is less clear (Kail, 1984). As a result, the use of verbal instructions can induce imagery as strong as emotional memories. This is documented in the physiological changes noted when children are encouraged to think in different ways (Lee & Olness, 1995). The capacity of children to show enhanced voluntary control of immune regulation through programmed imagining (suggestion) would be facilitated by the interdependence of imagination and memory (Persinger & De Sano, 1986).

Some practical questions that derive from research done in the area of psychoneuroimmunology are in clinical areas:

1. What stressors may predispose to streptococcal infections?
2. What stressors trigger recurrent herpes? Can their efforts be reversed via training in self-hypnosis?
3. Will anticipatory guidance for families include information about how parental distress impacts on the immune responses of their children?

Will we be able to recommend self-hypnosis practice for both children and parents to prevent undesirable immune responses?
4. How might immunosuppression or immunoenhancement be conditioned inadvertently in children? How could this be reversed?
5. How does winning (or losing) impact on immunity?
6. Is nonpharmacological treatment of warts less expensive than pharmacological treatment?

In all this we must resist the temptation to overstate clinical applications of psychoneuroimmunology research by making claims that are not grounded in sound data (Solomon, 1993).

CHAPTER SEVENTEEN

Teaching Child Hypnotherapy

The greatest of teachers, when his work is all done, the people (children) all say, "We have done it ourselves."
— OLD CHINESE PROVERB

In 1987 we were privileged to provide what we believe was one of the first Introductory Pediatric Hypnosis Workshops as part of the annual meeting of the Society for Behavioral Pediatrics (now the Society for Developmental and Behavioral Pediatrics [SDBP]), at the Disneyland Hotel in Anaheim, California. Disneyland seemed an especially appropriate place to promote the value of imagination to the healthy lives of children; and the workshop received excellent evaluations. Since then it has become a regular feature of the annual meeting of the SDBP. By the second year, 1988, we were asked to provide an "Intermediate"-level workshop training for those who had participated in the previous year's Introductory course and wanted to learn more. These companion workshops have continued; and at the 1994 annual meeting in Minneapolis, we added an "Advanced" Workshop for the first time. Over 60 child health professionals participated in the 1994 training; and over 250 have taken the SDBP hypnosis workshops since their inception in 1987.

WHY TEACH CHILD HYPNOTHERAPY?

As reflected in our review of the literature, in discussion of our and others' clinical experiences, and in our considerations and recommendations in this narrative, we have an abiding belief in the value of training children in cyberphysiologic strategies. Perhaps our only greater faith is in children themselves, in their intrinsic worth, their unabashed curiosity, their often

345

apparently limitless energy, and their potential. As childhood and adolescence are journeys toward mastery, and as relaxation/mental imagery (RMI), and self-hypnosis facilitate mastery, they are natural partners. And so we believe that all children ultimately should have the opportunity to learn these techniques so that they may apply them to foster their healthy growth and development and the realization of their potential. To continue to reach toward this dream, we have come to believe that hypnotherapy, like other diagnostic and therapeutic skills, should be part of the armamentarium of all health care professionals who work with children. Toward this end we began working with and teaching hypnosis skills to various child health professionals more than 20 years ago (Olness, 1977c).

WHO ARE THE LEARNERS?

Beyond our child patients and their parents, those to whom we have taught child hypnosis represent an ever-widening spectrum of those who provide health and illness care for children and their families. In Table 17.1, we note the spectrum of child physicians who have over the years sought our assistance with their patients and/or have availed themselves of training in clinical hypnosis either to better understand and facilitate our consultative efforts, or to employ clinical strategies themselves in integrating hypnosis into their practices. In Table 17.2, we note the variety of other child health care providers who have referred patients and/or sought training in pediatric hypnosis and hypnotherapy for the children and families with whom they work.

HISTORICAL PERSPECTIVES

We began many years ago teaching RMI skills to nurses on the inpatient units of a children's hospital (then Minneapolis Children's Health Center/Minne-

---

TABLE 17.1. Physicians Referring Patients for Child Hypnosis

Pediatricians	Pediatric surgeons
Pediatric subspecialists	General pediatric surgeons
Behavioral/developmental pediatricians	Orthopedists
Pediatric neurologists	Urologists
Pediatric gastroenterologists	Ophthalmologists
Pediatric pulmonologists	Ear, nose, and throat specialists
Pediatric intensivists	Family physicians
Pediatric emergency room physicians	Emergency room/urgent care physicians
Pediatric hematologists/oncologists	Child and adolescent psychiatrists
Pediatric nephrologists	Physical medicine and rehabilitation
Pediatric rheumatologists	specialists (physiatrists)
Allergists/immunologists	

TABLE 17.2. Child Health Professionals Seeking Training in Hypnosis/Hypnotherapy

Pediatric nurses
Pediatric nurse practitioners/associates
School nurses
Child psychologists (including school psychologists)
Clinical social workers (including school social workers)
Marital and family therapists
Occupational therapists
Physical therapists
Respiratory therapists
Child life specialists
Speech pathologists
Clergy (e.g., hospital chaplains)
Educators

apolis Children's Medical Center, now Children's Health Care–Minneapolis). As a natural extension of our work with individual children, nurses learned techniques to facilitate and reinforce what the children had been taught. Their greater and in some ways more natural accessibility to the children made this a "perfect fit"; and in the process, most nurses discovered that they were not as much learning new techniques as they were defining a structure and a nomenclature into which to fit and expand their natural orientation to caring, positive expectancies and flexibility to find the right words and strategy to meet the special or particular needs of a given child in a given predicament.

In the late 1970s and early 1980s, we extended our teaching and involvement of nursing personnel to the ambulatory setting and primarily to the emergency room, with specific workshop/seminar training for emergency room nursing staff. Challenged with the immediacy and urgency of saying and doing the things that will help the acutely ill and injured and highly stressed child (and family), nurses and other emergency department personnel focused on the special circumstances of hypnosis in emergencies (see Chapter 12; Kohen, 1986b).

Also beginning in the late 1970s, for 10 years we hosted a weekly hypnosis seminar for practitioners of clinical hypnosis. This Tuesday afternoon 4:30–5:30 P.M. slot provided a welcome ending to a day to which all participants looked forward. As an ongoing interdisciplinary "mutual supervision" group, it provided a forum for discussion of difficult cases (not limited to child hypnosis), an opportunity for sharing information learned from a recent conference or seminar, a safe proving ground for new ideas, a review of interesting articles or books, and an opportunity for group self-hypnosis practice for comfort, relaxation, and positive reinforcement. We have recently started similar monthly groups at the University of Minnesota and at Case Western Reserve University and strongly recommend this process for the values noted.

During the 1970s and 1980s while the interest and demand for education in clinical hypnosis grew nationally, and while regional American Society of Clinical Hypnosis (ASCH) Workshops and national ASCH and Society for Clinical and Experimental Hypnosis (SCEH) Workshops experienced increasing popularity, attention to the uniqueness of child hypnotherapy was inconsistent. While individual activism on national committees and organizational lobbying succeeded in including teaching in child hypnosis for Intermediate and Advanced Workshops, there was less success in consistently integrating training in child hypnosis to Introductory Workshops in Clinical Hypnosis. On a regional level, a 1- to 1½-hour presentation on child hypnosis and hypnotherapy has been a part of the University of Minnesota/Minnesota Society of Clinical Hypnosis Introductory course since the 1970s. This has not been true in consistent fashion either for Regional or National ASCH or SCEH workshops. The recently published Standards of Training in Clinical Hypnosis (Hammond & Elkins, 1994) note no requirement for training in child hypnosis other than to recommend that students in an Introductory course be made aware of the above-average hypnotizability of children from 9 to 12 years of age and of the Stanford Hypnotic Clinical Scale for Children.

It is also noted by contrast, however, that ASCH, SCEH, and the International Society of Hypnosis (ISH) have for the past 15 to 20 years provided opportunities in their Advanced Workshops for the presentation of "Advanced Pediatric Hypnosis" Workshops. Over the past 20 years, we have been privileged to teach in these workshops with an ever-growing number of pediatric, behavioral pediatric, and psychology colleagues.* Though this forum has been unique and commonly has attracted clinicians interested specifically in children, it has also been an immense challenge, as often participants represent a wide spectrum of prior knowledge and experience in child hypnosis. More often than not, however, most participants have been those who have had introductory and/or additional general clinical hypnosis training, and have clinical practices (medicine, psychology, dentistry) with a large per-

---

*We wish to acknowledge and honor our many colleagues with whom we have taught and learned over the years and to whom continuing learners can and should turn for information about continued research and additional workshop training. We have utilized our best self-hypnotic memories to include everyone and hope that anyone inadvertently left out will understand and forgive any unintended omission. We hope others have the opportunity to meet and learn from the writing and teaching of Franz Baumann, Gail Gardner (deceased), Stuart Anderson, William Cohen, Tim Culbert, Brooks Donald, Gary Elkins, Candace Erickson, Deb Fanurick, Bill Friedrich, Rebecca Kajander, Leora Kuttner, Linn LaClave, Sam LeBaron, Julie Linden, Clorinda Margolis, Anne McComb, Siegfried Mrochen, Don O'Grady (deceased), Lynne Powers, Jud Reaney, Judith Rhue, Mark Smith, Valerie Wall, Jim Warnke, Bill Wester, Graham Wicks, Elaine Wynne, Marty Young, and Lonnie Zeltzer.

centage of children; but they have had *no prior specific training in child hypnosis*. Such "Advanced Pediatric Hypnosis" workshops have often become, accordingly, very basic and quite introductory in nature.

These experiences led us to develop child clinician-specific training in clinical hypnosis, initially building on our knowledge and experience with general hypnosis workshop training and our training with hospital personnel.

In 1979, we taught an informational and descriptive 2-hour workshop on Pediatric Hypnosis at the Annual Meeting of the Ambulatory Pediatric Association (APA) (Atlanta, GA). We believe that this was the first such workshop to be taught as part of a major national pediatric meeting. A reprise of the same workshop was taught the following year at the APA Meeting in San Antonio, and similar workshops were taught by Dr. Olness at two annual meetings of the American Academy of Pediatrics.

In 1987, we were asked by the Child Life Staff and Hematology–Oncology Nursing staff of St. Paul Children's Hospital (now Children's Health Care–St. Paul) to provide training in pediatric clinical hypnosis specific to their needs. A 14-hour workshop/seminar was developed that we presented over 5 days (4 hours on Monday and Friday, and 2 hours each on Tuesday through Thursday), built into which was a commitment to provide ongoing supervision and review for 1 to 2 hours monthly. The success of that workshop training has been beyond our wildest dreams—monthly supervision (one morning a month for 1½ hours) has continued uninterrupted for the past 8 years.

CREATING AN INTEREST IN LEARNING

As we have utilized hypnotherapeutic strategies with our patients and observed what children are capable of doing and achieving via these strategies, we have resolved to bring this to the awareness of other professionals. Professionals with whom we have had contact have become aware of hypnosis and its potential value for children in a variety of ways, leading (some of) them to pursue further and formal training in pediatric hypnosis and hypnotherapy.

1. Medical students, pediatric residents, and family practice residents have observed us working with hypnosis with individual children patients as part of general pediatric learning rotations in our respective hospital inpatient or outpatient settings. Thus, by "accident" they may have witnessed hypnosis with a patient in the emergency room with an acute episode of asthma, an adolescent using hypnosis to help endure another bone marrow examination, a child practicing self-hypnosis for enuresis, or any of a myriad of other situations. Medical students at Case Western Reserve University have

the opportunity to choose an elective in clinical hypnosis, a course offering which is always full!

2. Pediatric residents (since 1988) on a obligatory month rotation in behavioral pediatrics have sat in with us during many sessions of pediatric hypnosis with a variety of patients and have also viewed videotapes of hypnotherapeutic interventions.

3. Pediatric and family practice residents as well as practicing clinicians have had the opportunity to do an "elective in pediatric hypnotherapy" at our respective institutions since 1977. These are usually limited to those who have already had Introductory workshop training in clinical hypnosis. One or two residents per year avail themselves of these opportunities.

4. Clinicians have had their interest piqued by the presentation of a "case conference" of one or several children who have benefited from hypnotherapy, and/or from a pediatric grand rounds describing clinical and/or research efforts in pediatric hypnosis.

5. Others have read reports of clinical cases or research, or review articles about applications of hypnosis in various mainstream pediatric journals.

6. Other professionals have had their curiosity and interest aroused by inquiries or urgings for information from their patients/families who either have heard of hypnosis or related self-regulation strategies helping someone they knew or have seen something in the media, which is once again arousing an interest in "alternative therapies" (Coleman & Gupin, 1993; Moyers, 1993).

A RECOMMENDED PLAN OF STUDY IN CHILD HYPNOSIS AND HYPNOTHERAPY

Just as we believe that there are many right ways—not merely one or two—to effectively do most things, we have also come to believe that certain approaches to learning child hypnosis and hypnotherapy seem to work. And so we commend them to the reader and clinician for consideration.

Education Theory

Unfortunately, the majority of child health professionals have not had formal training in educational theory. Most tend to teach by emulating teachers and educational processes that they themselves have experienced. Prior to planning an educational program, the professional should consider several important points:

1. Education derives from the Latin, *educere,* meaning to bring forth. Our task is to stimulate the learner, to encourage the learner, but not to cram in facts without attention to solid and tested principles of learning. This is especially true with respect to adult learners.

2. Who is the learner? How does he or she learn? There is much individual variability in learning styles. Some people learn best by watching, others by reading, some by listening, and still others by doing. When possible, the teacher should consider his or her own learning styles and ask about those of the students.

3. What are the overall goals for the educational experience? An example of a goal would be, "To increase the number of child health professionals who are knowledgeable regarding child hypnotherapy." A lesser goal but one that is often present is for the teacher "To gain experience as an educator in hypnotherapy."

4. What are the specific objectives for components of the program? The teacher must indicate these. An example would be, "The participant will be able to induce self-hypnosis easily."

5. What are the means of implementing the objectives? An example would be, "Each participant must have the opportunity to practice coaching eight colleagues into and through a hypnotic state." The teacher must consider what types of technical support will facilitate implementation of objectives, for example, slide projector, video examples, and so forth.

6. How will you know if you have achieved your goals and objectives? There must be an evaluation plan. These can be simple or detailed, but they must be reviewed and heeded. We believe such evaluations are most useful when they are bilateral. Thus, learners should receive feedback evaluation from teachers, for example, of how well they conduct a hypnotic induction and what language works well and what does not. And, teachers receive feedback from learners about all aspects of the teaching experience, from whether objectives have been met, to evaluation of the milieu, the handout materials, the technical support, and the style, demeanor, and attitude of the teacher. These are what lead ultimately to improved programs and improved teaching skills.

Ultimately the children are our best teachers, and we are at our best as teachers when we let our students and colleagues know that—and know how to learn from the children. As we work with them, our learning comes from their feedback: that is, asking them, "What works?" "What did you like the most?" "What helps?" "What did I say or do that you didn't like or didn't help you help yourself?" The best comes, therefore, from "doing," from making notes of how the process unfolded (written, mental, audiotaped, or videotaped notes) and then reviewing and discussing them, with our patients, our colleagues, our students, and our mentors.

Finally, the teacher must keep in mind an old Chinese saying, "The greatest of teachers, when his work is all done, the people all say, 'We have done it ourselves.' " Indeed that represents true success as a teacher.

Introductory Learning

Introductory learning in pediatric hypnosis should be in the context of a 3-day workshop either first in general clinical hypnosis and followed within 2 to 3 months by a 3-day workshop in pediatric hypnosis, or, preferably, first by a 3-day workshop in pediatric clinical hypnosis. Although we have known colleagues over the years who have learned in other formats, we believe that this approach provides the most effective beginning. As distinguished from a 10-week university course or an apprenticeship learning opportunity, the 3-day intensive workshop training model* affords the following advantages:

1. Curricular-based training over a specified period of time (3 days) with focused concentration
2. Exposure to several different, experienced faculty educators (representing behavioral and developmental pediatrics, pediatric psychology, pediatric social work, and pediatric nursing)
3. Opportunity for learning through a variety of proven educational experiences: didactic presentations, demonstrations (of hypnotic inductions, phenomena, techniques, language), modeling (by different faculty), videotape demonstrations, and small group practice sessions with supervision
4. Freedom (temporarily!) from distraction (other coursework, daily work, etc.)
5. Opportunity for informal learning, questions and answers, during "noninstructional" break time

The content of such an Introductory Workshop is reflected in the schedule of our 3-day SDBP Introductory Workshop, presented in Table 17.3.

Intermediate/Advanced/Continuing Learning in Pediatric Hypnotherapy

Some years ago, one of us (KO) developed a set of slides to focus the end of an introductory lecture and/or course in pediatric hypnosis as a guide for further learning. These form the outline of what we here present as a *menu of options* for ongoing training/(self-)education in pediatric hypnosis/hypnotherapy.

---

*Modeled after the SDBP Pediatric Clinical Hypnosis Workshop. Information available from the Society.

TABLE 17.3. **Introductory Workshop in Pediatric Clinical Hypnosis**

Day 1

8:00–8:30	Registration/continental breakfast and socialization
8:30–9:45	Introduction to hypnosis: Basic concepts—definition, history, theories, myths, and misconceptions
9:45–10:00	Break
10:00–10:45	Principles of induction of hypnosis: Induction demonstrations, presenting hypnosis to the patient
10:45–12:15	Small group practice (4–6 learners per faculty)
12:15–1:45	Lunch
1:45–2:45	Developmental issues and considerations
2:45–3:45	Videotapes of inductions—age and developmental variations
3:45–4:00	Break
4:00–5:30	Small group practice (4–6 learners per faculty)

Day 2

8:00–8:30	Continental breakfast/informal learning
8:30–9:30	Hypnosis: Application to anxiety
9:30–10:30	Preschool children: Hypnotic techniques and application to pain management in preschool children
10:30–10:45	Break
10:45–12:15	Small group practice (4–6 learners per faculty)
12:15–1:45	Lunch
1:45–3:00	Hypnosis for procedural and recurrent pain problems in older children and adolescents
3:00–3:45	Management of acute pain with hypnotic strategies
3:45–4:00	Break
4:00–5:30	Small group practice (4–6 learners per faculty)

Day 3

8:00–8:30	Continental breakfast/informal consultation with faculty
8:30–9:30	Hypnosis for common pediatric problems: Asthma, tics
9:30–9:45	Break
9:45–10:45	Hypnosis for common pediatric problems: Enuresis, encopresis, attentional disorders (e.g., ADHD)
10:45–12:15	Small group practice (4–6 learners per faculty)
12:15–1:45	Lunch
1:45–2:45	Physiological control with hypnosis
2:45–4:15	Small group practice (4–6 learners per faculty)
4:15–4:30	Break
4:30–5:15	Therapeutic dilemmas/questions and discussion
5:15–5:30	Wrap-up, evaluations, organizations, future study

1. After taking an introductory workshop, professionals should take a follow-up course no later than 3 to 6 months later. This could either be a second introductory course in pediatric hypnotherapy for the learner who desires additional opportunities for supervised small group practice, or an intermediate-level training such as available through the SDBP or as 1 to 2 workshops through ASCH. We also recommend that child health clinicians have solid grounding in adult hypnosis in order to be able to competently respond to questions about hypnosis from parents and other adults. Such training, available through ASCH, SCEH, or regional organizations such as the Minnesota Society of Clinical Hypnosis, could be taken either before or after an introductory child hypnosis course.

2. Practice the *personal use* of self-hypnosis daily for 2 to 3 months for relaxation, stress reduction, or some other personal need. We believe that such a personal experience with hypnosis affords the clinician an intimate understanding of its phenomenology and that this leads to greater effectiveness in presenting hypnosis to his or her patients.

3. Begin working with hypnosis in one or two specific areas, making sure they are areas in which the clinician is already comfortable and confident, if not expert, with the usual applicable diagnostic and therapeutic approaches.

4. Be certain — especially as psychotherapists — that the patient has had the usual / necessary diagnostic studies for their problem(s), especially if that patient is being referred expressly for hypnosis. This is critical in order to reduce or to avoid missed or misdiagnoses (Olness & Libbey, 1987).

5. Assess the patient's willingness to practice self-hypnosis (most patients / clients who don't or won't practice are still holding a belief that the change or ability for it somehow resides in their idealized or fantasized view of "the all-powerful therapist." It is, in turn, usually an unproductive and unsatisfying trap to buy into their fantasy that they need only "do it" (hypnosis) when they come to the office, and you "do it" to or for them.

6. Consider audiotaping and/or videotaping your work to analyze yourself. (See also #12.)

7. Consider using approaches, language style, and so forth, that take into account the patient's personality, interests, learning style, fears, knowledge, and experience.

8. Consider the family's knowledge, interest, and support, and with the patient agree whether they will or will not be involved, for example, in reminders to practice self-hypnosis.

9. *Be flexible and creative* — remember to ask the patient what was helpful and not helpful.

10. *Be permissive* — do not try to force ideas or imagery.

11. If uncertain how to proceed . . . call or ask a colleague for help as in any diagnostic and/or therapeutic enigma or dilemma.

12. Become involved in ongoing continuing education opportunities in hypnosis, both adult and pediatric.

The following sections focus on the variety of learning/teaching experiences in which we have been involved and found to be meaningful for us as educators and learners and for those working with and learning from us. Each methodology or forum is described and discussed briefly:

Independent Learning

Reading and reviewing videotapes and audiotapes of pediatric hypnotherapy are mainstays in providing ongoing information and stimulating our creativity. We believe we should all do this to complement and supplement our lifelong learning from our patients and other sources.

Independent Learning with a Mentor

Borrowed from our psychology colleagues, the methodology of Supervision or Clinical Supervision has seemed very well suited to pediatric hypnosis. As have our colleagues, we have conducted such experiences with many different kinds of learners, including nurse practitioners, pediatric residents, Fellows in behavioral pediatrics, practicing clinicians on "mini-Fellowships," and practicing clinical psychologists. Though they vary in specifics, common features of this very personal learning include:

1. *Long-term learning.* Commonly such supervision takes place over several months' time, often on a ½-day or 1-day per week basis.
2. *Individual patient/client care review/supervision.* Usually the learner is engaged in working with a patient or patients with hypnosis, and that process of diagnostic evaluation, treatment-plan evolution, and ongoing implementation of hypnotherapy is reviewed in step-by-step methodical fashion with one's mentor. For learning hypnosis, this process has the advantage of having the opportunity for precise review of process, language utilized, pacing/timing, and formulation of indirect and direct and formal and informal hypnotic behavior and suggestions through use and review of audiotapes or videotapes of patient encounters. This teaching is also beneficial to the mentor.

Group Supervision with a Mentor

Such arrangements allow for both personal and more diversified learning by bringing the perspective of several learners to a group, varying the types of problems encountered and discussed, and inevitably, encouraging more discussion and debate. It also tends to be more economically feasible. Such groups often meet monthly.

Group Mutual Supervision

These ongoing "study groups" or "seminars" have the advantage of bringing together professionals from different disciplines (e.g., pediatricians, nurse practitioners, social workers, nurses, psychologists, etc.) who are also at different stages in their own professional learning, expertise, comfort, and knowledge about hypnosis and hypnotherapy with children. Thus, rather than one "expert" teacher with many novices, the group becomes one of many teachers teaching one another, sharing responsibility from session to session for leadership, and perhaps for content, and style as well.

TEACHING TECHNIQUES, STRATEGIES, STYLES

In hypnosis as in any discipline, the nature, style, and strategy for effective teaching varies appropriately from teacher to teacher; and with the same teacher, from milieu to milieu and perhaps even from student to student. Approaches and strategies that seem to have served us best in the ongoing teaching of child hypnosis methodology beyond the introductory level include:

1. *Didactic presentations.* Such presentations should be brief, for example, 20 to 30 minutes, and be utilized primarily to introduce new ideas or material, such as application of hypnosis to an area not previously described, to present results of pediatric hypnosis research, or to offer case report examples and/or demonstrations as triggers for discussion and/or brainstorming.

2. *Small group practice and/or role-playing of specific case management.* We have found it very useful during intermediate and advanced workshops to prepare a series of five to seven case vignettes of common behavioral and/or medical pediatric problems with "trigger questions" for group consideration. Typically these might take the form of "A 7-year-old boy is brought by his parents for help with primary nocturnal enuresis. He is dry at night only once or twice a month, and parents are wondering what to do. Can hypnosis help him? How would you proceed? What would you say?" Or "A 12-year-old girl has had recurrent abdominal pain and occasional vomiting off and on for 4 years. She has had a negative evaluation by a pediatric gastroenterologist and now is missing more school. The problem seemed to get worse when she started junior high school. Is hypnosis appropriate? How

would you introduce it? What techniques might be effective?" With a mentor present to facilitate the discussion, the participants of a small group (four to six participants) would be encouraged to respond to these or other trigger cases, either through discussion, or through role playing of the case example. In the case of role playing and "doing" the recommended approach, the learning then resembles an advanced version of "small group practice" in which the clinician and subject—albeit in a role-playing situation—discuss the hypnotic experience after a 5- to 7-minute "practice," then additional members of the group are solicited for their impressions, and, finally, the mentor gets the proverbial "last word" before the group moves on to another case discussion/example, or another "practice pair." Commonly this evolves into discussion of one's own patients and dilemmas. Learners almost always give such experiences/opportunities high marks in feedback evaluations and discussions.

3. *Group review of videotape examples of hypnotic work.* This is a particularly effective technique especially when the teacher has previewed and/or edited the video(s) to allow for focus on and discussion of specific teaching points of various "teachable moments." These might include specific language used, pacing demonstrated, spontaneous hypnotic behavior before any "official" or "formal" induction, various hypnotic phenomena during trance, or the nature and structure of hypnotic suggestions.

4. *Individual review of videotape examples of individual's hypnotic work.* This form of supervised advanced learning is often the most powerful and important for many professionals. Though it seems on the surface to require a modicum of courage and self-confidence from a professional new to hypnosis to be willing to videotape his or her work with his or her new-found skill, at the same time it carries with it the strong promise of the highly positive reward of honest critique and feedback from experienced clinician(s)/teacher(s). Review of an individual's videotaped interview, preparation for hypnosis, and hypnotherapeutic intervention is an important, time- and labor-intensive endeavor with valuable outcomes. Such interactions are scrutinized carefully for all aspects of the professional/patient encounter, pre-, during, and post-hypnosis. Attention is paid rigorously to detail and subtleties in the interactional process, with feedback provided to the learner both positively and negatively regarding pre-hypnosis interview, induction, intensification, formulation of hypnotic suggestions, structure and use of language, post-hypnotic suggestions, termination of the trance, teaching of self-hypnosis, and closure of the interview. Feedback may be provided verbally and/or in written format; and time must be provided for discussion. The most commonly employed and most effective teaching strategies in this form of learning include positive and negative feedback (written and oral), modeling (by the mentor!), as well as discussion of certain behaviors/language, and, to a lesser degree, didactic instruction.

CHAPTER EIGHTEEN

Looking to the Future

We have brought together a variety of ideas concerning hypnotic responsiveness in childhood and the use of hypnotherapy in childhood disorders. In our attempt to integrate clinical observations with research studies, we have found that many have significant methodological shortcomings, including some of our own! The weight of evidence suggests that most children are responsive to hypnosis and that hypnotherapy can be useful in their treatment. At the same time, the data often raise more questions than they answer. There is a great deal of work still to be done.

Since the last edition of this book was published, the terms "alternative medicine," "alternative practitioners," and "alternative therapies" have entered the general vocabulary. Recent studies have documented that Americans use many types of alternative therapies and spend 26 billion dollars yearly on them (Eisenberg et al., 1993; Murray & Rubel, 1992; Spigelblatt, Laine-Ammara, Pless, & Guyver, 1994). Under pressure from Congress, the National Institutes of Health created an Office of Alternative Medicine in 1992. Its purpose is to facilitate excellent research on alternative medical therapies. Hypnosis falls under this alternative rubric.

Gellert (1994), in analyzing the credibility problem of alternative medical therapies, states that a critical factor is the tendency of alternative practitioners to "globalize" their therapies, that is, to advance them as cure-alls that can resolve all disease phenomena. He goes on to note that the experiential model engenders strong resistance from conventional medical practioners, although an initial empirical observation regarding an alternative therapy may have value. Dr. Gellert pleads for a sharpening of the focus of the experiential model through a narrowing of global explanations and expansion of conventional research interest. In this way, the alternative and conventional medical communities can gravitate toward the other's perspective.

Inasmuch as we are discussing research in an area categorized as alternative, it is essential that we avoid "globalization" and, if anything, design protocols with more care than we might in the conventional arena. We now present issues of research methodology, pointing out some technical considerations that should enhance the value of future research. Finally, we address specific problem areas in which we expect future research to provide clarification.

RESEARCH METHODOLOGY

Although we cannot attempt a full discussion of methodological issues in child hypnosis research, we would like to mention several problems that come up again and again in the studies previously cited. For a thorough review of the technical aspects of hypnosis research, we refer the reader to the excellent book edited by Fromm and Nash, *Contemporary Hypnosis Research* (1992); almost every chapter contains ideas that are relevant to child hypnosis research. Two other excellent books, *Behavioral Pediatrics: Research and Practice* by Russo and Varni (1982) and *Hypnotherapy of Pain in Children with Cancer* by LeBaron and Hilgard (1984), both describe specific protocols involving hypnosis with children. Another excellent monograph (Dienstfrey, 1992) on whether or not psychosocial influences on health can be demonstrated discusses significant methodological problems that relate to all research in the mind–body area.

Some of the recurrent design issues in protocols involving child hypnosis include controlling for individual variables, inability to develop double-blind crossover trials, contamination of subjects by other people during the course of a study, and the problems with standardization of a hynotic intervention.

With respect to individual variables, it is probable that we do not yet know all that are significant. We have noted that there are intrinsic differences in preferred mental imagery, in biobehavioral reactivity, in personality, and in learning styles. There are augmentors and reducers with respect to pain perceptions. There are vast differences among children in their past experiences that may make them more or less responsive to hypnotic interventions. Churchill, Persinger, and Thomas (1994) have described recent research indicating that some individuals are more responsive to geomagnetic field changes and that these changes impact on mental processing. Many of the studies we have cited have lumped school-age children and adolescents. We believe that age is an important variable and one that can be easily controlled in studies.

Individuals, including children, vary in preferred mental imagery and, rarely, one encounters a child who denies imagination altogether. If a standardized protocol mandates progressive relaxation cued to breathing or autogenic relaxation and the experimental subject is most comfortable with detailed visual imagery, he or she may find the instructions boring and dull and will be "turned-off" to the whole experiment. A child with superb auditory imagery and poor visual imagery is not going to respond well to prescribed focus on specific visual images. We have found repeatedly, to our dismay, that research review committees recommend that the intervention be constant for each child, and they request written descriptions of detailed instructions. The best way to handle this and also respond to individual preferences is to offer a protocol such as this: "The best way to go into hypnosis is to pretend you're in a favorite place doing what you like to do there, in a special, comfortable place. If you like you can imagine seeing things you enjoy seeing there or hearing things that you enjoy hearing or just feeling good, just the way you would feel if you were actually there."

We believe that protocols should control for differences in imagery preferences, personality type, and autonomic "fingerprints." This requirement often leads to a requirement for large numbers of subjects, which increases the cost and duration of studies.

Another research problem intrinsic to protocols involving hypnosis is that one cannot randomize interventions because the child who is in the hypnotic intervention group and the child who is in the resting or attention group will each know what group he or she is in. If one were to begin with a hypnotic intervention and then cross over to a medication, it would be impossible to prevent the subject from continuing the hypnotic intervention during the medication trial. It is true that sham biofeedback can be given but no one has developed a viable sham protocol for hypnotic inductions with children.

Perhaps a major problem encountered by many experts who have done research with hypnosis is the contamination of control groups. Children in control groups may either learn something about hypnosis by chance from other children or their parents or even from meeting someone in the waiting room who is in the experimental group. In the case of Santer's (1990) study of hypnosis in the emergency setting, parents were inadvertently giving subjects hypnotic inductions. Spontaneous hypnosis occurs frequently in children. Kohen (1986c) and Hall et al. (1992) have also had this problem in prospective, "controlled" studies. In one study (Plotnick et al., 1991), it was necessary that parents see the hypnosis induction protocol prior to providing consent. Although they were asked not to share this information with their children prior to the experiments, it is likely that some children learned in advance of the experiments.

Hypnotic Responsiveness

We have described hypnotic rating scales for children in Chapter 3. Although there has been some new research in the past decade (LeBaron et al., 1988;

Plotnick et al., 1991) including a fantasy scale, the existing scales do not allow predictions about which children might be most successful in the therapeutic application of hypnosis. It may be that there are other surrogate markers for hypnotic responsivity that we are missing. It is possible that the existing scales are unsuitable for children with certain personality traits, or learning styles, or with certain types of autonomic reactivity. We look for more sophisticated research on other correlates of hypnotic responsiveness and strongly urge our colleagues to continue research on the role of imagination in childhood hypnotic responsiveness.

Clinical Research

In the early to mid-1990s, we have been happy to note increasing numbers of clinical studies of hypnotherapy with children in print and to see them published in a variety of professional journals including journals of pediatrics, psychology, nursing, dentistry, and social work. Much good laboratory research with humans has evolved from clinical observations. The careful reporting of clinical observations is much needed in this area, and we encourage readers who are clinicians to do this. To the best of our knowledge, there is still a great lack of literature on applications of hypnosis with children in many areas. These include many types of procedures, dermatological problems, learning problems, ophthalmological problems, otolaryngological applications, child abuse, and in orthopedics. We hear clinical anecdotes from colleagues at workshops and meetings about creative, successful applications of hypnotherapy in some of these areas, but these need to be published. In all research studies, both negative and positive results should be reported, and there should be special attention to communicating effectively in oral presentations and in published reports. We recommend review of three papers on effective communication with colleagues in the field of hypnosis (Frankel, 1981; Fromm, 1981; Orne, 1981). The current abilities of computers to facilitate slide making has removed excuses for unreadable, dull slides. Information about hypnosis and hypnotherapy can be presented in ways that are both interesting and academically sound.

Consortium Research

In 1986 we began organizing a group of colleagues who were interested in designing consortium studies involving nonpharmacological therapy such as hypnotherapy and biofeedback. The initial hope was that such consortium studies could do what the Children's Cancer Study Group has done for many years, that is, assemble groups of comparable patients and study interventions more rapidly than would be possible at any one institution and by any one individual. We also hoped to overcome the frequent criticism that successful application of hypnotherapy and/or biofeedback was a phenomenon of individuals or settings. Initially, interested colleagues found times to meet and brainstorm research protocols at national scientific meetings. Later the W. T. Grant Foundation provided a few thousand dollars that allowed a planning meeting to be held in Cleveland in 1988. At this meeting, numerous possible protocols were discussed. Eventually, the group decided to focus on a protocol on nonpharmacological treatment of warts and a protocol on Tourette syndrome.

As is true with most protocols, it is far easier to write them than to obtain funding. Eventually, the wart protocol, involving seven institutions was funded by the Fetzer Foundation for a total of $50,000. It was evident that this could not cover investigator salaries, so all professional time was donated. In implementing the protocol, investigators found many unexpected complications. They learned that dermatologists had not established absolute classifications for describing warts and that there was no agreement on the immunological aspects of wart growth and regression. One of the investigators negotiated with the Edison Sensor Technology Center in Cleveland to design a wart sensor. The hope was that this sensor would allow some monitoring of physiological changes at the base of the wart that might be associated with or predict regression. This plan delayed the whole project. A sophisticated sensor was developed, but there were never enough sensors for each site. It turned out to be very complicated to get seven investigators at different sites to photograph warts in a comparable way. Thus, the initial study took 4 years instead of the projected 2 years (see Chapter 16)!

In spite of these difficulties, the consortium has learned a great deal and provides a basis for designing additional studies involving multiple institutions. The protocol for a comparison of hypnotherapy and Haldol in Tourette syndrome is long completed but has been turned down for funding several times. We continue to be supportive of such consortium research and encourage colleagues to get involved. One of the benefits is that younger, inexperienced researchers can learn about research from such collaborations.

TOPICS FOR FUTURE RESEARCH

Consciousness and Imagination

We have taken the position that hypnosis is an altered state of consciousness and that hypnotherapy is a treatment modality distinct from other forms of medical and psychological therapy that has unique benefits for many child patients. It is possible that we are wrong on both these points. It is possible that there is a generic common denominator in a number of cyberphysiologic strategies that remains to be defined. If we are right about hypnotherapy as a worthy treatment modality, we would hope to be able to increase the level of confidence of ourselves and our colleagues through research in several areas: the nature of consciousness in general; the nature of altered states of consciousness, how these are best achieved, and how they vary in terms of potential value; the nature of imagination and how imagery skills can be fostered and preserved; the process that connects changes in mental imaging to physiological responses.

Future research concerning child applications of hypnotherapy and related cyberphysiologic strategies must take into account why childhood imagery skills peak and subsequently fade as the child moves into adulthood. Imagery is intrinsic to child hypnotherapy; it is also an important part of child development, play patterns, creativity, and adult achievements.

Plato, in *The Republic*, was keenly aware of the tremendous influence of imaginative involvement on child development. He argued, for example, that children should be exposed to certain kinds of literature, drama, and music, whereas other kinds should be suppressed. Otherwise, children would learn inappropriate values and behave as adults in ways that would be harmful to themselves and to society. Plato may have been right; we certainly hear similar arguments today, especially with respect to children's television programming. Indeed, an important area for research relates to what types of images are triggered in young minds by television and the lag period from absorbing the image until acting on it.

It is one thing to restrict the focus of a child's imagination; it is something else to devalue imagination generally. While many people would agree with the former but not the latter, our society seems to be producing just the reverse situation. A plethora of images from constant access to television, headphones, and boomboxes are allowed children with few restrictions; yet many children are allowed no time and receive no direction or encouragement to enjoy their own creative images. Bronowski (1974) wrote: "All great civilizations have failed in one regard. They have limited the freedom of imagination of their young." This idea is old. William Blake, writing in 1788, lamented the loss of childhood imagination to the repressive forces of reason and expressed hope that "the real man, the Imagination" would be found again (Kazin, 1974, p. 83). Holton, in *The Creative Imagination* (1978), noted that antecedents of scientific discoveries made in adulthood were to be found in the childhood experiences of scientists. He provided many examples of this. Einstein, for example, as a child, imagined himself riding on a beam of light and tried to envision what the world would look like as he rode on that beam. He believed that this inspired his idea of the theory of relativity later in life.

We all think we know what imagination is, yet scientists are still trying to define it. There are many questions. Is imagination essentially a single process, or is it a set of discrete skills? Why does it persist in some people and drop out in others? Why do some people use it adaptively and others maladaptively? Since it appears to be of great value in dealing with certain potentially devastating situations, such as when one is a hostage or a prisoner of war, why don't we make a greater effort to teach people to preserve it, to use it for relatively minor problems as well as for major ones? Who should be the teachers, and how should they teach?

How is imagination related to eidetic imagery, a skill present in about 6% of children but only rarely in adults (R. N. Haber, 1980)? If imaginative skills facilitate hypnotic responsiveness, might it also be true that experience with hypnosis fosters the development and preservation of imaginative skills? Should all children be taught self-hypnosis? Are children who are familiar with self-hypnosis better able to adapt to life's challenges and to develop their own assets? Is creative use of imagination facilitated by reading or telling stories to children? Is it facilitated or thwarted by television, an important issue because the average preschooler in the United States watches television for more than 30 hours a week!

Links between Mental and Physiological Processes

There is now substantial evidence that voluntary changes in mental processing or imaging are associated with significant physiological changes even when the individual is not following a prescribed cyberphysiologic strategy. For example, hundreds of researchers and thousands of clinicians have noted that adults and children can deliberately increase and decrease peripheral temperature. How does this happen?

Every adult human body contains 100 trillion cells. These fundamental components of living things were first discovered in the 17th century. Since then, we have learned much about *what* happens inside cells but very little about how it happens. Researchers ponder why genes in individual cells appear to switch themselves on and off and perform differently in varying circumstances. For example, why does messenger ribonucleic acid (m-RNA) not always transmit the complete messages that it carries from deoxyribonucleic acid (DNA)? The whole issue of regulation of the function of the 100 trillion cells has thousands of scientists working. There is no clear explanation for how microtubules transmit instructions between cell nuclei and surfaces. Does some of the regulation of cell behavior evolve from messages of thoughts and/or mental images? We now know that cytokines, mediators of inflammation, are synthesized not only by immunocompetent cells that permeate the blood–brain barrier and enter the brain but also by microglia and by neurons. There are numerous cytokines, and they have many effects including the alteration of behavior and cognitive function. We know that both the amygdala and hippocampus have direct neural connections to hypothalamic nuclei and that they mediate affective and cognitive processes. How do the affective processes impact on the amygdala and hippocampus? What type of energy is associated with a thought? Are there specific cell receptors for this energy, and do they set off a conformational change that is passed along to an ion channel, setting off a cascade of movement from cell to cell and eventually to hypothalamic nuclei? Tracing transmission of thoughts to the cell and through cells and using that knowledge to alleviate the human condition must be a central task for the remainder of the 20th century and well into the next century.

Role of the Therapist in Hypnotherapy

It seems logical that mental processes — affect, imagery, and expectations — of therapists are related to treatment outcomes. For example, some studies (e.g., Rutter, 1980) have found a relationship between teacher expectations and student performance, independent of IQ levels. Many people have had the experience of feeling worse if a friend or neighbor says, "You don't look well. Are you sick?" What happens when the therapist anticipates a poor treatment outcome? What are the cues by which such an expectation gets communicated to a patient? The "hanging crepe phenomenon" first described as a problem in the medical profession by Siegler (1975) should be studied with regard to hypnotherapy.

What about chronobiology issues, fatigue, family concerns, and other variables in therapists? It is possible that we will develop objective measures of these variables that will enable us to decide that we should not work with children at certain times. Do some child hypnotherapists work more successfully with their patients than others? Which people are most suited to be therapists and which least? Should we discourage certain people from becoming child hypnotherapists? Should we be more selective in whom we accept for training?

How and to what extent should child hypnotherapists communicate their own imagery to patients? How should we foster and direct our own imaginative processes so as to be of maximal help to our patients?

There are essentially no answers to any of these questions that are relevant not only to hypnotherapy but to all therapeutic interactions with patients.

Role of the Child in Hypnotherapy

We hope that in future years a more prescriptive approach to hypnotherapy will be seen. By this we do not mean a "cookbook" approach but one basing diagnosis and treatment on data about important variables. More than many people now recognize, the design of a hypnotherapeutic approach for a particular child must take into account such factors as age; developmental level; verbal and imaginal fluency; activity level and other temperamental variables; personality factors such as motivation; internal–external locus of control; mechanisms of coping and defense; needs and conflicts; biobehavioral reactivity; anxiety level and the manner of its expression; learning styles and/or disabilities; and physical strengths. We must consider the child's role in the family, the school, and other social settings that have direct or indirect influences on treatment. We may find it important to measure autonomic responses and/or neurotransmitter levels before titering doses of hypnotherapy or making practice recommendations.

We already have some data suggesting that children respond differently to different kinds of hypnotic inductions. It is also likely that children respond differently to different kinds and amounts of hypnotherapeutic suggestions. Which children benefit most from direct suggestion? Which do better with more indirect, symbolic approaches? Which children need special emphasis on self-hypnosis? Which require more therapist contact? Which children do best with which therapists? Which children benefit most from treatment in groups and which from individual sessions?

When a child wants to master a problem, at what specific points is hypnotherapy likely to be helpful? If learning is state dependent (Tart, 1986), how can we insure that a review of learning will occur in a state comparable to that when it was first learned? For example, in a child with maladaptive anxiety regarding learning and performance, should we employ hypnotherapy before learning begins, during initial learning, during review of learned material, before performance, during performance, or at several of these points?

How can we predict these variations in response so that treatment programs can be designed more effectively and carried out with minimal cost of time and money?

THE FUTURE AND PROFESSIONAL HYPNOSIS ORGANIZATIONS

The Society for Clinical and Experimental Hypnosis (SCEH) and the American Society of Clinical Hypnosis (ASCH) have for many years provided forums for health care professonals who were interested in hypnotherapy. Increasingly, during the past decade, hypnosis and other cyberphysiologic strategies have been taught in other societies of health care professionals. The role of the ASCH and SCEH is changing somewhat, from providing only professional education to also providing public education and leadership with respect to ethical and public policy issues. An unfortunate fact of life for many clinicians, including those in child health who use hypnotherapy, is that reimbursement for hypnotherapy services is inadequate. Third-party and government payors, for example, are usually willing to pay for expensive procedures, such as MRI scans for children with migraine, or for untested medications, but they balk at reimbursement for training a child in self-hypnosis, a therapeutic intervention documented to be more effective than many medications. This now becomes an area in which the SCEH, ASCH, and other professional societies supporting nonpharmacological interventions can provide leadership and assistance to clinicians.

ART AND SCIENCE

As answers to questions mentioned in this chapter and to other questions not yet raised are learned, we will become better able to employ child hypnotherapy in the scientific context of prescriptive treatment. The application of approaches found to have particular value will be expanded, and useless approaches will be eliminated. Cultural changes may necessitate changes in approaches. We will learn how best to combine hypnotherapy with other treatment modalities. We will question basic assumptions and define new problems.

We believe that hypnotherapy will continue to involve art as well as science. Intuition and hunches may continue to be important; but we hope that scientific developments will lead to more creative and effective use of intuition. We also hope that tolerance for uncertainty will prevail.

Most of all, we hope that our synthesis of available observations and information will provide inspiration, clues, and nuggets for those who wish to expand the frontier of child hypnosis and hypnotherapy. The future involves a lot of hard work. It also contains the potential for excitement and satisfaction as we use our own skills to find better ways of allowing children to develop their potential to the fullest, to be all that they really are.

APPENDICES

Stanford Hypnotic Clinical Scale for Children

ARLENE MORGAN, Ph.D.
JOSEPHINE R. HILGARD, M.D., Ph.D.

MODIFIED FORM (AGES 4-8)

This form may be substituted for the child who cannot relax and does not like to close his or her eyes. Typically this will be the very young child (under 6 years of age, and occasionally 7 or 8 years) or the extremely anxious child. This form is similar to the standard version except for the active fantasy induction, a few changes in the wording of tests, and the omission of a post-hypnotic suggestion.

Induction

If Standard Form is used first, improvise transition.

I'd like to talk with you about how a person can use his imagination to do or feel different kinds of things. Do you know what I mean by imagination? *If necessary, explain:* Do you know what it's like to pretend things . . . to "make believe"? Do you ever pretend things or make believe that you are someone else?

When you can do anything you want to do, what do you do? That is, what are the things you like to do more than anything else in the world? *Probe for interests, for example, swimming, hiking, playing on the slide and merry-go-*

From Morgan and Hilgard (1979). With permission. Preliminary data are presented in Figure 3.3. The text for both the Modified Form and the Standard Form contains both *italicized* and nonitalicized material. The sentences in *italic type* are instructions to the hypnotist. Those in roman type are verbal instructions to the child.

round (playground), having a picnic, and so forth. Select a favorite activity and engage child in thinking about it. The picnic described here is an illustration.

Okay, let's do that right now.* Let's imagine [pretend] that we are on a picnic, and there's a big picnic basket right in front of us. What does the basket look like to you? How big is it? . . . I'm going to spread this bright yellow tablecloth on the grass here. . . . Why don't you take something out of the basket now? Tell me about it. . . . That's fine. . . . What else is in the basket? *Continue until a convincing fantasy is developed, or child shows total lack of involvement.*

You know, you can do lots of interesting things by thinking about it this way. It's like imagining [pretending] something so strongly that it seems almost real. How real did it seem to you? Good. Now let's try imagining some other things, okay?

1. Hand Lowering

Please hold your right [left] arm† straight out in front of you, with the palm up. *Assist if necessary.* Imagine that you are holding something heavy in your hand, like a heavy rock. Something very heavy. Shape your fingers around the heavy rock in your hand. What does it feel like? . . . That's good. . . . Now think about your arm and hand feeling more and more heavy, as if the rock were pushing down . . . more and more down . . . and as it gets heavier and heavier, the hand and arm begin to move down . . . down . . . heavier and heavier . . . moving . . . down, down, down . . . moving . . . moving . . . more and more down . . . heavier and heavier. . . . *Wait 10 seconds; note extent of movement.* That's fine. Now you can stop imagining there is a rock in your hand, and let your hand relax. . . . It is not heavy anymore. . . .

Score + if hand lowers at least 6 inches at end of 10 seconds.

2. Arm Rigidity

Now please hold your left [right] arm straight out and the fingers straight out, too. . . . That's right, your arm straight out in front of you, fingers straight out, too. . . . Think about making your arm very stiff and straight, very, very stiff. . . . Think about it as if you were a tree, and your arm is a strong branch

---

*It is not necessary for the child to close his or her eyes. Some children find it easier to imagine with their eyes closed. If closing eyes appears desirable, give child a choice: "You may close your eyes if you wish to, but keep them open if you'd rather."

†Either arm may be used for items 1 and 2; if, for example, one arm is immobilized, use other arm for both items.

of the tree, very straight and very strong, like the branch of a tree . . . so stiff that you can't bend it. . . . Try. . . . *Wait 10 seconds.* That's fine. . . . Now your arm is no longer like a branch of a tree. It is not stiff any longer. . . . Just let it relax again. . . .

   Score + if arm has bent less than 2 inches at end of 10 seconds.

3 and 4. Visual and Auditory Hallucination (TV)

What is your favorite TV program? For the occasional child who does not watch TV, substitute favorite movie and modify the instructions appropriately. Record response. You can watch that program right now if you want to, and I'll tell you how. When I count to three, you will see a TV in front of you, and you can watch (*name of program*). . . . Ready? One . . . two . . . three . . . do you see it?

If yes	*If no*
Is the picture clear? . . . Is it black and white, or is it in color? What's happening? Can you hear the program? . . . Is it loud enough. What are you hearing? . . . *Finally:* Now the program is ending. . . . The TV is disappearing. . . . It's gone now. . . . very good.	That's all right. . . . Sometimes it takes a little while to catch on how to do this. . . .

If eyes are open

Why don't you close your eyes for a moment and try to see it in your mind. . . . Sometimes it's easier to imagine things like this with your eyes closed. . . . *Continue:* Just wait a little while, and I think you'll start to see it pretty soon. *Wait 5 seconds.* There, what do you see now? What are you hearing? *If sees or hears, question as in left column above.*

If still no

That's okay. Just forget all about the TV. . . . We'll do something else. . . .

   Visual: Score + if child sees a program with sufficient detail to be comparable to actual viewing.
   Auditory: Score + if child reports hearing words, sound effects, music, etc.

5. Dream

Do you ever dream at night when you are asleep? *If child is puzzled, explain that a dream is like seeing things going on even when you are asleep.* I'd like you now to think about how you feel when you are just ready to go to sleep at night, and imagine that you are about to have a dream. . . . Just let a dream come into your mind . . . a dream just like the dreams that you have when you are asleep. . . . *If eyes are open:* Maybe you'd like to close your eyes while you do this. *Continue:* When I stop talking, in just a moment, you will have a dream, a very pleasant dream, just like when you are asleep at night. . . . Now a dream is coming into your mind. . . . *Wait 20 seconds.*

   The dream is over now, and I'd like you to tell me about it. *Record verbatim, probing as necessary for thoughts or images.* That's fine. You can forget about the dream now. . . . That's all for the dream. . . .

   Score + if child has an experience comparable to a dream, with some action.

6. Age Regression

Now I'd like you to think back to some very special time when you were younger than you are now . . . some time that you had a lot of fun . . . a special trip, perhaps, or a birthday party. Can you think of such a time? What was it? *Record target event.* All right, . . . now I'd like you to think about that time. . . . Think about being back there again. . . . In a little while you are going to feel just like you did on that day when (*specify target event*). I am going to count to five, and at the count of five, you will be right back there again . . . one . . . two . . . three . . . four . . . five. . . . You are now there. . . . Tell me about it. . . . Where are you? . . . What are you doing? . . . How old are you? . . . What are you wearing? . . . *Continue as appropriate and record responses.*

   That's fine. . . . Now you can stop thinking about that day and come right back to this day, in this room, with everything just as it was. Tell me how it seemed to be back at (*target event*). . . . Was it like being there, or did you just think about it? *How real was it?* That's fine. . . .

   Score + if child gives appropriate answers to questions and reports some experience of being there.

Termination

Well, you've done very well today. What was the most fun of the things I asked you to do? Is there anything else you'd like to talk about? . . . If there isn't, then we're all through.

Scoring Form

Name _____ Date _____ Total score _____

Age _____ Hypnotist _____

SUMMARY OF SCORES
(details on the pages that follow)

	Score (+ or −)
1. **Hand Lowering**	(1) _____
2. **Arm Rigidity**	(2) _____
3. **TV — Visual**	(3) _____
4. **TV — Auditory**	(4) _____
5. **Dream**	(5) _____
6. **Age Regression**	(6) _____
Total score	_____

Comments:

1. **Hand Lowering**   Score
   Describe movement:

   Score + if arm and hand lower at least 6 inches by end of
   10 seconds.   (1) _____

2. **Arm Rigidity**
   Describe movement:

   Score + if arm bends less than 2 inches by end of 10 seconds. (2) _____

3 and 4. Visual and Auditory Hallucination (TV)
   Program preferred:
   (3) Visual
       Do you see it?
       Is picture clear?
       Is it black and white or color?
       What's happening? (detail of action)

   Score + if child reports seeing a picture comparable to actual
   viewing.   (3) _____

   (4) Auditory
       Can you hear it?
       Is it loud enough?
       Sound reported (words, sound effects, music, etc.):

   Score + if child reports hearing some sound clearly.   (4) _____

5. **Dream**
   Verbatim account of dream:

   Score + if child has an experience comparable to a dream, with
   some action. This does not include vague, fleeting thoughts or
   feelings without accompanying imagery.   (5) _____

6. **Age Regression**   Score
   Target event:
   Where are you?
   What are you doing?

   How old are you?
   What are you wearing?
   How did it seem to be back there?

Was it like being there, or did you just think about it?

Other:

Score + if child gives appropriate responses and reports some
experience of being there.   (6) _____

                                        Total score   _____

STANDARD FORM (AGES 6-16)

Discussion of preconceived ideas that child and/or parent may have about hypnosis should precede administration of the scale. Be sure the meaning of the word "relax" is understood. If necessary, explain it in terms of "letting go" as when the hypnotist holds the child's wrist and lets it drop gently, or "feeling loose like a rag doll."

Induction

I'm going to help you learn some interesting things about imagination today. Most people say that it's fun [fascinating]. I will ask you to think of some different things, and we will see how your imagination works. Some people find it easier to imagine some things than other things. We want to find what is most interesting to you. Listen very carefully to me, and let's see what happens. Just be comfortable in the chair [bed], and let's imagine some things now. Please close your eyes so you can imagine these things better. . . . Now I'd like you to picture yourself floating in a warm pool of water. . . . What is it like? . . . And now can you picture yourself floating on a nice soft cloud in the air? . . . What is that like? . . .

   That's fine—just open your eyes. . . . Now I'd like to show you how you can feel completely relaxed and comfortable, because that makes it easier to imagine things, too. . . . I'm going to draw a little face on my thumbnail.* . . . Here it is. . . . *Hypnotist draws face on own thumbnail with red felt pen.* Let's put one on your thumb. Do you want to do it or shall I? *Hypnotist or child does so.* That's a good face! Now please hold your hand up in front of you like this— *assist child so that hand is in front, thumbnail facing him, with elbow not resting on anything*—and look at the little face [thumbnail], try to think only about the things I talk about, and let your body relax completely. . . . Let your whole body feel loose and limp and relaxed. . . . Relax completely . . . just let all the muscles in your body relax . . . relax completely. . . . Be as relaxed as you were while you were imagining that you were floating in the pool of water, or floating on a cloud. . . . Feel your body becoming more and more relaxed . . . more and more relaxed. . . . Your eyelids, too, are relaxing. They are starting to feel heavy. As you keep watching the face [thumbnail], your eyes feel heavier and heavier. . . . Your eyes are starting to blink a little, and that's a very good sign. That means you're relaxing really well. Just keep watching the face [thumbnail], your eyes feel heavier and heavier. . . . Your eyes are starting to blink a little, and that's a very good sign. That means you're relaxing really well. Just keep

---

*If drawing a face on thumbnail seems awkward for the older child, eliminate it and have him or her simply stare at the thumbnail. Substitute "thumbnail" for "little face" as indicated.

watching the face [thumbnail] and listening to my voice. . . . Already your eyelids feel heavy. Very soon they will feel so heavy that they will begin to close by themselves. . . . Let them close whenever they feel like it. And when they close, let them stay closed. . . . Even now, and your whole body is feeling so nice, so comfortable, completely relaxed. . . .

If child shows convincing evidence at any time of inability to relax, or unwillingness to let eyes close or remain closed, go to Modified Form.

Now I'm going to count from one to ten, and you will find your body becoming even more relaxed. . . . You will continue to relax as you listen to the counting . . . one . . . more and more relaxed, such a good feeling . . . two . . . three . . . more and more relaxed all the time, feeling so good . . . four . . . five . . . six . . . even more relaxed . . . and your eyes are feeling heavier, heavier. . . . It feels so good just to let go and relax completely . . . seven . . . eight . . . nine . . . VERY relaxed now . . . ten. . . .

If child is still holding hand up: Just let your hand relax completely, too. . . . Just let your eyes close and keep them closed while you listen to me. . . .

If eyes have not closed: Now please let your eyes close, and just relax completely. Just let your eyes close and keep them closed while you listen to me. . . .

For all children: And now as we go on, it will be very easy for you to listen to me because you are so relaxed and comfortable. If you can keep your eyes closed, you can imagine some things better, so why don't you let them stay closed. You'll be able to stay relaxed and talk to me when I ask you to. . . . Your are feeling very good. . . . Just keep listening to what I tell you and think about the things I suggest. Then let happen whatever you find is happening. . . . Just let things happen by themselves.

If eyes open at any time, request child gently to close them: Because imagination is easier that way.

1. Hand Lowering

Please hold your right [left] arm* straight out in front of you, with the palms up. *Assist if necessary.* Imagine that you are holding something heavy in your hand, like a heavy rock. Something very heavy. Shape your fingers around the heavy rock in your hand. What does it feel like? . . . That's good. . . . Now think about your arm and hand feeling heavier and heavier, as if the rock were pushing down . . . more and more down . . . and as it gets heavier and heavier, the hand and arm begin to move down . . . down . . . heavier and heavier . . . moving . . . down, down, down . . . moving . . . moving . . . more and more down . . . heavier and heavier. . . . *Wait 10 seconds; note extent of movement.*

---

*Either arm may be used for items 1 and 2; if, for example one arm is immobilized, use other arm for both items.

That's fine. Now you can stop imagining there is a rock in your hand, and let
your hand relax. . . . It is not heavy any more. . . .

    Score + if hand lowers at least 6 inches at end of 10 seconds.

2. Arm Rigidity

Now please hold your left [right] arm straight out and the fingers straight out,
too. . . . That's right, your arm straight out in front of you, fingers straight out,
too. . . . Think about making your arm very stiff and straight, very, very
stiff. . . . Think about it as if you were a tree, and your arm is a strong branch
of a tree . . . so stiff that you can't bend it. . . . That's right. . . . Now see how
stiff your arm is. . . . Try to bend it. . . . Try. . . . Try. . . . *Wait 10 seconds.*
That's fine. . . . Now your arm is no longer like a branch of a tree. It is not
stiff any longer. . . . Just let it relax again. . . .

    Score + if arm has bent less than 2 inches at end of 10 seconds.

3 and 4. Visual and Auditory Hallucination (TV)

It is easier to imagine what I am going to ask you to do if you keep your eyes
closed.

    What is your favorite TV program? *For the occasional child who does not
watch TV, substitute favorite movie and modify the instructions appropriately.
Record response.*

    You can watch that program right now if you want to, and I'll tell you
how. When I count to three, you will see a TV in front of you, and you can
watch (*name of program*). . . . Ready? One . . . two . . . three . . . do you see
it?

If yes	*If no*
Is the picture clear? . . . Is it black and white, or is it in color? What's happening? Can you hear the program? . . . Is it loud enough. What are you hearing? . . . *Finally:* Now the program is ending. . . . The TV is disappearing. . . . It's gone now . . . very good.	That's all right. . . . Sometimes it takes a little while to catch on how to do this. . . . Just wait a little while, and I think you'll start to see it pretty soon. *Wait 5 seconds.* There, what do you see now? What are you hearing? *If sees or hears, question as in left column above.*

If eyes are open

That's okay. Just forget all about the TV. . . . We'll do something else. . . . Just relax and keep listening to my voice. . . .

Visual: Score + if child sees a program with sufficient detail to be comparable to actual viewing.
Auditory: Score + if child reports hearing words, sound effects, music, etc.

5. Dream

Do you dream at night when you are asleep? *If child is puzzled, explain that a dream is like seeing things going on even when you are asleep.* I'd like you to think about how you feel when you are just ready to go to sleep at night, and imagine that you are about to have a dream. . . . Just let a dream come into your mind, . . . a dream just like the dreams that you have when you are asleep. . . . When I stop talking, in just a moment, you will have a dream, a very pleasant dream, just like the dreams you have when you are asleep at night. . . . Now a dream is coming into your mind. . . . *Wait 20 seconds.*

The dream is over now, and I'd like you to tell me about it. *Record verbatim, probing as necessary for thoughts or images.* That's fine. You can forget about the dream now, and just relax. Just relax completed and let your whole body feel good. . . .

Score + if child has an experience comparable to a dream, with some action.

6. Age Regression

Now I'd like you to think back to some very special time when you were younger than you are now. Some time that happened last year, or maybe when you were even younger than that . . . a special trip, perhaps, or a birthday party. Can you think of such a time? What was it? *Record target event.* All right, . . . now I'd like you to think about that time. . . . Think about being younger and smaller. . . . In a little while you are going to feel just like you did on that day when (*specify target event*). I am going to count to five, and at the count of five, you will be right back there again . . . one . . . two . . . three . . . four . . . five. . . . You are now there. . . . Tell me about it. . . . Where are you? What are you doing? How old are you? Look at yourself and tell me what you're wearing. *Continue as appropriate and record responses.*

That's fine. . . . Now you can stop thinking about that day and come right back to today, in this room, with everything just as it was. Tell me how it seemed to be back at (*target event*). . . . Was it like being there, or did you just think about it? How real was it? Did you feel smaller? . . . That's fine. . . . Just relax completely again now. . . .

Score + if child gives appropriate answers to questions and reports some experience of being there.

7. Post-hypnotic Response

That's it . . . very relaxed . . . feeling so good, so comfortable . . . so relaxed. . . . In a moment I will ask you to take a deep breath and open your eyes and feel wide awake, so we can talk a little about the things we have done today. . . . However, while we are talking, I will clap my hands two times, like this—*demonstrate*. When you hear me clap, you will immediately close your eyes and go right back to feeling just the way you do now . . . completely relaxed. . . . You'll be surprised at how easy it is to let your eyes close, and let your whole body relax completely again, when you hear the handclap . . . relaxed and comfortable, just as you are now. . . . All right, then . . . now take a deep breath and open your eyes. . . . That's fine. . . . Maybe you'd like to stretch just a little so you'll feel alert. . . . You've done very well at imagining these things. . . . Which of the things that I asked you to think about was the most fun? *After approximately 20 seconds, clap hands. Note response.*

   Score + if child closes eyes and exhibits characteristics of relaxation.

   Do you feel relaxed? Do you feel as relaxed as you did before, before I asked you to open your eyes? . . . That's fine. Now I'm going to count from five to one, and when I get to one, you will open your eyes and feel wide awake again, and you will know that our imagining things together is over for today. Okay, then . . . five . . . four . . . three . . . two . . . one . . . very good. How do you feel now? Let's talk a little about the other things we did today. *Remind child of specific items so that he recalls all suggestions.* Now I'm going to clap my hands again, and this time it will not make you drowsy and relaxed. *Clap hands, record response, and be sure that child is fully alert.*

Termination

You've done very well today. What was the most fun of the things I asked you to do? Is there anything else you'd like to talk about? . . . If there isn't, then we're all through.

Scoring Form

Name _____ Date _____ Total score _____

Age _____ Hypnotist _____

SUMMARY OF SCORES
(details on the pages that follow)

		Score (+ or −)
1.	**Hand Lowering**	(1) _____
2.	**Arm Rigidity**	(2) _____
3.	**TV — Visual**	(3) _____
4.	**TV — Auditory**	(4) _____
5.	**Dream**	(5) _____
6.	**Age Regression**	(6) _____
7.	**Post-hypnotic Response**	(7) _____
	Total score	_____

Comments:

1. Hand Lowering   Score
   Describe movement:

   Score + if arm and hand lower at least 6 inches by end of
   10 seconds.   (1) _____

2. Arm Rigidity
   Describe movement:

   Score + if arm bends less than 2 inches by end of 10 seconds.   (2) _____

3 and 4. Visual and Auditory Hallucination (TV)
   Program preferred:
   (3) Visual
       Do you see it?
       Is picture clear?
       Is it black and white or color?
       What's happening? (detail of action)

   Score + if child reports seeing a picture comparable to actual
   viewing.   (3) _____

   (4) Auditory
       Can you hear it?
       Is it loud enough?
       Sound reported (words, sound effects, music, etc.):

   Score + if child reports hearing some sound clearly.   (4) _____

5. Dream
   Verbatim account of dream:

   Score + if child has an experience comparable to a dream, with
   some action. This does not include vague, fleeting thoughts or
   feelings without accompanying imagery.   (5) _____

6. **Age Regression**   Score
   Target event:
   Where are you?
   What are you doing?

   How old are you?
   What are you wearing?
   Look at yourself and tell me what you're wearing.
   How did it seem to be back there?

   Was it like being there, or did you just think about it?

   Did you feel smaller?
   Other:

   Score + if child gives appropriate responses and reports some
   experience of being there.   (6) _____

7. **Post-hypnotic Response**
   Response to handclap:
   Did child close eyes?
   Appear to relax?
   Do you feel relaxed?
   As relaxed as before?
   Discussion of specific items:

   Response to handclap after suggestion removed:

   Score + if child closed eyes and relaxed at initial handclap (7) _____

                                                   Total score   _____

Rainbow Babies
and Children's Hospital
General Academic Pediatrics
Imagery/Discomfort Questionnaire

General Information

1. Child's name _____
   Preferred name or nickname _____
   Any special pronunciation _____

2. Mother's name _____
   Address   _____
                   _____

3. Father's name _____
   Address   _____
                   _____

4. Child's age _____ Birth date _____

5. Names and ages of siblings:
   Brothers _____ Sisters _____

6. Child's primary physician (pediatrician/family doctor):
   Doctor's name _____
   Address   _____
                 _____

   Phone ( ) _____

7. Child's other physician:
   Doctor's name _____
   Address   _____
                 _____

   Phone ( ) _____

The following questions are for child or teen-ager to answer:

8. What kind of things make you laugh most frequently?
   ____ Jokes   ____ Silly play   ____ Stories
   ____ Cartoons/comics   ____ Other _____

9. What is your favorite place away from home? (Check one)
   ____ Park   ____ Forest/woods   ____ City streets
   ____ Beach   ____ Ocean   ____ Playground
   ____ Mountains   ____ Lake   ____ Friend's house
   ____ Desert   ____ River   ____ Zoo
   ____ Cabin   ____ School
   ____ Other _____

10. What activity is most fun for you? Circle the most fun activity and check
    four others:
    ____ Reading   ____ Gymnastics   ____ Soccer
    ____ Watching TV   ____ Running   ____ Skiing/x-country
    ____ Listening to music ____ Football   ____ Doing puzzles
    ____ Playing with   ____ Walking/hiking ____ Chess/checkers
         toys/dolls   ____ Swimming   ____ Baseball
    ____ Computer games/   ____ Canoeing   ____ Basketball
         programs   ____ Fishing   ____ Hockey
    ____ Daydreaming   ____ Boating   ____ Playing with pets
    ____ Playing a musical ____ Hunting   ____ Cub Scouts/
         instrument   ____ Studying   Brownies
    ____ Water skiing   ____ Going to the zoo ____ Board games
    ____ Gardening   ____ Sledding   ____ Skiing downhill
    ____ Dancing   ____ Other (describe) _____
    ____ School   _____
    ____ Playing with friends

11. What do you do best? (Check one)
    ____ School work   ____ Art   ____ Writing
    ____ Dance   ____ Sports   ____ Camping
    ____ Music   ____ Reading
    ____ Other (describe) _____

Your Discomfort/Pain

12. Select and describe what is most distressing to you at this time. If possible,
    choose only one:
    ____ Pain   ____ Anxiety   ____ Fatigue
    ____ Nausea/vomiting   ____ Loss of appetite
    ____ Other (describe) _____

13. If possible, please shade in the specific area(s) where you have this distress:

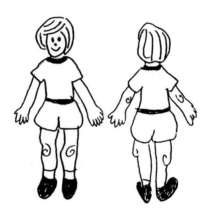

14. Do you have other distress at the same time?

_____ Yes   _____ No

If yes, please indicate:

_____ Stomachache	_____ Diarrhea	_____ Drowsiness
_____ Nausea	_____ Vomiting	_____ Dizziness
_____ Fear	_____ Sweating	_____ Headache
_____ Loss of appetite	_____ Sneezing	_____ Running nose
_____ Tired/no energy	_____ Sadness	

_____ Pain (describe) _____

_____ Other (describe) _____

15. Tell me what you do or how you act when you are . . .

Afraid/anxious _____

Happy _____

Frustrated _____

16. My distress feels . . . (Check all that apply)

_____ Sharp	_____ Sensitive	_____ Blah!
_____ Stabbing	_____ Intense	_____ Sickening
_____ Jabbing	_____ Itchy	_____ Exhausting
_____ Achy	_____ Gnawing	_____ Throbbing
_____ Pulsing/shooting	_____ Tight	_____ Dull
_____ Out of control	_____ Wretched	_____ Suffocating
_____ Stinging	_____ Fearful	_____ Hot/burning
_____ Twisting	_____ Hopeless	

17. The color of my distress is usually . . .

_____ Purple	_____ Yellow	_____ Black
_____ Blue	_____ Orange	_____ White
_____ Green	_____ Red	_____ Other _____

18. The shape of my distress is usually . . .
    ____ Circle   ____ Square   ____ Big blot
    ____ Rectangle   ____ Triangle   ____ Jagged
    ____ Other _____

19. My distress occurs . . .
    ____ Constantly   ____ Occasionally   ____ Once a day
    ____ 1–3 times a week ____ 4–5 times a week   ____ Several times
                                                                              daily

20. My discomfort . . .
    ____ Wakes me up in the middle of the night
    ____ Makes me mad
    ____ Keeps me from falling asleep
    ____ Other (describe) _____

21. My distress and discomfort keep me from . . . (Check the top three)
    ____ Going to school   ____ Having more energy
    ____ Doing my homework   ____ Eating
    ____ Concentrating in school   ____ Watching TV
    ____ Playing outside   ____ Being on the team
    ____ Playing with my pets   ____ Baseball
    ____ Reading   ____ Football
    ____ Playing with my friends   ____ Soccer
    ____ Participating in sports   ____ Basketball
    ____ Riding my bike   ____ Hockey
    ____ Sleeping over at friend's house   ____ Volleyball
    ____ Playing my music   ____ Tennis
    ____ Concentrating better   ____ Swimming
    ____ Feeling better   ____ Track
    ____ Watching TV or movies   ____ Gymnastics
    ____ Other (describe) _____

22. What is your favorite color? (Check one)
    ____ Red   ____ Purple   ____ Brown
    ____ Blue   ____ Green   ____ Orange
    ____ Yellow   ____ Pink   ____ Other (describe)
                                                                                        _____

23. What is your favorite musical type?
    ____ Rock   ____ Country   ____ Classical
    ____ Easy listening   ____ Folk   ____ New Age
    ____ Rap   ____ Other (describe) _____

24. Do you like to play imagery games?
    ____ Yes   ____ No

25. Can you imagine a smell?   ____ Yes   ____ No

26. Can you imagine a song?   ____ Yes   ____ No
    If yes, which song? _____

27. Can you imagine a taste?   ____ Yes   ____ No
    If yes, which taste? _____

28. Can you imagine the feeling of being in the bathtub or in a swimming pool?
    ____ Yes   ____ No

29. Can you imagine the feeling of petting a dog or cat?
    ____ Yes   ____ No

APPENDIX C

Enuresis Questionnaire

Name of child _____ Date _____
Age of child _____ Filled out by _____
(years and months) Relationship _____
Birth date _____

Please circle appropriate choice:
Y = Yes; N = No; DK = Don't Know

Y N DK   1. Did your child ever have dry beds? If so, when did he or she begin wetting the bed?

Y N DK   2. Did some frightening or upsetting event happen before he or she began bedwetting? If so, what and when?

_____   3. At what age did your child have complete bowel control?

Y N DK   4. Is your child constipated frequently, or does he or she have irregular, hard bowel movements?

Y N DK   5. Is there any stool soiling?

Y N DK   6. Does your child wet during the daytime now? If so, how often?

Y N DK   7. Does your child have the feeling that he or she is dribbling during the day?

Y N DK   8. Does your child have the feeling that he or she must get to the bathroom immediately when he or she feels the urge to go?

_____   9. How often does your child go to the bathroom (to urinate) during the day?

_____   10. How many nights a week does your child have dry beds?

Y   N   DK   11. Is your child aware of any special time he or she is certain that he or she will wet the bed? If so, when?

Y   N   DK   12. Does your child ever fall asleep suddenly during the daytime?

Y   N   DK   13. Does anyone tease him or her about wet beds? If so, when?

Y   N   DK   14. Do you punish him or her for bedwetting?

Y   N   DK   15. Does your child have any allergies such as hayfever, eczema, asthma, food or drug intolerance? If so, which one(s) and for how long?

Y   N   DK   16. Did your child have any allergies when younger which have since disappeared? If so, which one(s), when, and for how long?

Y   N   DK   17. Does your child take any medications at any time for any reason? If so, which one(s), when, and how often?

Y   N   DK   18. Do any of your child's brothers and/or sisters wet the bed at night? If so, who and what age(s)?

Y   N   DK   19. Do any of your child's brothers and/or sisters have allergies now or in the past? If so, who and which one(s)?

_____   20. Who washes wet bedclothing?

Y   N   DK   21. Have you tried any treatment plans to cure betwetting? If so, what were they?

Y   N   DK   22. Does your child drink any caffeine-containing drinks?

APPENDIX D

Instruction Form for Parents: Bedwetting (Enuresis)

Your child is practicing self-regulation for control of bedwetting, and it is important that you enhance your child's self-confidence and learning in the following ways:

- You should ensure that there will be a quiet spot available every evening where your child can practice the relaxation exercise.
- In general, the best time for practice is shortly before bedtime; however, if your child is one who is exceedingly tired and ready to fall asleep as soon as he or she gets into bed, practice should be immediately after supper or at some other convenient time between suppertime and bedtime.
- Your child should practice while sitting on the bed, on the floor, or in a comfortable chair in the room designated for practice. Although it is perfectly all right to practice in bed he or she should not lie down.
- Ideally, a half-dollar—which can be a reminder to practice—should be available where your child is likely to see it.
- *You should not remind your child to practice!* This is hard for many parents to follow because we naturally remind our children to do many things. However, bladder control is entirely the child's responsibility, and we must recognize this. The only aid you can give is to provide a reminder—put the coin in a conspicuous spot, tie a colored string around a toothbrush, tape the calendar on the wall, etc.
- If your child does not practice, please tell his or her pediatrician, but not in the child's presence. Also let the pediatrician know if there are family stresses, such as the death of a pet, the absence of a parent, or anxiety over school.
- Your child may have been told to ask you to help draw a funny face on his or her thumbnail. This gives your child something to focus on during the relaxation exercise. If your child asks you to do this, please oblige. Please don't remind him or her that it's "time to draw the face on the thumb now."

- Please encourage your child to make follow-up calls to the pediatrician as requested. We feel these are very important to successful outcome.
- Please don't put diapers, plastic pants, or even "pull-ups" on your child when he or she is practicing bladder control, because doing so tells your child that you don't expect he or she will succeed.
- Please don't wake your child at night to use the bathroom.

Behavioral/Developmental Pediatrics Questionnaire

While your child is waiting in the waiting room, if he or she has not already done so, our staff would like the child to draw a picture of his or her family. We will provide pencils, crayons, or pens if he or she prefers. It is helpful to have a basis with which to open conversation with your child. If your child does not wish to do this, we do not insist.

We would appreciate your taking the time to complete this questionnaire. It will aid us in determining your child's treatment program. All of the questions are optional, but please answer as many as you can.

Child's name _____ Nickname _____
Age _____ Date of birth _____
Home address _____
Home phone number _____ Parent's work number _____

1. With whom does your child live? Please check.
   ____ Mother   ____ Father   ____ Grandparent   ____ Other
   How many: Sisters _____ Age(s) _____
                Brothers _____ Age(s) _____

2. List all medications that the child's mother received during pregnancy.
   _____
   _____

3. List all medications that you can remember your child having received since birth. (We realize that you may not be able to recall them all.)
   _____
   _____
   _____
   _____

 4. How do you rate your child's health? _____

 5. What foods does your child like? _____

 6. What foods does your child dislike? _____
    _____

 7. How many hours of sleep per night does your child need? _____

 8. Has your child ever had any negative experiences in the office of a doctor
    or dentist or in a hospital? If so, please describe. _____
    _____

 9. How does your child act when afraid? _____
    _____

10. What measures do you use to help your child with fears? _____
    _____
    _____

11. What coping measures does your child use? _____
    _____
    _____

12. What are your child's strengths? What is he or she good at? _____
    _____
    _____

13. What are your child's favorite activities? _____
    _____
    _____

14. How do you believe your child learns best? By watching? By reading? By
    listening? Some other way? _____

15. What music does your child like? _____

16. What tasks does your child like to do at home? _____
    _____

17. What tasks does your child not like to do at home? _____
    _____

18. Does your child have a regular job? _____ If so, what? _____

19. Does your child spend money immediately or save it? _____

20. What are your child's weaknesses? _____
    _____

21. What are your child's fears? _____

22. Is there anything your child is trying to accomplish right now that he or she feels is very important? _____

23. Have there been any stressful events lately that you think might have affected your child? _____

24. Have there been any exciting, happy, or proud events lately? If so, please describe. _____

25. Who are the significant adults for your child besides his or her parents? (For example, which relative, neighbor, teacher, or Sunday school teacher?) _____

26. How does your child get along with other family members? _____

27. In general, how do you feel about your child? _____

28. In general, how do you think your child feels about him- or herself? ___

29. What is your dream for your child? _____

30. If your child goes to school, please summarize his or her last school report card. _____

Please add anything additional you would like us to know in order to best help you and your child. _____

_____   _____
Signature of person completing this form   Date

Guidelines for Therapists: Evaluating Persistent Somatic Complaints in Children

1. Evaluate yourself with respect to personal and family physiological responses to stress. Be aware of how your own problems or symptoms may affect interpretation of a patient's symptoms.

2. Make thoughtful choices concerning approach to a child and his or her family.

   - Find out the family's previous experiences with child health professionals.
   - Record the age, developmental stage, likes, dislikes, and interests of the child. Begin with nonsensitive areas, if possible, focusing on some of the child's strengths and successes.
   - Determine familial psychophysiological responses with simple questions (e.g., How does your body react when you get nervous?).
   - What have been the primary ailments of four biological grandparents, aunts, or uncles, if known?
   - What events or situations are clearly stressful for the parents?
   - How aware is the child of his or her parents' likes, dislikes, work, and so on?
   - What is the family's daily life style? Details such as wake-up times, menus, parent work schedules, chronic illness in family, and hobbies are important.
   - What is the child's learning style? Parents usually have some idea about this.

3. Consider cultural norms that may be related to the symptoms.

4. Be certain that a careful physical examination and appropriate lab and X-ray diagnostics are done.

5. Be certain that the complaints are not the result of a medication that the child is taking.

6. Is it possible to videotape the child at home in segments over several weeks (in order to desensitize him or her to the camera)? Audiotaping is a suitable alternative.

7. Use a statement such as that recommended by Dr. Morris Green: "In seeing many children with _____ pain, I've found it sometimes due to physical causes, sometimes to stresses, and sometimes to both. But pain is pain no matter what the cause, so it's my practice to examine all possibilities thoroughly."

8. Remain as case manager for your patient or make sure he or she has one. If you have many patients with persistent somatic complaints, maintain a tickler or process file that you check frequently.

9. Maintain a tolerance for uncertainty. Be *sure* before concluding that the cause of symptoms is primarily psychogenic.

APPENDIX G

Hypnotherapeutic Suggestions Useful for Patients with Tic Disorders and Tourette Syndrome

- **Imagery** of favorite place/activity
- **Progressive relaxation** (*Note:* Relaxation from toe to head may be more useful and effective, as it purposefully begins as far away as possible from the face and head, the most common sites of tics.)
- **Stop sign imagery** (e.g., "Notice the tic right *before* it comes and put the stop sign up in your mind.")
- **Transfer the tic** to a more acceptable place in the body (e.g., "Let the feeling of the tic about to happen [implies awareness] go all the way down to and out your fingertips or down to your big toe[s], and twitch as much as it wants to [dissociation] there.")
- **Lower the intensity/frequency** (combine self-monitoring scales of, e.g., 1–5, 1–10, 1–12, with self-regulation of those scales; e.g., "Push the elevator button to ride down from 7 to 2.")
- **Store the associated anxiety/stress trigger away** (e.g., bury the anxiety or put it in a "safe place" somewhere—implied control)
- **"Save" the tics** (implies control and modulation) until a more acceptable time (e.g., after school/work, in private)
- **Metaphoric stories for control** (e.g. quarterback who gives all members of the team instructions on how, when, where to move; control of music "movements," movement of bow on a violin, etc.)
- **Future projection** (e.g., to a time without tics, such as "Mirror in your mind of when you are older")
- **Trip around body to find the *twitch switch*,** turn it down/off

Expectation Models for Asthma

Negative Expectation Model for Asthma

IMMUNOLOGIC & NON-IMMUNOLOGIC TRIGGERS

- Respiratory Viral Infections
- Exercise
- Environmental Allergens
- Emotional Stress
- Temperature Change
- Barometric Pressure Change
- Air Pollution

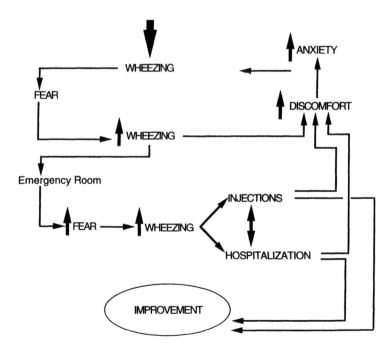

Positive Expectation Model for Asthma

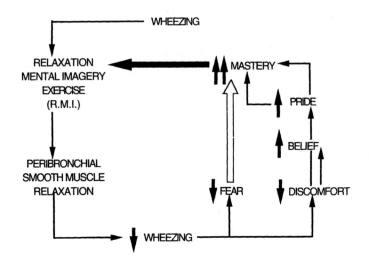

References

Achmon, J., Granek, M., Golomb, M., & Hart, J. (1989). Behavioral treatment of essential hypertension: A comparison between cognitive therapy and biofeedback of heart rate. *Psychosomatic Medicine, 51,* 152–164.

Adams, J. A., & Weaver, S. J. (1986). Self-esteem and perceived stress in young adolescents with chronic disease: Unexpected findings. *Journal of Adolescent Health Care, 7,* 173–177.

Ader, R. (Ed.). (1981). *Psychoneuroimmunology.* New York: Academic Press.

Ader, R. (1989). Conditioned immune responses and pharmacotherapy. *Arthritis Care Research, 2,* S58–S64.

Ader, R. (Ed.). (1991). *Psychoneuroimmunology* (2nd ed.). New York: Academic Press.

Agle, D. (1975). Psychological factors in hemophilia: The concept of self-care. *Annals of the New York Academy of Sciences, 240,* 221–225.

Alpert, J. J. (1975). Accidental stresses: Stressful accidents [Audiotape]. *Pediatric Audio Digest Foundation, 219*(2).

Ambrose, G. (1952). Nervous control of sweating. *Lancet, 1,* 926.

Ambrose, G. (1961). *Hypnotherapy with children* (2nd ed.). London: Staples.

Ambrose, G. (1963). Hypnotherapy for children. In J. M. Schneck (Ed.), *Hypnosis in modern medicine* (3rd ed.). Springfield, IL: Charles C Thomas.

Ambrose, G. (1968). Hypnosis in the treatment of children. *American Journal of Clinical Hypnosis, 11,* 1–5.

American Academy of Pediatrics. (1990). Report of the consensus conference on the management of pain in childhood cancer. *Pediatrics* (Suppl.), *86,* 813–834.

American Psychiatric Association. (1994). *Diagnostic and statistical manual of mental disorders* (4th ed.). Washington, DC: Author.

Anand, K. (1990). The biology of pain perception in newborn infants. In D. Tyler & E. Krane (Eds.), *Advances in pain research and therapy: Vol. 15. Pediatric pain* (pp. 113–122). New York: Raven Press.

Anderson, F. M. (1975). Occult spinal dysraphism: A series of 73 cases. *Pediatrics, 55,* 826–835.

Andolsek, K., & Novik, B. (1980). Procedures in family practice: Use of hypnosis with children. *Journal of Family Practice, 10,* 503–507.

Andrasik, F., Blanchard, E. B., Edlund, S. B., & Rosenblum, E. L. (1982). Autogenic feedback in the treatment of two children with migraine headache. *Child and Family Behavioral Therapy, 4,* 13–23.

Andrasik, F., & Holroyd, K. A. (1980). Test of specific and non-specific effects in the biofeedback treatment of tension headache. *Journal of Consulting and Clinical Psychology, 48,* 575–586.

Antitch, J. L. S. (1967). The use of hypnosis in pediatric anesthesia. *Journal of the American Society of Psychosomatic Dentistry and Medicine, 14,* 70–75.

Apley, J. (1977). Psychosomatic aspects of gastrointestinal problems in children. *Clinics in Gastroenterology, 6,* 311–320.

Aronoff, G. M., Aronoff, S., & Peck, L. W. (1975). Hypnotherapy in the treatment of bronchial asthma. *Annals of Allergy, 34,* 356–362.

Aronson, D. M. (1986). The adolescent as hypnotist: Hypnosis and self-hypnosis with adolescent psychiatric inpatients. *American Journal of Clinical Hypnosis, 28,* 163–169.

Bakken, E. (1988). *Cyberphysiology.* Minneapolis: Archaeus Project.

Baldwin, J. M. (1891). Suggestion in infancy. *Science, 17,* 113–117.

Banerjee, S., Srivastav, A., & Palan, B. M. (1993). Hypnosis and self-hypnosis in the management of nocturnal enuresis: A comparative study with imipramine therapy. *American Journal of Clinical Hypnosis, 36*(2), 113–119.

Barber, T. X. (1979). Suggested ("hypnotic") behavior: The trance paradigm versus an alternative paradigm. In E. Fromm & R. E. Shor (Eds.), *Hypnosis: Developments in research and new perspectives* (2nd ed., pp. 217–271). Hawthorne, NY: Aldine.

Barber, T. X., & Calverley, D. S. (1963). "Hypnotic-like" suggestibility in children. *Journal of Abnormal and Social Psychology, 66,* 589–597.

Barber, T. X., & Hahn, K. W., Jr. (1962). Physiological and subjective responses to pain producing stimulation under hypnotically-suggested and waking imagined "analgesia." *Journal of Abnormal and Social Psychology, 65,* 411–418.

Barbour, J. (1980). Medigrams: Self hypnosis and asthma. *American Family Physician, 21,* 173.

Barr, M., Pennebaker, J. W., & Watson, D. (1988). Improving blood pressure estimation through internal and environmental feedback. *Psychosomatic Medicine, 50,* 37–45.

Bartlett, E. E. (1968). A proposed definition of hypnosis with a theory of its mechanism of action. *American Journal of Clinical Hypnosis, 11,* 69–73.

Basmajian, J. V. (1989). *Biofeedback: Principles and practice for clinicians.* Baltimore: Williams & Wilkins.

Bass, J. L., Christoffel, K. K., Widome, M., Boyle, W., Scheidt, P., Stanwick, R., & Roberts, K. (1993). Childhood injury prevention counseling in primary care settings: A critical review of the literature. *Pediatrics, 92*(4), 544–550.

Bauchner, H. C., Howland, J., & Adair, R. (1988). The impact of pediatric asthma education on morbidity: Assessing the evidence [Abstract]. *American Journal of Diseases of Children, 142*(4), 398–399.

Baumann, F. (1970). Hypnosis and the adolescent drug abuser. *American Journal of Clinical Hypnosis, 13,* 17–21.

Baumann, F. W., & Hinman, F. (1974). Treatment of incontinent boys with non-obstructive disease. *Journal of Urology, 111,* 114–116.

Beahrs, J. O., Harris, D. R., & Hilgard, E. R. (1970). Failure to alter skin inflammation by hypnotic suggestion in five subjects with normal skin reactivity. *Psychosomatic Medicine, 32,* 627–631.

Belsky, J., & Khanna, P. (1994). The effects of self-hypnosis for children with cystic fibrosis: A pilot study. *American Journal of Clinical Hypnosis, 36,* 282–292.

Bensen, V. B. (1971). One hundred cases of post-anesthetic suggestion in the recovery room. *American Journal of Clinical Hypnosis, 14,* 9–15.

Benson, H. (1990). *The relaxation response* (2nd ed.). New York: Avon Books.

Berger, H. G., Honig, P. J., & Liebman, R. (1977). Recurrent abdominal pain: Gaining control of the symptom. *American Journal of Diseases of Children, 131,* 1340–1344.

Bernick, S. M. (1972). Relaxation, suggestion, and hypnosis in dentistry: What the pediatrician should know about children's dentistry. *Clinical Pediatrics, 11,* 72–75.

Bernstein, N. R. (1963). Management of burned children with the aid of hypnosis. *Journal of Child Psychology and Psychiatry, 4,* 93–98.

Bernstein, N. R. (1965). Observations on the use of hypnosis with burned children on a pediatric ward. *International Journal of Clinical and Experimental Hypnosis, 13,* 1–10.

Betcher, A. M. (1960). Hypnosis as an adjunct in anesthesiology. *New York State Journal of Medicine, 60,* 816–822.

Bierman, S. F. (1989). Hypnosis in the emergency department. *American Journal of Emergency Medicine, 7,* 238–242.

Black, S., Humphrey, J. H., & Niven, J. S. (1963). Inhibition of the Mantoux reaction by direct suggestion under hypnosis. *British Medical Journal, 6,* 1649–1652.

Blanchard, E. B. (1990). Biofeedback treatments of essential hypertension. *Biofeedback and Self-Regulation, 15,* 209–228.

Blanton, J., & Johnson, L. J. (1991). Using computer assisted biofeedback to help children with attention-deficit hyperactivity disorder to gain self-control. *Journal of Special Education Technology, 11*(1), 49–56.

Blessing-Moore, J., Fritz, G., & Lewiston, N. J. (1985). Self-management programs for childhood asthma—a review. *Chest, 87*(1), 107S–110S.

Boswell, L. K., Jr. (1962). Pediatric hypnosis. *British Journal of Medical Hypnotism, 13,* 4–11.

Bowers, K. S., & LeBaron, S. L. (1986). Hypnosis and hypnotizability: Implications for clinical intervention. *Hospital and Community Psychiatry, 37,* 457–467.

Bowers, P., & London, P. (1965). Developmental correlates of role playing ability. *Child Development, 30,* 499–508.

Boyce, W. T., Chesney, M., Kaiser, P., Alkon, A., Eisenhardt, M., Chesterman, E., & Tschann, J. (1990). Development of a protocol for measuring cardiovascular response to stress in pre-school children. *Journal of Developmental and Behavioral Pediatrics, 11*(4), 214.

Boyce, W. T., Chesterman, E. A., Martin, N., Folkman, S., Cohen, F., & Wara, D. (1993). Immunologic changes occurring at kindergarten entry predict respiratory illnesses after the Loma Prieta earthquake. *Journal of Developmental and Behavioral Pediatrics, 14,* 196–203.

Braid, J. (1855). *The physiology of fascination and the critics criticized.* Manchester, England: Grant & Co.

Braid, J. (1960). *Neurypnology; or the rationale of nervous sleep* [Revised as *Braid on hypnotism,* 1889]. New York: Julian Press. (Original work published 1843)

Bramwell, J. M. (1956). *Hypnotism: Its history, practice and theory* [Reissued with new introduction]. New York: Julian Press. (Original work published 1903)

Bronowski, J. (1974). *The ascent of man.* Boston: Little, Brown.

Broome, M. E., Lillis, P. P., McGahee, T. W., & Bates, T. (1992). The use of distraction and imagery with children during painful procedures. *Oncology Nursing Forum, 19,* 499–502.

Brown, B. (1974). *New mind: New body.* New York: Harper & Row.

Browning, C. W., Quinn, L. H., & Crasilneck, H. B. (1958). The use of hypnosis in suppressing amblyopia of children. *American Journal of Ophthalmology, 46,* 53–67.

Buchanan, A., & Clayden, G. (1992). *Children who soil: Assessment and treatment.* Chichester, England: Wiley.

Burke, E. J., & Andrasik, F. (1989). Home vs. clinic-based biofeedback treatment for pediatric migraine: Results of treatment through one-year follow-up. *Headache, 29,* 434–440.

Buske-Kirschbaum, A., Kirschbaum, C., Stierle, H., Lehnert, H., & Hellhammer, D. (1992). Conditioned increase of natural killer cell activity in humans. *Psychosomatic Medicine, 54,* 123–132.

Call, J. D. (1976). Children, parents, and hypnosis: A discussion. *International Journal of Clinical and Experimental Hypnosis, 24,* 149–155.

Carey, S., & Diamond, R. (1980). Maturational determination of the developmental course of face encoding. In D. Caplan (Ed.), *Biological studies of mental processes.* Cambridge, MA: MIT Press.

Carson, D. K., Council, J. R., & Schauer, R. W. (1991). The effectiveness of a family asthma program for children and parents. *Children's Health Care, 20*(2), 114–119.

Chakravarty, K., Pharoah, P. D. P., Scott, D. G. I., & Barker, S. (1992). Erythromelalgia — the role of hypnotherapy. *Postgraduate Medical Journal, 68,* 44–46.

Chandrasena, R. (1982). Hypnosis in the treatment of viral warts. *Psychiatric Journal of the University of Ottawa, 7,* 135–137.

Cheek, D. B. (1959). Unconscious perception of meaningful sounds during surgical anesthesia as revealed under hypnosis. *American Journal of Clinical Hypnosis, 1,* 101–113.

Chesney, M. A., Agras, W. S., Benson, H., Blumenthal, J. A., Engel, B. T., Foreyt, J. P., Kaufmann, P. G., Levenson, R. M., Pickering, T. G., Randall, W. C., & Schwartz, P. J. (1987). Task Force 5: Nonpharmacologic approaches to the treatment of hypertension. *Circulation, 76*(Suppl. 1), 104–109.

Christopherson, E. R., Finney, J. W., & Friman, P. C. (Eds.). (1986). Prevention in primary care [Special issue]. *Pediatric Clinics of North America, 33,* 743–1009.

Churchill, D. R., Persinger, M. A., & Thomas, A. W. (1994). Geophysical variables and behavior: Increased geomagnetic activity and decreased pleasantness of spontaneous narratives for percipients but not agents. *Perceptual and Motor Skills, 79,* 387–392.

Cioppa, F. J., & Thal, A. D. (1975). Hypnotherapy in a case of juvenile rheumatoid arthritis. *American Journal of Clinical Hypnosis, 18,* 105–110.

Clawson, T. A., Jr., & Swade, R. H. (1975). The hypnotic control of blood flow and pain: The cure of warts and the potential for the use of hypnosis in the treatment of cancer. *American Journal of Clinical Hypnosis, 17,* 160–169.

Clayden, G. S., & Lawson, J. (1976). Investigation and management of longstanding chronic constipation in childhood. *Archives of Diseases of Childhood, 51,* 918–923.

Cohen, M. W. (1975). Enuresis. *Pediatric Clinics of North America, 22,* 545–560.

Coleman, D., & Gupin, J. (Eds.). (1993). *Mind body medicine.* Yonkers, NY: Consumer Reports Books.

Collison, D. R. (1970). Hypnotherapy in the management of nocturnal enuresis. *Medical Journal of Australia, 1,* 52–54.

Collison, D. R. (1975). Which asthmatic patients should be treated by hypnotherapy? *Medical Journal of Australia, 1*(25), 776–781.

Cooper, L. M., & London, P. (1966). Sex and hypnotic susceptibility in children. *International Journal of Clinical and Experimental Hypnosis, 14,* 55–60.

Cooper, L. M., & London, P. (1971). The development of hypnotic susceptibility: A longitudinal (convergence) study. *Child Development, 42,* 487–503.

Cooper, L. M., & London, P. (1976). Children's hypnotic susceptibility, personality, and EEG patterns. *International Journal of Clinical and Experimental Hypnosis, 24,* 140–148.

Cooper, W., Shafter, W. L., & Tyndall, C. S. (1986). Shortening labor with hypnosis as an adjunct to Lamaze [Abstract]. *American Journal of Clinical Hypnosis, 28,* 193.

Cotanch, P., Hockenberry, M., & Herman, S. (1985). Self-hypnosis as antiemetic therapy in children receiving chemotherapy. *Oncology Nursing Forum, 12,* 41–46.

Cousins, N. (1976). Anatomy of an illness (as perceived by the patient). *New England Journal of Medicine, 295,* 1458–1463.

Crasilneck, H. B., & Hall, J. A. (1970). The use of hypnosis in the rehabilitation of complicated vascular and post-traumatic neurological patients. *International Journal of Clinical and Experimental Hypnosis, 28,* 145–159.

Crasilneck, H. B., & Hall, J. A. (1973). Clinical hypnosis in problems of pain. *American Journal of Clinical Hypnosis, 15,* 153–161.

Crasilneck, H. B., & Hall, J. A. (1975). *Clinical hypnosis: Principles and applications.* New York: Grune & Stratton.

Crasilneck, H. B., & Hall, J. A. (1985). *Clinical hypnosis: Principles and applications* (2nd ed.). New York: Grune & Stratton.

Crasilneck, H. B., McCranie, E. J., & Jenkins, M. T. (1956). Special indications for hypnosis as a method of anesthesia. *Journal of the American Medical Association, 162,* 1606–1608.

Creer, T. L., Stein, R. E. K., Rappaport, L., & Lewis, C. (1992). Behavioral consequences of illness: Childhood asthma as a model. In P. C. Scheidt & D. Bacchi (Eds.), Research in behavioral pediatrics. *Pediatrics* (Suppl.), *80* (5, Pt. 2), 808–815.

Crowther, J. (1983). Stress management training and relaxation imagery in the treatment of essential hypertension. *Journal of Behavioral Medicine, 6,* 169–186.

Culbert, T., Reaney, J., & Kohen, D. P. (1994). Cyberphysiologic strategies in children: The biofeedback–hypnosis interface. *International Journal of Clinical and Experimental Hypnosis, 42*(2), 97–117.

Culbertson, F. M. (1989). A four-step hypnotherapy model for Gilles de la Tourette's syndrome. *American Journal of Clinical Hypnosis, 31*(4), 252–256.

Cullen, S. C. (1958). Current comment and case reports: Hypno-induction techniques in pediatric anesthesia. *Anesthesiology, 19,* 279–281.

Dahlquist, L. M., Gil, K. M., Armstrong, F. D., Ginsburg, A., & Jones, B. (1985). Behavioral management of children's distress during chemotherapy. *Journal of Behavior Therapy and Experimental Psychiatry, 16,* 325–329.

Daniels, E. (1962). The hypnotic approach in anesthesia for children. *American Journal of Clinical Hypnosis, 4,* 244–248.

Davidson, M., & Wasserman, R. (1966). The irritable colon of childhood. *Journal of Pediatrics, 69,* 1027–1038.

Diamond, H. H. (1959). Hypnosis in children: The complete cure of forty cases of asthma. *American Journal of Clinical Hypnosis, 1,* 124–129.

Diego, R. V. (1961). Hypnosis in the treatment of the asthmatic child. *Bulletin of the Tulane Medical Society, 20,* 307–313.

Dientsfrey, H. (Ed.). (1992). Can we demonstrate important psychosocial influences on health? *Advances: The Journal of Mind–Body Health, 8,* 5–45.

Dikel, W., & Olness, K. (1980). Self-hypnosis, biofeedback, and voluntary peripheral temperature control in children. *Pediatrics, 66,* 335–340.

Dodge, J. A. (1976). Recurrent abdominal pain in children. *British Medical Journal, 1,* 385–387.

Doleys, D. M. (1977). Behavioral treatments for nocturnal enuresis in children: A review of the literature. *Psychological Bulletin, 84,* 30–54.

Domangue, B. B., Margolis, C. G., Lieberman, D., & Kaji, H. (1985). Biochemical correlates of hypnoanalgesia in arthritic pain patients. *Journal of Clinical Psychiatry, 46,* 235–238.

Edel, J. W. (1959). Nosebleed controlled by hypnosis. *American Journal of Clinical Hypnosis, 2,* 89–90.

Edwards, S. D., & van der Spuy, H. I. (1985). Hypnotherapy as a treatment for enuresis. *Journal of Child Psychology and Psychiatry, 26,* 161–170.

Ehrlich, R. M. (1974). Diabetes mellitus in childhood. *Pediatric Clinics of North America, 21,* 871–884.

Eisenberg, D. M., Kessler, R. C., Foster, C., Norlock, F. E., Calkins, D. R., & Delbanco, T. L. (1993). Unconventional medicine in the United States. *New England Journal of Medicine, 328,* 246–252.

Eland, J. M., & Anderson, J. E. (1977). The experience of pain in children. In A. Jacox (Ed.), *Pain: A source book for nurses and other health professionals.* Boston: Little, Brown.

Elinoff, V. (1993). Remission of dysphagia in a 9 year old treated in a family practice office setting. *American Journal of Clinical Hypnosis, 35,* 205–208.

Elliotson, J. (1843a). Cases of cures by mesmerism. *The Zoist, 1,* 161–208.

Elliotson, J. (1843b). *Numerous cases of surgical operations without pain in the mesmeric state.* Philadelphia: Lea & Blanchard.

Engel, J. M., Rapoff, M. A., & Pressman, A. R. (1992). Long-term follow-up of relaxation training for pediatric headache disorders. *Headache, 32,* 152–156.

Engstrom, D. R. (1976). Hypnotic susceptibility, EEG alpha, and self-regulation. In G. E. Schwartz & D. Shapiro (Eds.), *Consciousness and self-regulation* (Vol. 1). New York: Plenum Press.

Erickson, C. J. (1991). Applications of cyberphysiologic techniques in pain management. *Pediatric Annals, 20,* 145–156.

Erickson, M. H. (1958a). Naturalistic techniques of hypnosis. *American Journal of Clinical Hypnosis, 1,* 3–8.

Erickson, M. H. (1958b). Pediatric hypnotherapy. *American Journal of Clinical Hypnosis, 1,* 25–29.

Erickson, M. H. (1959). Further techniques of hypnosis: Utilization techniques. *American Journal of Clinical Hypnosis, 2,* 3–21.

Erickson, M. H. (1962). The identification of a secure reality. *Family Process, 1,* 294–303.

Ewart, C. K., Harris, W. L., Iwata, M. M., Coates, T. J., Bullock, R., & Simon, B. (1987). Feasibility and effectiveness of school-based relaxation in lowering blood pressure. *Health Psychology, 6,* 399–416.

Ewin, D. (1992). Hypnotherapy for warts (Verucca vulgaris): 41 consecutive cases with 33 cures. *American Journal of Clinical Hypnosis 35*(1), 1–10.

Faigel, H. C. (1983). Learning disabilities in adolescents with high IQ scores. *Developmental and Behavioral Pediatrics, 4,* 11–15.

Falck, F. J. (1964). Stuttering and hypnosis. *International Journal of Clinical and Experimental Hypnosis, 12,* 67–74.

Feldman, G. M. (1976). The effect of biofeedback training on respiratory resistance of asthmatic children. *Psychosomatic Medicine, 38,* 27–34.

Felt, B., Hall, H., Coury, D., Kohen, D., Broffmann, G., Berman, B., & Olness, K. (1994, November). *A prospective comparison of self-hypnosis and topical treatment in the management of juvenile warts* [Abstract]. Paper presented at the meeting of the Psychoneuroimmunology Society, Key Biscayne, FL.

Fitzgerald, M., Millard, C., & McIntosh, N. (1988). Hyperalgesia in premature infants. *Lancet, 1,* 292.

Fleisher, D. R. (1976). The diagnosis and treatment of disorders of defecation in children. *Pediatric Annals, 5,* 700–722.

Flodmark, A. (1986). Augmented auditory feedback as an aid in gait training of the cerebral-palsied child. *Developmental Medicine and Child Neurology, 28,* 147–155.

Fowler-Kerry, S. (1990). Adolescent oncology survivors' recollection of pain. In D. Tyler & E. Krane (Eds.), *Advances in pain research and therapy: Vol. 15. Pediatric pain* (pp. 365–371). New York: Raven Press.

Francis, P. W. J., Krastins, I. R. B., & Levison, H. (1980). Oral and inhaled salbutamol in the prevention of exercise induced bronchospasm. *Pediatrics, 66,* 103–108.

Frankel, F. H. (1981). Reporting hypnosis in the medical context: A brief communication. *International Journal of Clinical and Experimental Hypnosis, 29,* 10–14.

Frankel, F. H., & Perry, C. W. (Eds.). (1994). Hypnosis and delayed recall: Part 1 [Special issue]. *International Journal of Clinical and Experimental Hypnosis, 42*(4), 259–446.

Freyschuss, U., Hjemdahl, P., Juhlin-Dannfelt, A., & Linde, B. (1988). Cardiovascular and sympathoadrenal responses to mental stress: Influence of beta blockade. *American Journal of Physiology, 255,* 1443–1451.

Friedrich, W. N. (1991). Hypnotherapy with traumatized children. *International Journal of Clinical and Experimental Hypnosis, 39*(2), 67–81.

Frischholz, E. J., & Tryon, W. W. (1980). Hypnotizability in relation to the ability to learn thermal biofeedback. *American Journal of Clinical Hypnosis, 23,* 53–56.

Fromm, E. (1972). Ego activity and ego passivity in hypnosis. *International Journal of Clinical and Experimental Hypnosis, 20,* 238–251.

Fromm, E. (1977). An ego-psychological theory of altered states of consciousness. *International Journal of Clinical and Experimental Hypnosis, 25,* 372–387.

Fromm, E. (1979). The nature of hypnosis and other altered states of consciousness: An ego-psychological theory. In E. Fromm & R. E. Shor (Eds.), *Hypnosis: Developments in research and new perspectives* (2nd ed., pp. 81–103). Hawthorne, NY: Aldine.

Fromm, E. (1981). How to write a clinical paper: A brief communication. *International Journal of Clinical and Experimental Hypnosis, 29,* 5–9.

Fromm E., & Gardner, G. G. (1979). Ego psychology and hypnoanalysis: An integration of theory and technique. *Bulletin of the Menninger Clinic, 43,* 413–423.

Fromm, E., & Hurt, S. W. (1980). Ego-psychological parameters of hypnosis and altered states of consciousness. In G. D. Burrows & L. Dennerstein (Eds.), *Handbook of hypnosis and psychosomatic medicine* (pp. 13–27). New York: Elsevier/North-Holland Biomedical Press.

Fromm, E., & Nash, M. R. (Eds.). (1992). *Contemporary hypnosis research.* New York: Guilford Press.

Gaal, J. M., Goldsmith, L., & Needs, R. E. (1980, November). *The use of hypnosis, as an adjunct to anesthesia, to reduce pre- and post-operative anxiety in children.* Paper presented at the annual meeting of the American Society of Clinical Hypnosis, Minneapolis.

Gallwey, W. T. (1974). *The inner game of tennis.* New York: Random House.

Gallwey, W. T., & Kriegel, B. (1977). *Inner skiing.* New York: Random House.

Gardner, G. G. (1973). Use of hypnosis for psychogenic epilepsy in a child. *American Journal of Clinical Hypnosis, 15,* 166–169.

Gardner, G. G. (1974a). Hypnosis with children. *International Journal of Clinical and Experimental Hypnosis, 22,* 20–38.

Gardner, G. G. (1974b). Parents: Obstacles or allies in child hypnotherapy? *American Journal of Clinical Hypnosis, 17,* 44–49.

Gardner, G. G. (1976a). Attitudes of child health professionals toward hypnosis: Implications for training. *International Journal of Clinical and Experimental Hypnosis, 24,* 63–73.

Gardner, G. G. (1976b). Childhood, death, and human dignity: Hypnotherapy for David. *International Journal of Clinical and Experimental Hypnosis, 24,* 122–139.

Gardner, G. G. (1977a). Hypnosis with infants and preschool children. *American Journal of Clinical Hypnosis, 19,* 158–162.

Gardner, G. G. (1977b). The rights of dying children: Some personal reflections. *Psychotherapy Bulletin, 10,* 20–23.

Gardner, G. G. (1978a). Hypnotherapy in the management of childhood habit disorders. *Journal of Pediatrics, 92,* 838–840.

Gardner, G. G. (1978b). The use of hypnotherapy in a pediatric setting. In E. Gellert (Ed.), *Psychosocial aspects of pediatric care.* New York: Grune & Stratton.

Gardner, G. G. (1980). Hypnosis with children: Selected readings. *International Journal of Clinical and Experimental Hypnosis, 28,* 289–293.

Gardner, G. G. (1981). Teaching self-hypnosis to children. *International Journal of Clinical and Experimental Hypnosis, 29,* 300–312.

Gardner, G. G., & Hinton, R. M. (1980). Hypnosis with children. In G. D. Burrows & L. Dennerstein (Eds.), *Handbook of hypnosis and psychosomatic medicine.* New York: Elsevier/North-Holland Biomedical Press.

Gardner, G. G., & Tarnow, J. D. (1980). Adjunctive hypnotherapy with an autistic boy. *American Journal of Clinical Hypnosis, 22,* 173–179.

Garfield, C. (1985). *Peak performance.* New York: Warner. (Original work published 1984)

Gay, M., Blager, F., Bartsch, K., Emergy, C. F., Rosenstiel-Gross, A. K., & Spears, J. (1987). Psychogenic habit cough: Review and case reports. *Journal of Clinical Psychiatry, 48*(12), 483–486.

Gellert, G. (1994). Global explanations and the credibility problem of alternative medicine. *Advances: The Journal of Mind–Body Health, 10,* 60–67.

Gerrard, J. W., Jones, B., Shokier, M. K., & Zaleski, A. (1971). Allergy and urinary infections: Is there an association? *Pediatrics, 48,* 994–995.

Gevgen, P. J., Mullally, D. I., & Evans, R. (1980). Third national survey of prevalence of asthma among children in the United States 1976. *Pediatrics, 81*(1), 1–7.

Gildston, P., & Gildston, H. (1992). Hypnotherapeutic intervention for voice disorders related to recurring juvenile laryngeal papillomatosis. *International Journal of Clinical and Experimental Hypnosis, 40*(2), 74–87.

Glenn, T. J., & Simonds, J. F. (1977). Hypnotherapy of a psychogenic seizure disorder in an adolescent. _American Journal of Clinical Hypnosis, 19,_ 245–250.

Glicklich, L. B. (1951). An historical account of enuresis. _Pediatrics, 8,_ 859–876.

Goldsmith, H. (1962). Chronic loss of bowel control in a nine-year-old child. _American Journal of Clinical Hypnosis, 4,_ 191–193.

Goldstein, A., & Hilgard, E. R. (1975). Lack of influence of the morphine antagonist naloxone on hypnotic analgesia. _Proceedings of the National Academy of Sciences, 72,_ 2041–2043.

Good, R. A. (1981). Interactions of the body's major networks: Foreword. In R. Ader (Ed.), _Psychoneuroimmunology_ (pp. xviii–xix). New York: Academic Press.

Gould, R. (1972). _Child studies through fantasy: Cognitive–affective patterns in development._ New York: Quadrangle Books.

Gray, J. A. (1987). _The psychology of fear and stress._ Cambridge, England: Cambridge University Press.

Green, E., & Green, A. (1989). _Beyond biofeedback._ Fort Wayne, IN: Knoll Publishers.

Green, L. (1994). Touch and visualization to facilitate a therapeutic relationship in an intensive care unit—a personal experience. _Intensive and Critical Care Nursing, 10,_ 51–57.

Greene, R. J., & Reyher, J. (1972). Pain tolerance in hypnotic analgesic and imagination states. _Journal of Abnormal Psychology, 79,_ 29–38.

Greene, W. A., Jr., & Miller, G. (1958). Psychological factors and reticuloendothelial disease. IV. Observations on a group of children and adolescents with leukemias: An interpretation of disease development. _Psychosomatic Medicine, 10,_ 124–144.

Grollman, E. (1991). _Talking about death: A dialogue between parent and child._ Boston: Beacon Press.

Gross, M. (1984). Hypnosis in the therapy of anorexia hysteria. _American Journal of Clinical Hypnosis, 26,_ 175–181.

Grynkewich, M. A. (1994). _The use of mental imagery strategies to improve school performance._ Unpublished manuscript, University of Arizona.

Gualtieri, C. T., Koriath, U., Van Bourgondien, M., & Saleeby, N. (1983). Language disorders in children referred for psychiatric services. _Journal of the American Academy of Child Psychiatry, 22,_ 165–171.

Gustke, S. S. (1973, October). _Alterations in in vitro coagulation during hypnosis in hemophiliacs._ Paper presented at the annual meeting of the American Society of Clinical Hypnosis, Toronto.

Haber, C. H., Nitkin, R., & Shenker, L. R. (1979). Adverse reactions to hypnotherapy in obese adolescents: A developmental viewpoint. _Psychiatric Quarterly, 51,_ 55–63.

Haber, R. N. (1980). Eidetic images are not just imaginary. _Psychology Today, 14,_ 72–82.

Hall, H. R., Minnes, L., & Olness, K. (1993). The psychophysiology of voluntary immunomodulation. _International Journal of Neuroscience, 69,_ 221–234.

Hall, H. R., Minnes, L., Tosi, M., & Olness, K. (1992). Voluntary modulation of neutrophil adhesiveness using a cyberphysiologic strategy. *International Journal of Neuroscience, 63,* 287–297.

Halley, F. M. (1991). Self-regulation of the immune system through biobehavioral strategies. *Biofeedback and Self-Regulation, 16,* 55–74.

Halpern, W. I. (1977). The treatment of encopretic children. *Journal of the American Academy of Child Psychiatry, 16,* 478–499.

Hammond, D. C., & Elkins, G. R. (1994). *Standards of training in clinical hypnosis.* Des Plaines, IA: American Society of Clinical Hypnosis.

Haslam, D. R. (1969). Age and the perception of pain. *Psychonomic Science, 15,* 86.

Hatch, J. P., Borcherding, S., & Norris, L. K. (1990). Cardiopulmonary adjustments during operant heart rate control. *Psychophysiology, 27,* 641–648.

Hatzenbuehler, L. C., & Schroeder, H. E. (1978). Desensitization procedures in the treatment of childhood disorders. *Psychological Bulletin, 85,* 831–844.

Heimel, A. (1978, September 28). Use of hypnosis in pediatric clinical practice: A report of 68 patients [Abstract]. *Proceedings of the Northwestern Pediatric Society,* Minneapolis.

Heitkemper, T., Layne, C., & Sullivan, D. M. (1993). Brief treatment of children's dental pain and anxiety. *Perceptual and Motor Skills, 76,* 192–194.

Henderson, W. R., Shelhamer, J. H., Reingold, D. B., Smith, L. J., Evans, R. III, & Kaliner, M. (1979). Alpha-adrenergic hyper-responsiveness in asthma. *New England Journal of Medicine, 300,* 642–647.

Hendricks, C. G., & Wills, R. (1975). *The centering book.* New York: Transpersonal Books.

Henoch, E. (1994). Lectures on diseases of children. In *A handbook for physicians and students* (special ed., *The classics of pediatrics library;* pp. 257–258). New York: Gryphon Editions.

Hewson Bower, B. (1995). *Psychological treatment decreases colds and flu in children by increasing salivary immunoglobin A.* PhD thesis, Murdoch University, Perth, Western Australia.

Hilgard, E. R. (1971). Hypnosis and childlikeness. In J. P. Hill (Ed.), *Minnesota symposia on child psychology* (Vol. 5). Minneapolis: Lund Press.

Hilgard, E. R. (1977). *Divided consciousness: Multiple controls in human thought and action.* New York: Wiley.

Hilgard, E. R., & Hilgard, J. R. (1975). *Hypnosis in the relief of pain.* Los Altos, CA: William Kaufman.

Hilgard, E. R., Weitzenhoffer, A. M., Landes, J., & Moore, R. K. (1961). The distribution of susceptibility to hypnosis in a student population: A study using the Stanford Hypnotic Susceptibility Scale. *Psychological Monographs, 75*(8, Whole No. 512).

Hilgard, J. R. (1970). *Personality and hypnosis: A study of imaginative involvement.* Chicago: University of Chicago Press.

Hilgard, J. R., & Hilgard, E. R. (1962). Developmental–interactive aspects of hypnosis: Some illustrative cases. *Genetic Psychology Monographs, 66,* 143–178.

Hilgard, J. R., & LeBaron, S. (1982). Relief of anxiety and pain in children with cancer: Quantitative measures and qualitative clinical observations in a flexible approach. *International Journal of Clinical and Experimental Hypnosis, 30,* 417–442.

Hilgard, J. R., & Morgan, A. H. (1978). Treatment of anxiety and pain in childhood cancer through hypnosis. In F. H. Frankel & H. S. Zamansky (Eds.), *Hypnosis at its bicentennial: Selected papers.* New York: Plenum Press.

Hindi-Alexander, M. C. (1985). Decision-making in asthma self-management. *Chest* (Suppl.), *87*(1), 100S–102S.

Hinman, F., Jr., & Baumann, F. W. (1976). Complications of vesicoureteral operations from incoordination of micturition. *Journal of Urology, 116,* 638–643.

Hobbie, C. (1989). Relaxation techniques for children and young people. *Journal of Pediatric Health Care, 3,* 83–87.

Hockenberry, M. J., & Cotanch, P. H. (1985). Hypnosis as adjuvant antiemetic therapy in childhood cancer. *Nursing Clinics of North America, 20,* 105–107.

Hogan, M., Olness, K., & MacDonald, J. (1985). The effects of hypnosis on brainstem auditory responses in children. *American Journal of Clinical Hypnosis, 27*(3), 91–94.

Holton, G. (1978). *The creative imagination.* New York: Cambridge University Press.

Hopayian, R. (1984). A brief technique of hypnoanesthesia for children in a casualty department. *Anaesthesia, 39,* 1139–1141.

Houts, A. C. (1982). Relaxation and thermal feedback of childhood migraine headache: A case study. *American Journal of Clinical Biofeedback, 5,* 154–157.

Hull, C. L. (1933). *Hypnosis and suggestibility: An experimental approach.* New York: D. Appleton-Century.

Hunter, S. H., Russel, H. L., Russell, E. D., & Zimmerman, R. L. (1976). Control of fingertip temperature increases via biofeedback in learning-disabled and normal children. *Perceptual and Motor Skills, 43,* 743–755.

Hurwitz, T. D., Mahowald, M. W., Schenck, C. H., Schluter, J. L., & Bundlie, S. R. (1991). A retrospective outcome study and review of hypnosis as treatment of adults with sleepwalking and sleep terror. *Journal of Nervous and Mental Disease, 179,* 228–233.

Illovsky, J. (1963). An experience with group hypnosis in reading disability in primary behavior disorders. *Journal of Genetic Psychology, 102,* 61–67.

Illovsky, J., & Fredman, N. (1976). Group suggestion in learning disabilities of primary grade children: A feasibility study. *International Journal of Clinical and Experimental Hypnosis, 24,* 87–97.

Irwin, C. E., Cataldo, M. F., Matheny, A. P., & Peterson, L. (1992). Health consequences of behaviors: Injury as a model. In P. C. Scheidt & D. Bacchi (Eds.), Research in behavioral pediatrics. *Pediatrics* (Suppl.), *80*(5, Pt. 2), 798–807.

Jacknow, D. S., Tschann, J. M., Link, M. P., & Boyce, W. T. (1994). Hypnosis in the prevention of chemotherapy-related nausea and vomiting in children: A prospective study. *Journal of Developmental and Behavioral Pediatrics, 15,* 258–264.

Jacobs, L. (1962). Hypnosis in clinical pediatrics. *New York State Journal of Medicine, 62,* 3781–3787.

Jacobs, L. (1964). Sleep problems of children: Treatment by hypnosis. *New York State Journal of Medicine, 64,* 629–634.

Jacobs, L., & Jacobs, J. (1966). Hypnotizability of children as related to hemispheric reference and neurological organization. *American Journal of Clinical Hypnosis, 8,* 269–274.

Jacobs, T. J., & Charles, E. (1980). Life events and the occurrence of cancer in children. *Psychosomatic Medicine, 42,* 11–24.

Jampolsky, G. G. (1970). Use of hypnosis and sensory motor stimulation to aid children with learning problems. *Journal of Learning Disabilities, 3,* 570–575.

Jampolsky, G. G. (1975, October). *Hypnosis in the treatment of learning problems.* Paper presented at the 27th annual scientific meeting of the Society for Clinical and Experimental Hypnosis, Chicago.

Jay, S. M., Ozolins, M., Elliott, C. H., & Caldwell, S. (1983). Assessment of children's distress during painful medical procedures. *Health Psychology, 2,* 133–147.

Johnson, L. S., Johnson, D. L., Olson, M. R., & Newman, J. P. (1981). The uses of hypnotherapy with learning disabled children. *Journal of Clinical Psychology, 37,* 291–299.

Jones, C. W. (1977). Hypnosis and spinal fusion by Harrington instrumentation. *American Journal of Clinical Hypnosis, 19,* 155–157.

Jung, F. F., & Ingelfinger, J. R. (1993). Hypertension in childhood and adolescence. *Pediatrics in Review, 14,* 169–179.

Kaffman, M. (1968). Hypnosis as an adjunct to psychotherapy in child psychiatry. *Archives of General Psychiatry, 18,* 725–738.

Kagan, J. (1994). *Galen's prophecy.* New York: Basic Books.

Kail, R. (1984). *The development of memory in children* (2nd ed.). New York: W. H. Freeman.

Katz, E. R., Kellerman, J., & Siegel, S. E. (1980). Behavioral distress in children with cancer undergoing medical procedures: Developmental considerations. *Journal of Consulting and Clinical Psychology, 48,* 356–365.

Katz, E. R., Sharp, B., Kellerman, J., Marston, A. R., Hershman, J. M., & Siegel, S. E. (1982). Beta-endorphin immunoreactivity and acute behavioral distress in children with leukemia. *Journal of Nervous and Mental Disease, 170,* 72–77.

Kazin, A. (Ed.). (1974). *The portable Blake.* New York: Viking Press.

Kellerman, J. (1981). Hypnosis as an adjunct to thought-stopping and covert reinforcement in the treatment of homicidal obsessions in a twelve-year-old boy. *International Journal of Clinical and Experimental Hypnosis, 29,* 128–135.

Kelly, L. J. (1976, October). *Hypnosis and children in the emergency department.* Paper presented at the annual meeting of the American Society of Clinical Hypnosis, Chicago.

Kelsey, D., & Barron, J. N. (1958). Maintenance of posture by hypnotic suggestion in patients undergoing plastic surgery. *British Medical Journal, 1,* 756.

Kemmer, F. W., Bisping, R., Steingruber, H. J., Baar, H., Hardtmann, F., Schlaghecke, R., & Berger, M. (1986). Psychological stress and metabolic control in patients with type I diabetes mellitus. *New England Journal of Medicine, 314,* 1078–1084.

Khan, A. U. (1977). Effectiveness of biofeedback and counterconditioning in the treatment of bronchial asthma. *Journal of Psychosomatic Research, 21,* 97–104.

Khan, A. U., Staerk, M., & Bonk, C. (1974). Hypnotic suggestibility compared with other methods of isolating emotionally-prone asthmatic children. *American Journal of Clinical Hypnosis, 17,* 50–53.

Kiecolt-Glaser, J. K., Glaser, R., Stain, E. C., & Stout, J. C. (1985). Modulation of cellular immunity in medical students. *Journal of Behavioral Medicine, 9,* 5–21.

King, N., Cranstoun, F., & Josephs, A. (1989). Emotive imagery and children's night-time fears: A multiple baseline design evaluation. *Journal of Behavior Therapy and Experimental Psychiatry, 20*(2), 125–135.

King, N. J., & Montgomery, R. B. (1980). Biofeedback-induced control of human peripheral temperature: A critical review of the literature. *Psychological Bulletin, 88,* 738–752.

Koe, G. G. (1989). Hypnotic treatment of sleep terror disorder: A case report. *American Journal of Clinical Hypnosis, 32*(1), 36–40.

Kohen, D. P. (1980a, May). *Hypnotherapy in a child with asthma.* Videotape presented at the annual meeting of the Ambulatory Pediatric Association, San Antonio, TX.

Kohen, D. P. (1980b). Relaxation–mental imagery (hypnosis) and pelvic examinations in adolescents. *Journal of Behavioral and Developmental Pediatrics, 1,* 180–186.

Kohen, D. P. (1982, October). *Use of relaxation/mental imagery in an 11½ year old boy with asthma.* Videotape presented to the American Society of Clinical Hypnosis, Denver, CO.

Kohen, D. P. (1986a). The value of relaxation/mental imagery (self-hypnosis) to the management of children with asthma: A cyberphysiologic approach. *Topics in Pediatrics, 4*(1), 11–18.

Kohen, D. P. (1986b). Applications of relaxation/mental imagery (self-hypnosis) in pediatric emergencies. *International Journal of Clinical and Experimental Hypnosis, 34*(4), 283–294.

Kohen, D. P. (1986c). Applications of relaxation/mental imagery (self-hypnosis) to the management of asthma: Report of behavioral outcomes of a two-year, prospective controlled study [Abstract]. *American Journal of Clinical Hypnosis, 28,* 196.

Kohen, D. P. (1987a). A biobehavioral approach to managing childhood asthma. *Children Today, 16*(2), 6–10. (DHHS Pub. No. [OHDS] 87-30014)

Kohen, D. P. (1987b). *Self-hypnosis in the management of chronic headaches—interview and demonstration (Kate)* [Videotape]. Minneapolis: Behavioral Pediatrics, Minneapolis Children's Medical Center.

Kohen, D. P. (1987c, April). *Use of relaxation/mental imagery in a 17 year old boy with asthma.* Videotape presented to the Society for Behavioral Pediatrics, Anaheim, CA.

Kohen, D. P. (1990). A hypnotherapeutic approach to enuresis. In D. C. Hammond (Ed.), *Handbook of hypnotic suggestions and metaphors* (pp. 489–493). New York: W. W. Norton.

Kohen, D. (1991). Applications of relaxation/mental imagery (self-hypnosis) for habit problems. *Pediatric Annals, 20*(3), 136–144.

Kohen, D. P. (1992, July). *Hypnotherapeutic management of pediatric trichotillomania: Experience with five children.* Paper presented to the 12th International Congress of Hypnosis, International Society of Hypnosis, Jerusalem, Israel.

Kohen, D. P. (1993). Entspannung und mentales Vorstellungstraining (Selbsthypnose) als Hilfe zur Selbshilfe für Kinder mit Asthma [Helping children with asthma help themselves with relaxation/mental imagery (self-hypnosis). In S. Mrochen, K. L. Holtz, & B. Trenkle (Eds.), *Die Pupille des Bettnassers: Hypnotherapeutische Arbeit mit Kindern und Jugendlichen [The eye in the middle of the crater—on child hypnosis]* (pp. 212–235). Heidelberg: Carl Auer.

Kohen, D. P. (1994, March 15). *Self-regulation by children and adolescents with cystic fibrosis: Applications of relaxation/mental imagery (self-hypnosis).* Paper presented to the 36th annual scientific meeting of the American Society of Clinical Hypnosis, Philadelphia.

Kohen, D. P. (1995a, January, 19). *Childhood grief and mourning: Applications of hypnotherapy.* Paper presented to the Minnesota Society of Clinical Hypnosis, Minneapolis.

Kohen, D. P. (1995b). Ericksonian communication and hypnotic strategies in the management of tics and Tourette syndrome in children and adolescents. In S. R. Lankton & J. K. Zeig (Eds.), *Ericksonian monographs: No. 10. Difficult contexts for therapy* (pp. 117–142). New York: Brunner/Mazel.

Kohen, D. P. (1995c). Relaxation/mental imagery (self-hypnosis) for childhood asthma: Behavioral outcomes in a prospective, controlled study. *Hypnos— Swedish Journal of Hypnosis in Psychotherapy and Psychosomatic Medicine and the Journal of the European Society of Hypnosis in Psychotherapy and Psychosomatic Medicine, 22,* 132–144.

Kohen, D. P. (1995d). Coping with the stress of Tourette syndrome in children and adolescents: Use of self-hypnosis techniques. *Australian Journal of Clinical and Experimental Hypnosis, 23,* 145–157.

Kohen, D. P. (in press). Teaching children with asthma to help themselves with relaxation/mental imagery (self-hypnosis). In W. J. Matthews (Ed.), *The evolution of brief therapy: An annual publication of the Milton H. Erickson Foundation.* New York: Brunner/Mazel.

Kohen, D. P., & Botts, P. (1987). Relaxation-imagery (self-hypnosis) in Tourette syndrome: Experience with four children. *American Journal of Clinical Hypnosis, 29*(4), 227–237.

Kohen, D. P., Colwell, S. O., Heimel, A., & Olness, K. N. (1984). The use of relaxation/mental imagery (self-hypnosis) in the management of 505 pediatric behavioral encounters. *Journal of Developmental and Behavioral Pediatrics, 5*(1), 21–25.

Kohen, D. P., Mahowald, M. W., & Rosen, R. R. (1992). Sleep terror disorder in children: The role of self-hypnosis in management. *American Journal of Clinical Hypnosis, 34*(4), 233–244.

Kohen, D. P., & Olness, K. N. (1987). Child hypnotherapy: Uses of therapeutic communication and self-regulation for common pediatric situations. *Pediatric Basics, 46,* 4–10.

Kohen, D. P., & Olness, K. (1993). Hypnotherapy with children. In J. Rhue, S. J. Lynn, & I. Kirsch (Eds.), *Handbook of clinical hypnosis* (pp. 357–381). Washington, DC: American Psychological Association.

Kohen, D. P., & Ondich, S. (1992, July). *Children's self-regulation of cardiovascular function with relaxation mental imagery (self-hypnosis): Report of a controlled study.* Paper presented at the 12th International Congress of Hypnosis, Jerusalem, Israel.

Kohen, D. P., & Wynne, E. R. (1988, August). *A preschool family asthma education program: Uses of storytelling, imagery, and relaxation.* Paper presented at the 11th International Congress of Hypnosis and Psychosomatic Medicine, The Hague, The Netherlands.

Kolko, D. J., & Rickard-Figueroa, J. L. (1985). Effects of video games on the adverse corollaries of chemotherapy in pediatric oncology patients: A single-case analysis. *Journal of Counseling and Clinical Psychology, 53,* 223–228.

Kolvin, I. (Ed.). (1973). *Bladder control and enuresis.* Philadelphia: Lippincott.

Konig, P. (1978). Pharmacologic management of childhood asthma. *Advances in Asthma and Allergy, 5,* 3.

Korn, E. R., & Johnson, K. (1978, October). *Hypnosis and imagery in rehabilitation of a brain damaged patient.* Paper presented at the annual meeting of the American Society of Clinical Hypnosis, St. Louis.

Kosslyn, S. M., Margolis, J. A., Barrett, A. M., Goldknopf, E. J., & Daly, P. F. (1990). Age differences in imagery abilities. *Child Development, 61,* 995–1010.

Kotses, H., Harver, A., Segreto, J., Glaus, K. D., Creer, T. L., & Young, G. A. (1991). Long term effects of biofeedback-induced facial relaxation on measures of asthma severity in children. *Biofeedback and Self-Regulation, 16,* 1–22.

Kotses, H., & Miller, D. J. (1987). The effects of changes in facial muscle tension on respiratory resistance. *Biological Psychology, 25,* 211–219.

Kramer, R. L. (1989). The treatment of childhood night terrors through the use of hypnosis: A case study: A brief communication. *International Journal of Clinical and Experimental Hypnosis, 37,* 283–284.

Krippner, S. (1966). The use of hypnosis with elementary and secondary school children in a summer reading clinic. *American Journal of Clinical Hypnosis, 8,* 261–266.

Kroger, W. S., & DeLee, S. T. (1957). Use of hypnoanesthesia for cesarean section and hysterectomy. *Journal of the American Medical Association, 163,* 442–444.

Krojanker, R. J. (1969). Human hypnosis, animal hypnotic states, and the induction of sleep in infants. *American Journal of Clinical Hypnosis, 11,* 178–179.

Kübler-Ross, E. (1969). *On death and dying.* New York: Macmillan.

Kübler-Ross, E. (1974). *Questions and answers on death and dying.* New York: Macmillan.

Kuttner, L. (1986). *No fears . . . no tears: Children with cancer coping with pain* [Videotape and manual]. Vancouver, BC: Canadian Cancer Society.

Kuttner, L. (1988). Favorite stories: A hypnotic pain reduction technique for children in acute pain. *American Journal of Clinical Hypnosis, 30*(4), 289–295.

Kuttner, L. (1989). Management of young children's acute pain and anxiety during invasive medical procedures. *Pediatrician, 16,* 39–44.

Kuttner, L. (1991). Helpful strategies in working with preschool children in pediatric practice. *Pediatric Annals, 20*(3), 120–127.

LaBaw, W. L. (1973). Adjunctive trance therapy with severely burned children. *International Journal of Child Psychotherapy, 2,* 80–92.

LaBaw, W. L. (1975). Autohypnosis in hemophilia. *Haematologia, 9,* 103–110.

LaBaw, W., Holton, C., Tewell, K., & Eccles, D. (1975). The use of self-hypnosis by children with cancer. *American Journal of Clinical Hypnosis, 17,* 223–238.

Labbe, E., & Williamson, D. A. (1983). Temperature biofeedback in the treatment of children with migraine headaches. *Journal of Pediatric Psychology, 8,* 317–326.

LaClave, L., & Blix, S. (1989). Hypnosis in the management of symptoms in a young girl with malignant astrocytoma: A challenge to the therapist. *International Journal of Clinical and Experimental Hypnosis, 37*(1), 6–14.

LaGrone, R. (1993). Hypnobehavioral therapy to reduce gag and emesis with a 10-year-old pill swallower. *American Journal of Clinical Hypnosis, 36*(2), 132–136.

Laguaite, J. K. (1976). The use of hypnosis with children with deviant voices. *International Journal of Clinical and Experimental Hypnosis, 24,* 98–104.

Landsberg, L., & Young, J. B. (1978). Fasting, feeding, and regulation of the sympathetic nervous system. *New England Journal of Medicine, 198,* 1293–1301.

Lawlor, E. D. (1976). Hypnotic intervention with "school phobic" children. *International Journal of Clinical and Experimental Hypnosis, 24,* 74–86.

Lazar, B. S. (1977). Hypnotic imagery as a tool in working with a cerebral palsied child. *International Journal of Clinical and Experimental Hypnosis, 25,* 78–87.

Lazar, B. S., & Jedliczka, Z. T. (1979). Utilization of manipulative behavior in a retarded asthmatic child. *American Journal of Clinical Hypnosis, 21,* 287–292.

LeBaron, S. L. (1983). Fantasies of children and adolescents: Implications for behavioral intervention in chronic illness. In D. R. Copeland, B. Pfefferbaum, & A. Storall (Eds.), *The mind of the child who is said to be sick.* Springfield, IL: Charles C Thomas.

LeBaron, S., & Hilgard, J. R. (1984). *Hypnotherapy of pain in children with cancer.* Los Altos, CA: William Kaufmann.

LeBaron, S., & Zeltzer, L. (1984). Assessment of acute pain and anxiety in children and adolescents by self-reports, observer reports, and a behavior checklist. *Journal of Consulting and Clinical Psychology, 52,* 729–738.

LeBaron, S., & Zeltzer, L. (1985a). Pediatrics and psychology: A collaboration that works. *Journal of Developmental and Behavioral Pediatrics, 6,* 157–161.

LeBaron, S., & Zeltzer, L. K. (1985b). The role of imagery in the treatment of dying children and adolescents. *Journal of Developmental Behavioral Pediatrics, 6,* 252–258.

LeBaron, S., Zeltzer, L., & Fanurik, D. (1988). Imaginative involvement and hypnotic susceptibility in childhood. *International Journal of Clinical and Experimental Hypnosis, 36,* 284–295.

Lee, L., & Olness, K. (1995). Impact of imagery changes on autonomic reactivity in children [Abstract]. *Archives of Pediatrics and Adolescent Medicine, 149,* 47.

Lee, S. W. (1991). Biofeedback as a treatment for childhood hyperactivity: A critical review of the literature. *Psychological Reports, 68,* 163–192.

Leffert, F. (1980). The management of acute severe asthma. *Journal of Pediatrics, 96,* 1.

Lehrer, P. M., Sargunaraj, D., & Hochron, S. (1992). Psychological approaches to the treatment of asthma. *Journal of Consulting and Clinical Psychology, 60*(4), 639–643.

Leventhal, J. M. (1984). Psychosocial assessment of children with chronic physical disease. *Pediatric Clinics of North America, 31,* 71–86.

Levine, M. D. (1982). Encopresis: Its potentiation, evaluation, and alleviation. *Pediatric Clinics of North America, 29*(2), 315–330.

Levitan, A. A., & Harbaugh, T. E. (1992). Hypnotizability and hypnoanalgesia: Hypnotizability of patients using hypnoanalgesia during surgery. *American Journal of Clinical Hypnosis, 34*(4), 223–226.

Lewenstein, L. N. (1978). Hypnosis as an anesthetic in pediatric ophthalmology. *Anesthesiology, 49,* 144–145.

Locke, S. E., Ransil, B. J., Zachariae, R., Molay, F., Tollins, K., Covino, N. A., & Danforth, D. (1994). Effect of hypnotic suggestion on the delayed-type hypersensitivity response. *Journal of the American Medical Association, 272,* 47–52.

Loening-Baucke, V. (1990). Modulation of abnormal defecation dynamic by biofeedback treatment in chronically constipated children with encopresis. *Journal of Pediatrics, 116,* 214–222.

London, P. (1962). Hypnosis in children: An experimental approach. *International Journal of Clinical and Experimental Hypnosis, 10,* 79–91.

London, P. (1963). *Children's Hypnotic Susceptibility Scale.* Palo Alto, CA: Consulting Psychologists Press.

London, P. (1965). Developmental experiments in hypnosis. *Journal of Projective Techniques and Personality Assessment, 29,* 189–199.

London, P. (1966). Child hypnosis and personality. *American Journal of Clinical Hypnosis, 8,* 161–168.

London, P. (1976). Kidding around with hypnosis. *International Journal of Clinical and Experimental Hypnosis, 24,* 105–121.

London, P., & Cooper, L. M. (1969). Norms of hypnotic susceptibility in children. *Developmental Psychology, 1,* 113–124.

London, P., & Madsen, C. H., Jr. (1968). Effect of role playing on hypnotic susceptibility in children. *Journal of Personality and Social Psychology, 10,* 66–68.

Look, Y. K., Choy, D. C., & Kelly, J. M., Jr. (1965). Hypnotherapy in strabismus. *American Journal of Clinical Hypnosis, 7,* 335–341.

Lubar, J. F. (1991). Discourse on the development of EEG diagnostics and biofeedback for attention-deficit/hyperactivity disorders. *Biofeedback and Self-Regulation, 16,* 201–226.

Lucas, O. N. (1965). Dental extractions in the hemophiliac: Control of the emotional factors by hypnosis. *American Journal of Clinical Hypnosis, 7,* 301–307.

Luparello, T., Leist, N., Lourie, C. H., & Sweet, P. (1970). Interaction of psychologic stimuli and pharmacologic agents on airway reactivity in asthmatic subjects. *Psychosomatic Medicine, 32,* 509–513.

Lynch, W. C., Hama, H., Kohn, S., & Miller, N. E. (1976). Instrumental control of peripheral vasomotor responses in children. *Psychophysiology, 13,* 219–221.

MacQueen, G. M., Marshall, J., Perdue, M. Siegel, S., & Bienenstock, J. (1989). Pavlovian conditioning of rat mucosal mast cells to secrete rat mast cell protease II. *Science, 243,* 83–85.

Madrid, A. D., & Barnes, S. v. d. H. (1991). A hypnotic protocol for eliciting physical changes through suggestions of biochemical responses. *American Journal of Clinical Hypnosis, 34*(2), 122–128.

Madsen, C. H., Jr., & London, P. (1966). Role playing and hypnotic susceptibility in children. *Journal of Personality and Social Psychology, 3,* 13–19.

Margolis, H. (1990). Relaxation training: A promising approach for helping exceptional learners. *International Journal of Disability, Development, and Education, 37*(3), 215–234.

Marion, R. J., Creer, T. L., & Reynolds, R. V. C. (1985). Direct and indirect costs associated with the management of childhood asthma. *Annals of Allergy, 54,* 31–34.

Marino, R. V. (1994). Facilitation of extubation with physician-assisted cyber-physiologic ventilatory stabilization: Common sense, compassion, and sensitivity really enhance outcomes! *Archives of Pediatrics and Adolescent Medicine, 148,* 545.

Marmer, M. J. (1959). Hypnosis as an adjunct to anesthesia in children. *AMA Journal of Diseases of Children, 97,* 314–317.

Marshall, S., Marshall, H. H., & Richards, P. L. (1973). Enuresis: An analysis of various therapeutic approaches. *Pediatrics, 52,* 813–817.

Mason, R. O. (1897). Educational uses of hypnotism: A reply to Prof. Lightner Witmer's editorial in *Pediatrics* for January 1, 1897. *Pediatrics, 3,* 97–105.

Mattson, A. (1975). Psychologic aspects of childhood asthma. *Pediatric Clinics of North America, 22*(1), 77–89.

McKnight-Hanes, C., Myers, D. R., Dushku, J. C., & Davis, H. C. (1993). The use of behavior management techniques by dentists across practitioner type, age, and geographic region. *Pediatric Dentistry, 15*(4), 267–271.

Mead, M. (1949). *Male and female: A study of the sexes in a changing world.* New York: William Morrow.

Mellor, N. H. (1960). Hypnosis in juvenile delinquency. *General Practitioner, 22*, 83–87.

Menkes, M. S., Matthews, K. A., Krantz, D. S., Lundburg, U., Mead, L. A., Qagish, B., Liang, K. Y., Thomas, C. B., & Pearson, T. A. (1989). Cardiovascular reactivity to the cold pressor test as a predictor of hypertension. *Hypertension, 14*, 524–530.

Messerschmidt, R. (1933a). Responses of boys between the ages of five and sixteen years to Hull's postural suggestion test. *Journal of Genetic Psychology, 43*, 405–421.

Messerschmidt, R. (1933b). The suggestibility of boys and girls between the ages of six and sixteen years. *Journal of Genetic Psychology, 43*, 422–437.

Meyer, R., & Haggerty, R. (1962). Streptococcal infections in families: Factors altering individual susceptibility. *Journal of Pediatrics, 29*, 539–549.

Miles, M. (1971). *Annie and the old one.* Boston: Little, Brown.

Miller, N. E. (1969). Learning of visceral and glandular responses. *Science, 163*, 434–445.

Miller, N. E. (1985). Some professional and scientific problems and opportunities for biofeedback. *Biofeedback and Self Regulation, 10*, 3–24.

Mirvish, I. (1978). Hypnotherapy for the child with chronic eczema: A case report. *South African Medical Journal, 54*, 410–412.

Mohlman, H. J. (1973). Thumbsucking. In *A syllabus on hypnosis and a handbook of therapeutic suggestions.* Des Plaines, IL: American Society of Clinical Hypnosis Education and Research Foundation.

Moore, C. L. (1980, November). *Hypnotherapy with parents of asthmatic children.* Paper presented at the annual meeting of the American Society of Clinical Hypnosis, Minneapolis.

Moore, R. K., & Cooper, L. M. (1966). Item difficulty in childhood hypnotic susceptibility scales as a function of item wording, repetition, and age. *International Journal of Clinical and Experimental Hypnosis, 14*, 316–323.

Moore, R. K., & Lauer, L. W. (1963). Hypnotic susceptibility in middle childhood. *International Journal of Clinical and Experimental Hypnosis, 11*, 167–174.

Moore, W. E. (1946). Hypnosis in a system of therapy for stutterers. *Journal of Speech Disorders, 11*, 117–122.

Morgan, A. H. (1973). The heritability of hypnotic susceptibility in twins. *Journal of Abnormal Psychology, 82*, 55–61.

Morgan, A. H. (1974). *Hypnotizability in children as a function of the nature of the suggestion item.* Paper presented at the 82nd meeting of the American Psychological Association, New Orleans.

Morgan, A. H., & Hilgard, E. R. (1973). Age differences in susceptibility to hypnosis. *International Journal of Clinical and Experimental Hypnosis, 21*, 78–85.

Morgan, A. H., & Hilgard, E. R. (1979). The Stanford Hypnotic Clinical Scale for Children. *American Journal of Clinical Hypnosis, 21*, 148–169.

Morgan, A. H., Hilgard, E. R., & Davert, E. C. (1970). The heritability of hypnotic susceptibility of twins: A preliminary report. *Behavior Genetics, 1*, 213–224.

Morgan, W. P. (1980). Hypnosis and sports medicine. In G. D. Burrows & L. Dennerstein (Eds.), *Handbook of hypnosis and psychosomatic medicine.* New York: Elsevier/North-Holland Biomedical Press.

Moskowitz, C. B. (1991). The primary dystonias of childhood. *Journal of Neuroscience Nursing, 23,* 175–178.

Mott, T. (Ed.). (1994). Editorial: The use of recovered memories outside of therapy [Special issue on hypnosis and memory]. *American Journal of Clinical Hypnosis, 36*(3), 161–162.

Moyers, B. (1993). *Healing and the mind.* New York: Doubleday.

Mullinix, J. M., Norton, B. J., Hack, S., & Fishman, M. A. (1978). Skin temperature biofeedback and migraine. *Headache, 17,* 242–244.

Murphy, J. K., Alpert, B. S., & Walker, S. S. (1991). Stability of ethnic differences in children's pressor responses during three annual examinations. *American Journal of Hypertension, 4,* 630–634.

Murphy, L. (1962). *The widening world of childhood: Paths toward mastery.* New York: Basic Books.

Murray, R. H., & Rubel, A. J. (1992). Physicians and healers—unwitting partners in health care. *New England Journal of Medicine, 326,* 61–64.

Mutter, C. B. (1990). Hypnosis with defendants: Does it really work? *American Journal of Clinical Hypnosis, 32*(4), 257–262.

Nash, J., Neilson, P. D., & O'Dwyer, N. J. (1989). Reducing spasticity to control muscle contracture of children with cerebral palsy. *Developmental Medicine and Child Neurology, 31*(4), 471–480.

Neiburger, E. J. (1976). Waking hypnosis through sensory confusion: 302 cases of dental prophylaxis. *Journal of the American Society of Psychosomatic Dentistry and Medicine, 23,* 88–98.

Neiburger, E. J. (1978). Child response to suggestion: Study of age, sex, time, and income levels during dental care. *Journal of Dentistry for Children, 45,* 396–402.

Nixon, H. H. (1964). Review: Hirschprung's disease. *Archives of Diseases in Childhood, 39,* 109–115.

Noll, R. B. (1994). Hypnotherapy for warts in children and adolescents. *Journal of Developmental and Behavioral Pediatrics, 15,* 170–173.

Nowlis, D. P. (1969). The child rearing antecedents of hypnotic susceptibility and of naturally occurring hypnotic-like experience. *International Journal of Clinical and Experimental Hypnosis, 17,* 109–120.

O'Connell, S. (1985). Hypnosis in terminal care: Discussion paper. *Journal of the Royal Society of Medicine, 78,* 122–125.

Olness, K. (1975). The use of self-hypnosis in the treatment of childhood nocturnal enuresis: A report on forty patients. *Clinical Pediatrics, 14,* 273–279.

Olness, K. (1976). Autohypnosis in functional megacolon in children. *American Journal of Clinical Hypnosis, 19,* 28–32.

Olness, K. (1977a). *Comparison of hypnotherapy and biofeedback in management of fecal soiling in children.* Paper presented at the annual meeting of the Society for Clinical and Experimental Hypnosis, Los Angeles.

Olness, K. (1977b). How to help the wet child and the frustrated parents. *Modern Medicine, 45,* 42–46.

Olness, K. (1977c). In-service hypnosis education in a children's hospital. *American Journal of Clinical Hypnosis, 20,* 80–83.

Olness, K. (1981a). Hypnosis in pediatric practice [Monograph]. *Current Problems in Pediatrics, 12,* 3–47.

Olness, K. (1981b). Imagery (self-hypnosis) as adjunct care in childhood cancer: Clinical experience with 25 patients. *American Journal of Pediatric Hematology/Oncology, 3,* 313–321.

Olness, K. (1985a). Hypnotherapy: A useful tool for busy pediatricians. *Contemporary Pediatrics, 66–78.*

Olness, K. (1985b). Little people, images, and child health. *American Journal of Clinical Hypnosis, 27,* 169–174.

Olness, K. (1989). Relaxation–mental imagery, applications to developmental and behavioral medicine. In M. Gottlieb & J. E. Williams (Eds.), *Advances in developmental and behavioral pediatrics* (pp. 233–246). New York: Plenum Press.

Olness, K. (1990a). Pediatric psychoneuroimmunology: Hypnosis as a possible mediator: Potentials and problems. In R. Van Dyck et al. (Eds.), *Hypnosis: Current theory, research, and practice* (pp. 71–81). Amsterdam: Free University Press.

Olness, K. (1990b). Reflex sympathetic dystrophy syndrome: Treatment of children with cyberphysiologic strategies. *Swedish Journal of Hypnosis in Psychotherapy and Psychosomatic Medicine, 17,* 15–18.

Olness, K., & Ader, R. (1992). Conditioning as an adjunct in the pharmacotherapy of lupus erythematosus. *Journal of Developmental and Behavioral Pediatrics, 13,* 124–125.

Olness, K., & Agle, D. (1981). *The enhancement of mastery in the child with hemophilia, via imagery-relaxation exercises (self-hypnosis) and biofeedback techniques* [Monograph]. National Hemophilia Association.

Olness, K., & Conroy, M. (1985). A pilot study of voluntary control of transcutaneous PO_2 by children. *International Journal of Clinical and Experimental Hypnosis, 33,* 1–5.

Olness, K., Culbert, T., & Uden, D. (1989). Self-regulation of salivary immunoglobulin A by children. *Pediatrics, 83,* 66–71.

Olness, K., Fallon, J., Coit, A., Fry, G., & Bassford, M. (1974). *Group hypnotherapy in management of obesity in teenage girls.* Paper presented at the annual meeting of the American Society of Clinical Hypnosis, New Orleans.

Olness, K., & Gardner, G. G. (1978). Some guidelines for uses of hypnotherapy in pediatrics. *Pediatrics, 62,* 228-233.

Olness, K., & Hall, M. (1985). Behavioral considerations in leukemia management. In C. Pochedley (Ed.), *Acute lymphoid leukemia in children.* New York: Masson Publishing USA.

Olness, K., & Immershein, R. (1977, May). *Association of nocturnal enuresis and allergy* [Abstract]. Paper presented to the Ambulatory Pediatric Association, Washington, DC.

Olness, K., & Kohen, D. (1984).Suggestion and hypnotherapy in pediatric practice (Pts. I–II). In C. L. Tishler & M. T. Plaisted (Eds.), *Feelings and their medical significance* (pp. 13–20, 26). Columbus, OH: Ross Laboratories.

Olness, K., & Libbey, P. (1987). Unrecognized biologic bases of behavioral symptoms in patients referred for hypnotherapy. *American Journal of Clinical Hypnosis, 30,* 1–8.

Olness, K., & MacDonald, J. (1987). Headaches in children. *Pediatrics in Review, 8,* 307–311.

Olness, K., MacDonald, J., & Uden, D. (1987). A prospective study comparing self-hypnosis, propranolol, and placebo in management of juvenile migraine. *Pediatrics, 79,* 593–597.

Olness, K., McParland, F. A., & Piper, J. (1980). Biofeedback: A new modality in the management of children with fecal soiling. *Journal of Pediatrics, 96,* 505–509.

Olness, K., & Rusin, W. (1990). Cyberphysiology in children and its relationship to self-regulatory control. In L. P. Lipsitt & L. I. Mitnick (Eds.), *Loss of self-regulatory control: Its causes and consequences* (pp. 241–256). Norwood, NJ: Ablex Press.

Olness, K., & Singher, L. (1989). Five year follow-up of 61 children taught cyberphysiologic strategies as adjunct management in cancer. *Topics in Pediatrics, 7,* 2–6.

Olton, D. S., & Noonberg, A. R. (1980). *Biofeedback: Clinical applications in behavioral medicine.* Englewood Cliffs, NJ: Prentice-Hall.

Orne, M. T. (1959). The nature of hypnosis: Artifact and essence. *Journal of Abnormal and Social Psychology, 58,* 277–299.

Orne, M. T. (1981). The why and how of a contribution to the literature: A brief communication. *International Journal of Clinical and Experimental Hypnosis, 29,* 1–4.

Orne, M. T. (Ed.). (1990). Forensic hypnosis [Special issue]. *International Journal of Clinical and Experimental Hypnosis, 38*(4), 219–319.

Osterhaus, S. O. L., & Passchier, J. (1993). Effects of behavioral psychophysiological treatment on school children with migraine in a non-clinical setting: Predictors and process variable. *Journal of Pediatric Psychology, 18,* 697–715.

Osterhaus, S. O. L., Passchier, J., van der Helm-Hylkema, H., de Jong, K. T., Orlebeke, J. F., de Grauw, A. J. C., & Dekker, P. H. (1993). Effects of behavioral psychophysiological treatment on schoolchildren with migraine in a nonclinical setting: Predictors and process variables. *Journal of Pediatric Psychology, 18,* 697–715.

Owens-Stively, J., McCain, D., & Wynne, E. (1986). *Childhood constipation and soiling: A practical guide for parents and children.* Minneapolis: Behavioral Pediatrics Program, Minneapolis Children's Medical Center.

Patel, C., & Marmot, M. G. (1987). Stress management, blood pressure, and quality of life. *Journal of Hypertension, 5*(Suppl. 1), 21–28.

Pederson, C. (1993). *Ways to feel comfortable* [Videotape and companion booklet]. Minneapolis: University of Minnesota, School of Nursing.

Perloff, M. M., & Spiegelman, J. (1973). Hypnosis in the treatment of a child's allergy to dogs. *American Journal of Clinical Hypnosis, 15,* 269–272.

Persinger, M. A. (1987). *The neuropsychological bases of the God experience.* New York: Praeger.

Persinger, M. A., & De Sano, C. F. (1986). Temporal lobe signs: Positive correlations with imaginings and hypnosis induction profiles. *Psychological Reports, 58,* 347–350.

Petrie, A. (1967). *Individuality in pain and suffering.* Chicago: University of Chicago Press.

Petty, G. L. (1976). Desensitization of parents to tantrum behavior. *American Journal of Hypnosis, 19,* 95–97.

Plotnick, A. B., Payne, P. A., & O'Grady, D. J. (1991). Correlates of hypnotizability in children: Absorption, vividness of imagery, and social desirability. *American Journal of Clinical Hypnosis, 34,* 51–58.

Porges, S. W., Matthews, K. A., & Pauls, D. L. (1992). The biobehavioral interface in behavioral pediatrics. In P. C. Scheidt & D. Bacchi (Eds.), Research in behavioral pediatrics. *Pediatrics* (Suppl.), *80*(5, Pt. 2), 789–797.

Portes, P. R., Best, S. M., Sandhu, D., & Cuentas, T. (1992). Relaxation training effects on anxiety and academic performance. *Journal of the Society for Accelerative Learning and Teaching, 17,* 117–148.

Prichard, A., & Taylor, J. (1989). Creative writing and visual imagery activities in an experimental reading program. *Journal of the Society for Accelerative Learning and Training, 14*(4), 297–310.

Puskarich, C. A., Whitman, S., Dell, J., Hughes, J. R., Rosen, A. J., & Hermann, B. P. (1992). Controlled examination of effects of progressive relaxation training on seizure reduction. *Epilepsia, 33*(4), 675–680.

Puskar, K. R., & Mumford, K. (1990). The healing power. *Nursing Times, 86*(33), 50–52.

Rachelefsky, G. S., Lewis, C. E., & DeLaSota, A. (1985). ACT (asthma care training) for kids; a childhood asthma self-management program. *Chest* (Suppl.), *87*(1), 98S–100S.

Rachelefsky, G. S., & Siegel, S. (1985). Asthma in infants and children-treatment of childhood asthma: Part II. *Journal of Allergy and Clinical Immunology, 76*(3), 409–425.

Rakos, R. F., Grodek, M. V., & Mack, K. K. (1985). The impact of a self-administered behavioral intervention program in pediatric asthma. *Journal of Psychosomatic Research, 29*(1), 101–108.

Ratner, H., Gross, L., Casas, J., & Castells, S. (1990). A hypnotherapuetic approach to the improvement of compliance in adolescent diabetes. *American Journal of Clinical Hypnosis, 32,* 154–159.

Reaney, J. (1994, August). *Tommy's blankets and flying bed: Hypnosis and a dying child.* Paper presented at the 1994 Asia–Pacific Congress of Hypnosis, Cairns, North Queensland, Australia.

Reaney, J., Chang, P., & Olness, K. (1978, April). The use of relaxation and visual imagery in children with asthma. *Proceedings of the Ambulatory Pediatric Association,* p. 28.

Reiff, M. I., Banez, G. A., & Culbert, T. P. (1993). Children who have attentional disorders: Diagnosis and evaluation. *Pediatrics in Review, 14*(12), 455–465.

Rhue, J. W., & Lynn, S. J. (1991). Storytelling, hypnosis and the treatment of sexually abused children. *International Journal of Clinical and Experimental Hypnosis, 39*(4), 198–214.

Rhue, J. W., & Lynn, S. J. (1993). Hypnosis and storytelling in the treatment of child sexual abuse: Strategies and procedures. In J. W. Rhue, S. J. Lynn,

& I. Kirsch (Eds.), *Handbook of clinical hypnosis* (pp. 455–478). Washington, DC: American Psychological Association.

Rhue, J. W., Lynn, S. J., & Kirsch, I. (Eds.). (1993). *Handbook of clinical hypnosis.* Washington, DC: American Psychological Association.

Rickert, V. I., & Jay, S. M. (1994). Psychosomatic disorders: The approach. *Pediatrics in Review, 15,* 448–454.

Ritterman, M. K. (1982). Hemophilia in context: Adjunctive hypnosis for families with a hemophiliac member. *Family Practice, 21,* 469–476.

Roberts, A. H., Schuler, J., Bacon, J. G., Zimmerman, R. L., & Patterson, R. (1975). Individual differences and autonomic control, absorption, and the unilateral control of skin temperature. *Journal of Abnormal Psychology, 84,* 272–279.

Rogeness, G. A., Javors, M. S., & Pliszka, S. (1992). Neurochemistry and child and adolescent psychiatry. *Journal of the American Academy of Child and Adolescent Psychiatry, 31,* 765–781.

Ross, D. M., & Ross, S. A. (1984). Childhood pain: The school-aged child's viewpoint. *Pain, 20,* 179–191.

Ruch, J. C. (1975). Self-hypnosis: The result of heterohypnosis or vice-versa? *International Journal of Clinical and Experimental Hypnosis, 23,* 282–304.

Rusin, W. (1988, May). *Home biofeedback of taped stories or music for children with encopresis* [Abstract]. Paper presented to the Ambulatory Pediatric Association, Washington, DC.

Rusin, W., & Wynne, E. (1987, April). *Stress reduction intervention program in grade school children using computer game feedback.* Paper presented to the Society for Behavioral Pediatrics, Washington, DC.

Russo, D., & Varni, J. W. (Eds.). (1982). *Behavioral pediatrics: Research and practice.* New York: Plenum Press.

Rutter, M. (1980). School influences on children's behavior and development. *Pediatrics, 65,* 208–220.

Santer, L. (1990a). *Imagery use during laceration repair in children.* Paper presented at the annual scientific meeting of the Society for Clinical and Experimental Hypnosis, Tucson, AZ.

Sarbin, T. R. (1950). Contributions to role-taking theory: I. Hypnotic behavior. *Psychological Review, 57,* 225–270.

Sarles, R. M. (1975). The use of hypnosis with hospitalized children. *Journal of Clinical Child Psychology, 4,* 36–38.

Savedra, M. C., Tesler, M. D., Holzemer, W. L., & Ward, J. A. (1989). *Adolescent Pediatric Pain Tool (APPT) preliminary user's manual.* San Francisco: University of California Press.

Schecter, N. L., Berde, C. B., & Yaster, M. (Eds.). (1993). *Pain in infants, children, and adolescents.* Baltimore: Williams & Wilkins.

Schecter, N. L., Bernstein, B. A., Beck, A., Hart, L., & Sherzer, L. (1991). Individual differences in children's response to pain: Role of temperament and parental characteristics. *Pediatrics, 87,* 171–177.

Scherr, M. S., & Crawford, P. L. (1978). Three-year evaluation of biofeedback techniques in the treatment of children with chronic asthma in a summer camp environment. *Annals of Allergy, 41,* 288–292.

Schleifer, S. J., Scott, B., Stein, M., & Keller, S. E. (1986). Behavioral and developmental aspects of immunity. *Journal of the American Academy of Child Psychiatry, 26,* 751–763.

Schmitt, B. D. (1990). Nocturnal enuresis: Finding the treatment that fits the child. *Contemporary Pediatrics, 2,* 70–97.

Schowalter, J. E. (1994). Fears and phobias. *Pediatrics in Review, 15,* 384–388.

Scott, D. L. (1969). Hypnosis as an aid to anesthesia in children. *Anesthesia, 24,* 643–644.

Scott, D. L., & Holbrook, L. A. (1981). Hypnotic psychotherapy and cosmetic surgery. *British Journal of Plastic Surgery, 34,* 478.

Secter, I. I. (1973). Thumbsucking. In *A syllabus on hypnosis and a handbook of therapeutic suggestions.* Des Plaines, IL: American Society of Clinical Hypnosis Education and Research Foundation.

Secter, I. I., & Gelberd, M. B. (1964). Hypnosis as a relaxant for the cerebral palsied patient. *American Journal of Clinical Hypnosis, 6,* 364–365.

Shaw, S. I. (1959). A survey of the management of children in hypnodontia. *American Journal of Clinical Hypnosis, 1,* 155–162.

Sheffer, A. L. (Chair, Expert Panel). (1991). *National Asthma Education Program. Expert panel report. Guidelines for the diagnosis and management of asthma* (Pub. No. 91-3042). Washington, DC: U.S. Department of Health and Human Services, Public Health Service.

Shertzer, C. L., & Lookingbill, D. P. (1987). Effects of relaxation therapy and hypnotizability in chronic urticaria. *Archives of Dermatology, 123,* 913–916.

Shor, R. E. (1960). The frequency of naturally occurring "hypnotic-like" experiences in the normal college population. *International Journal of Clinical and Experimental Hypnosis, 8,* 151–163.

Shor, R. E., & Orne, E. C. (1962). *The Harvard Group Scale of Hypnotic Susceptibility, form A.* Palo Alto, CA: Consulting Psychologists Press.

Shor, R. E., Orne, M. T., & O'Connell, D. N. (1962). Validation and cross-validation of a scale of self-reported personal experiences which predicts hypnotizability. *Journal of Psychology, 53,* 55–75.

Shuck, A. U., & Ludlow, B. L. (1984). Effects of suggestibility on learning by retarded and nonretarded students. *Psychological Reports, 54,* 663–666.

Siegler, M. (1975). Pascal's wager and the hanging of crepe. *New England Journal of Medicine, 293,* 853–857.

Silber, S. (1968). Encopresis: Rectal rebellion and anal anarchy? *Journal of the American Society of Psychosomatic Dentistry and Medicine, 15,* 97–106.

Silber, S. (1973). Fairy tales and symbols in hypnotherapy of children with certain speech disorders. *International Journal of Clinical and Experimental Hypnosis, 21,* 272–283.

Singer, J. L. (1973). *The child's world of make-believe: Experimental studies of imaginative play.* New York: Academic Press.

Singer, J. L. (1974). *Imagery and daydream methods in psychotherapy and behavior modification.* New York: Academic Press.

Smith, G. G., Crasilneck, H. B., & Browning, C. W. (1961). A follow-up study of suppression amblyopia in children previously subjected to hypnotherapy. *American Journal of Ophthalmology, 52,* 690–693.

Smith, G. R., McKenzie, J. M., Marmer, D. J., & Steele, R. W. (1985). Psychologic modulation of the human immune response to varicella zoster. *Archives of Internal Medicine, 145,* 2110–2112.

Smith, J. M., & Burns, C. L. C. (1960). The treatment of asthmatic children by hypnotic suggestion. *British Journal of Diseases of the Chest, 54,* 78–81.

Smith, M. S. (1983). Acute psychogenic stridor in an adolescent athlete treated with hypnosis. *Pediatrics, 72,* 247–248.

Smith, M. S. (1991). Biofeedback. *Pediatric Annals, 20,* 128–134.

Smith, M. S., Womack, W. M., & Pertik, M. (1987). Temperature feedback and hypnotic ability in children and adolescents. *International Journal of Medicine and Health, 3,* 91–99.

Smith, S. D., Trueworthy, R. C., Klopovich, P. M., Vats, T. S., & Snodgrass, W. (1984). Management of children with isolated testicular leukemia. *Cancer, 54,* 2854–2858.

Sokel, B., Devane, S., & Bentovim, A. (1991). Getting better with honor: Individualized relaxation / self-hypnosis techniques for control of recalcitrant abdominal pain in children. *Family Systems Medicine, 9,* 83–91.

Sokel, B. S., Devane, S. P., Bentovim, A., & Milla, P. J. (1990). Self-hypnotherapeutic treatment of habitual reflex vomiting. *Archives of Disease in Childhood, 65,* 627–628.

Sokel, B., Lansdown, R., & Kent, A. (1990). The development of a hypnotherapy service for children. *Child Care and Health Development, 16,* 227–233.

Solomon, G. F. (1993). Whither psychoneuroimmunology? A new era of immunology, of psychosomatic medicine, and of neuroscience. *Brain, Behavior, and Immunity, 7,* 352–366.

Solovey de Milechnin, G. (1955). Conduct problems in children and hypnosis. *Diseases of the Nervous System, 16,* 249–253.

Solovey, G., & Milechnin, A. (1959). Concerning the treatment of enuresis. *American Journal of Clinical Hypnosis, 3,* 22–30.

Southam, M. A., Agras, W. S., Taylor, C. B., & Kraemer, H. C. (1982). Relaxation training: Blood pressure lowering during the working day. *Archives of General Psychiatry, 39,* 715–717.

Spanos, N. P., Lush, N. I., Smith, J. E., & deGroh, M. M. (1986). Effects of two hypnotic induction procedures on overt and subjective responses to two measures of hypnotic susceptibility. *Psychological Reports, 59,* 1227–1230.

Spanos, N. P., Stenstrom, R. J., & Johnston, J. C. (1988). Hypnosis, placebo, and suggestion in the treatment of warts. *Psychosomatic Medicine, 50,* 245–260.

Spevack, M., Vost, M., Maheux, V., & Bestercezy, A. (1978). Group passive relaxation exercises in asthma. *Pediatric News, 12,* 14.

Spigelblatt, L., Laine-Ammara G., Pless, B., & Guyver, A. (1994). The use of alternative medicine by children. *Pediatrics, 94,* 811–814.

Stabler, B., Gibson, F. W., Jr., & Cutting, D. S. (1973). Parents as therapists: An innovative community-based model. *Professional Psychology, 4,* 397–402.

Stam, H. J., & Spanos, N. P. (1980). Experimental designs, expectancy effects, and hypnotic analgesia. *Journal of Abnormal Psychology, 89,* 751–762.

Stanton, H. E. (1979). Short-term treatment of enuresis. *American Journal of Clinical Hypnosis, 22,* 103–107.

Staples, L. M. (1973). Thumbsucking. In *A syllabus on hypnosis and a hand-book of therapeutic suggestions*. Des Plaines, IL: American Society of Clinical Hypnosis Education and Research Foundation.

Starfield, B. (1982). Behavioral pediatrics and primary health care. *Pediatric Clinics of North America, 29*, 377–390.

Stein, C. (1963). The clenched fist technique as a hypnotic procedure in clinical psychotherapy. *American Journal of Clinical Hypnosis, 6*, 113–119.

Sternlicht, M., & Wanderer, Z. W. (1963). Hypnotic susceptibility and mental deficiency. *International Journal of Clinical and Experimental Hypnosis, 11*, 104–111.

Stukát, K. G. (1958). *Suggestibility: A factorial and experimental analysis*. Stockholm: Almquist & Wiksell.

Surman, O. S., Gottlieb, S. K., & Hackett, T. P. (1972). Hypnotic treatment of a child with warts. *American Journal of Clinical Hypnosis, 15*, 12–14.

Taboada, E. L. (1975). Night terrors in a child treated with hypnosis. *The American Journal of Clinical Hypnosis, 17*, 270–271.

Tansey, M. A. (1993). Ten year stability of EEG biofeedback results for a hyperactive boy who failed fourth grade perceptually impaired class. *Biofeedback and Self-Regulation, 18*(1), 33–44.

Tart, C. (1986). *Waking up: Overcoming the obstacles to human potential*. Boston: New Science Library.

Tasini, M. F., & Hackett, T. P. (1977). Hypnosis in the treatment of warts in immunodeficient children. *American Journal of Clinical Hypnosis, 19*, 152–154.

Thomas, L. (1979). On warts. In *The medusa and the snail* (pp. 76–81). New York: Viking Press.

Thompson, K. F. (1963). A rationale for suggestion in dentistry. *American Journal of Clinical Hypnosis, 5*, 181–186.

Thorne, D. E., & Fisher, A. G. (1978). Hypnotically suggested asthma. *International Journal of Clinical and Experimental Hypnosis, 26*, 92–103.

Tilton, P. (1980). Hypnotic treatment of a child with thumbsucking, enuresis and encopresis. *American Journal of Clinical Hypnosis, 22*, 238–240.

Tinterow, M. M. (1970). *Foundations of hypnosis: From Mesmer to Freud*. Springfield, IL: Charles C Thomas.

Torem, M. S. (1987). Ego-state therapy for eating disorders. *American Journal of Clinical Hypnosis, 20*, 94–103.

Torem, M. S. (1991). Eating disorders. In W. C. Wester & D. O'Grady (Eds.), *Clinical hypnosis with children* (pp. 230–257). New York: Brunner/Mazel.

Traphagen, V. (1959). A survey of attitudes toward hypnotherapy with children. *American Journal of Clinical Hypnosis, 2*, 138–142.

Tromater, F. T. (1961). *Some developmental correlates of hypnotic susceptibility*. Unpublished master's thesis, University of Illinois, Urbana.

Trustman, R., Dubovsky, S., & Titley, R. (1977). Auditory perception during general anesthesia — myth or fact? *International Journal of Clinical and Experimental Hypnosis, 25*, 88–105.

Tucker, K. R., & Virnelli, F. R. (1985). The use of hypnosis as a tool in plastic surgery. *Plastic and Reconstructive Surgery, 76*, 140–146.

U. S. Department of Health and Human Services. (1992). *Acute pain manage-*

ment: Operative or medical procedures and trauma (Clinical practice guide, AHCPR Pub. No. 92-0032). Rockville, MD: Agency for Health Care Policy and Research, U.S. Public Health Service.

Vadurro, J. F., & Butts, P. A. (1982). Reducing the anxiety and pain of childbirth through hypnosis. *American Journal of Nursing, 82,* 620–623.

Valente, S. M. (1991). Clinical hypnosis with school-age children. *Archives of Psychiatric Nursing, 4,* 131–136.

Valente, S. M. (1991). Using hypnosis with children for pain management. *Oncology Nursing Forum, 18,* 699–704.

Van der Does, A. J. W., Van Dyck, R., & Spijker, R. E. (1988). Hypnosis and pain in patients with severe burns: A pilot study. *Burns, 14*(5), 399–404.

Van Rood, Y. R., Bogaards, M., Goulmy, E., & van Houwelingen, H. C. (1993). The effects of stress and relaxation on the in vitro immune response in man: A meta-analytic study. *Journal of Behavioral Medicine, 16,* 163–181.

Varni, J. W., & Gilbert, A. (1982). Self-regulation of chronic arthritic pain and long-term analgesic dependence in a hemophiliac. *Rheumatology and Rehabilitation, 22,* 171–174.

Varni, J. W., Katz, E. R., & Dash, J. (1982). Behavioral and neurochemical aspects of pediatric pain. In D. C. Russo & J. W. Varni (Eds.), *Behavioral pediatrics: Research and practice.* New York: Plenum Press.

Varni, J. W., Thompson, K. L., & Hanson, V. (1987). The Varni–Thompson Pediatric Pain Questionnaire. I. Chronic musculoskeletal pain in juvenile rheumatoid arthritis. *Pain, 28,* 27–38.

Viorst, J. (1971). *The tenth good thing about Barney.* New York: Atheneum.

Wakeman, R. J., & Kaplan, J. Z. (1978). An experimental study of hypnosis in painful burns. *American Journal of Clinical Hypnosis, 21,* 3–12.

Walco, G. A., Varni, J. W., & Ilowite, N. T. (1992). Cognitive–behavioral pain management in children with juvenile rheumatoid arthritis. *Pediatrics, 89*(6), 1075–1079.

Wang, Y., & Morgan, W. P. (1992). The effect of imagery perspectives on the psychophysiological responses to imagined exercise. *Behavior and Brain Research, 52,* 167–174.

Wangensteen, O. H. (1962). New operative techniques in intestinal obstructions. *Wisconsin Medical Journal, 62,* 159–169.

Watkins, J. G. (1962, August). [Hypnotherapy American Psychological Association post-doctoral institute course, Brooklyn, NY.]

Wechsler, D. (1949). *Wechsler Intelligence Scale for Children.* New York: Psychological Corporation.

Weitzenhoffer, A. M. (1959). A bibliography of hypnotism in pediatrics. *American Journal of Clinical Hypnosis, 2,* 92–95.

Weitzenhoffer, A. M., & Hilgard, E. R. (1959). *Stanford Hypnotic Susceptibility Scale, forms A and B.* Palo Alto, CA: Consulting Psychologists Press.

Werder, D. S., & Sargent, J. D. (1984). A study of childhood headache using biofeedback as a treatment alternative. *Headache, 24,* 122–126.

West, N., Oakes, L., & Hinds, P. S. (1994). Measuring pain in pediatric oncology ICU patients. *Journal of Pediatric Oncology Nursing, 11,* 64–68.

White, E. B. (1952). *Charlotte's web.* New York: HarperCollins.

Whittam, E. H. (1993). Terminal care of the dying child: Psychosocial implications of care. *Cancer, 71,* 3450–3462.

Whorwell, P. J., Prior, A., & Colgan, S. M. (1987). Hypnotherapy in severe irritable bowel syndrome: Further experience. *Gut, 28,* 423–425.

Wiggins, S. L., & Brown, C. W. (1968). Hypnosis with two pedicle graft cases. *International Journal of Clinical and Experimental Hypnosis, 16,* 215.

Williams, D. T. (1979). Hypnosis as a therapeutic adjunct. In J. D. Noshpitz (Ed.), *Basic handbook of child psychiatry* (Vol. 3). New York: Basic Books.

Williams, D. T., & Singh, M. (1976). Hypnosis as a facilitating therapeutic adjunct in child psychiatry. *Journal of the American Academy of Child Psychiatry, 15,* 326–342.

Winkelstein, L. B., & Levinson, J. (1959). Fulminating preeclampsia with cesarean section performed under hypnosis. *American Journal of Obstetrics and Gynecology, 78,* 420–423.

Witmer, L. (1897). The use of hypnotism in education. *Pediatrics, 3,* 23–27.

Woody, R. H., & Billy, H. T. (1970). Influencing the intelligence scores of retarded and nonretarded boys with clinical suggestion. *American Journal of Clinical Hypnosis, 12,* 268–271.

Woody, R. H., & Herr, E. L. (1967). Mental retardation and clinical hypnosis. *Mental Retardation, 5,* 27–28.

Wright, M. E. (1960). Hypnosis and child therapy. *American Journal of Clinical Hypnosis, 2,* 197–205.

Wright, M. E., with Wright, B. A. (1987). *Clinical practice of hypnotherapy.* New York: Guilford Press.

Young, M. H., & Montano, R. J. (1988). A new hypnobehavioral method for the treatment of children with Tourette's disorder. *American Journal of Clinical Hypnosis, 31,* 97–106.

Young, M. H., Montano, R. J., & Goldberg, R. (1991). Self-hypnosis, sensory cueing, and response prevention: Decreasing anxiety and improving written output of a preadolescent with learning disabilities. *American Journal of Clinical Hypnosis, 34,* 129–136.

Zahm, D. N. (1990). Hypnosis in the treatment of Tourette syndrome. In C. D. Hammond (Ed.), *Handbook of hypnotic suggestions and metaphors* (pp. 501–502). New York: W. W. Norton.

Zeltzer, L., Dash, J., & Holland, J. P. (1979). Hypnotically induced pain control in sickle cell anemia. *Pediatrics, 64,* 533–536.

Zeltzer, L., & LeBaron, S. (1984). *Stanford Hypnotic Clinical Scale for Children—Revised (SHCS-C-R).* Unpublished data.

Zeltzer, L., LeBaron, S., & Zeltzer, P. M. (1984a). The effectiveness of behavioral intervention for reducing nausea and vomiting in children and adolescents receiving chemotherapy. *Journal of Clinical Oncology, 2,* 683–690.

Zeltzer, L., LeBaron, S., & Zeltzer, P. M. (1984b). Paradoxical effects of prophylactic phenothiazine antiemetics in children receiving chemotherapy. *Journal of Clinical Oncology, 2,* 936–940.

Author Index

433

Subject Index